Textbook of
Pharmaceutical
Dispensing

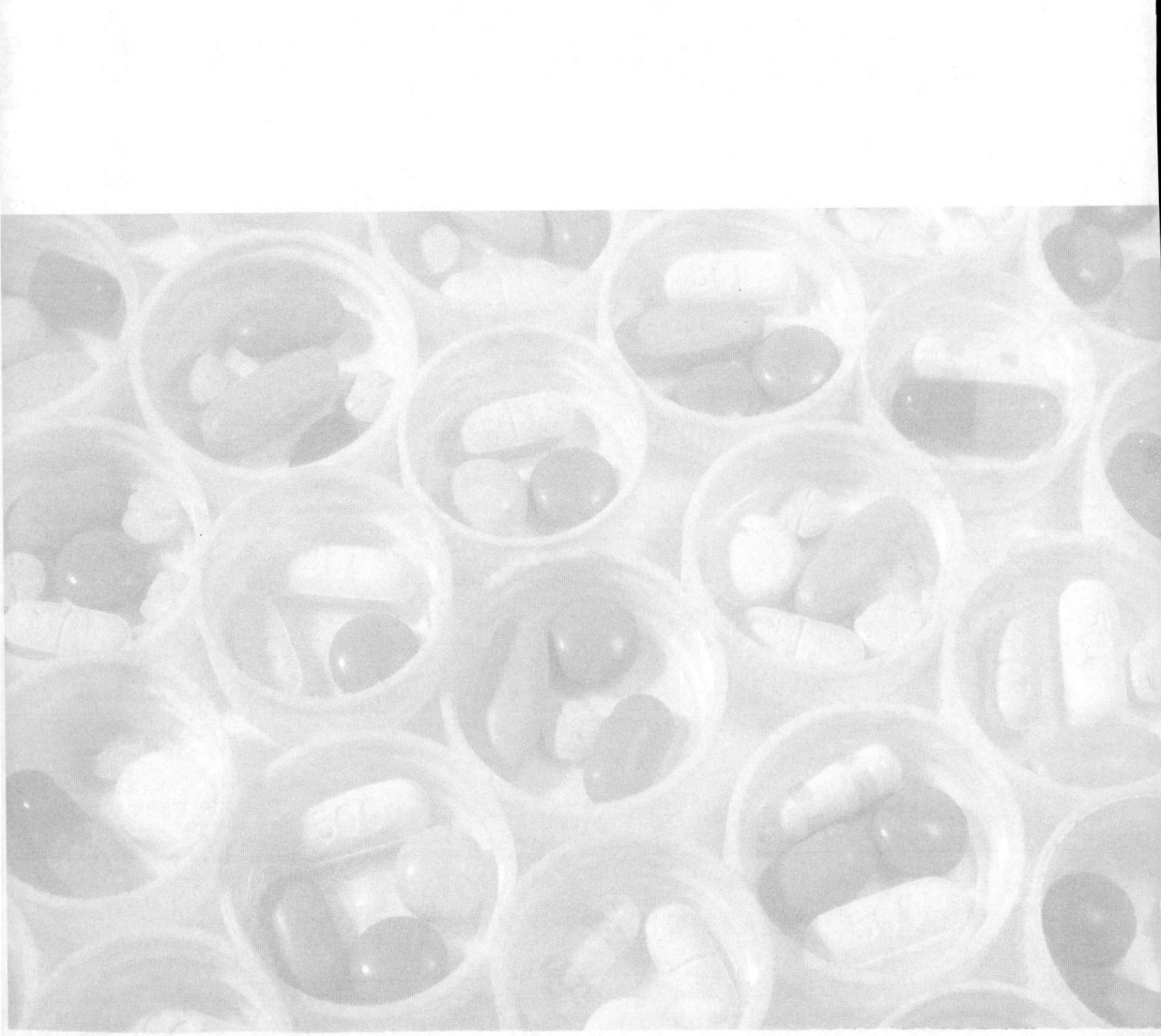

Textbook of
Pharmaceutical
Dispensing

Amit K Goyal M Pharm, PhD
Associate Professor

Goutam Rath M Pharm
Associate Professor

RK Narang M Pharm
Associate Professor

Department of Pharmaceutics
ISF College of Pharmacy
Moga, Punjab

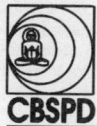

CBSPD

CBS Publishers & Distributors Pvt Ltd

New Delhi • Bengaluru • Chennai • Kochi • Kolkata • Lucknow • Mumbai
Hyderabad • Jharkhand • Nagpur • Patna • Pune • Uttarakhand

Textbook of
Pharmaceutical
Dispensing

ISBN: 978-81-239-2201-0

Copyright © Authors and Publisher

First Edition: 2012
  Reprint: 2017, 2019, 2023

Published by **Satish Kumar Jain** and produced by **Varun Jain** for

CBS Publishers & Distributors Pvt Ltd
4819/XI Prahlad Street, 24 Ansari Road, Daryaganj, New Delhi 110 002, India.
Ph: 011-23289259, 23266861, 23266867   Website: www.cbspd.com
Fax: 011-23243014   e-mail: delhi@cbspd.com;

Corporate Office: 204 FIE, Industrial Area, Patparganj, Delhi 110 092
Ph: 011-4934 4934   Fax: 011-4934 4935
                                        e-mail: publishing@cbspd.com; publicity@cbspd.com

Branches

- **Bengaluru:** Seema House 2975, 17th Cross, KR Road, Banasankari 2nd Stage, Bengaluru 560 070, Karnataka, India
  Ph: +91-80-26771678/79   Fax: +91-80-26771680   e-mail: bangalore@cbspd.com
- **Chennai:** 7, Subbaraya Street, Shenoy Nagar, Chennai 600 030, Tamil Nadu, India
  Ph: +91-44-26680620, 26681266   Fax: +91-44-42032115   e-mail: chennai@cbspd.com
- **Kochi:** 42/1325, 1326, Power House Road, Opp KSEB, Power House, Ernakulam Kochi 682 018, Kerala, India
  Ph: +91-484-4059061-65,67   Fax: +91-484-4059065   e-mail: kochi@cbspd.com
- **Kolkata:** 147, Hind Ceramics Compound, 1st Floor, Nilgunj Road, Belghoria, Kolkata-700056, West Bengal, India
  Ph: +033-25633055, 033-25633056   e-mail: kolkata@cbspd.com
- **Lucknow:** Basement, Khushnuma Complex, 7 Meerabai Marg (Behind Jawahar Bhawan),Lucknow-226001, UP, India
  Ph: +0522-4000032   e-mail: tiwari.lucknow@cbspd.com
- **Mumbai:** PWD Shed, Gala no 25/26, Ramchandra Bhatt Marg, Next to JJ Hospital Gate no. 2, Opp. Union Bank of India, Noorbaug, Mumbai-400009, Maharashtra, India
  Ph: 022-66661880/89   e-mail: mumbai@cbspd.com

Representatives

- Hyderabad   0-9885175004
- Patna   0-9334159340
- Jharkhand   0-9811541605
- Pune   0-9623451994
- Nagpur   0-9421945513
- Uttarakhand   0-9716462459

Printed at Glorious Printers, Delhi, India

Preface

Pharmaceutical dispensing is a branch of pharmacy that continues to play the crucial role of drug development. Compounding and dispensing pharmacists develop the pharmaceutical formulations for new drugs so that the active ingredients are effective, stable, easy to use, and acceptable to patients. It is an integral element of the pharmaceutical profession that involves the rational design, compounding, and dispensing of dosage forms to ensure the required biological and physical performances of the therapeutic agent. Thus, dispensing pharmacist is expected to have knowledge of several pharmaceutical disciplines, including prescription handing and processing, pharmaceutical incompatibilities, drug interaction, pharmacological action, compounding, dispensing, patient-counseling and community pharmacy. This book provides interesting reading for those involved in community pharmacy and product development. This contemporary book is specifically tailored to meet the needs of a broader audience, particularly to include the students undertaking programs in pharmacy/pharmaceutical science, medicine and other branches of biomedical/clinical sciences.

The content of this textbook is designed in the newer way that provides basic information on the main aspects of pharmacy in a relatively simple but practical manner. The primary objective of the text is to provide insight into the theoretical and practical aspects of pharmaceutical compounding and dispensing of various dosage forms like emulsions, suspensions, solutions, mixtures, ointments, powders, and suppositories. In particular, the text aims to deliver the essential information concerning the dispensing of these dosage forms in a format that will hopefully aid the understanding and hence remove the complexities of the various topics. Under each class there are several subclasses and several principles of preparation are to be understood. The contents of this text have also been included handling and processing of prescription, incompatibility studies, pharmaceutical calculation and community pharmacy. The primary objective of this textbook is to ease the perceived difficulties of this subject and, hopefully, illustrate the significance of pharmaceutical dispensing and the unique role of the pharmacist in the development of medicines. This exciting textbook discusses the plethora of examples related to prescription, incompatibility, compounding and dispensing of therapeutic drugs.

Authors from their selected areas present a balanced view of the science and its application. Their insights will surely prove useful to the pharmacy students as well as practising pharmacists involved in the development or dispensing of existing and next generation drug products. This simple and user-friendly textbook presents dispensing pharmacy in a way that has never been presented before.

Amit K Goyal
Goutam Rath
RK Narang

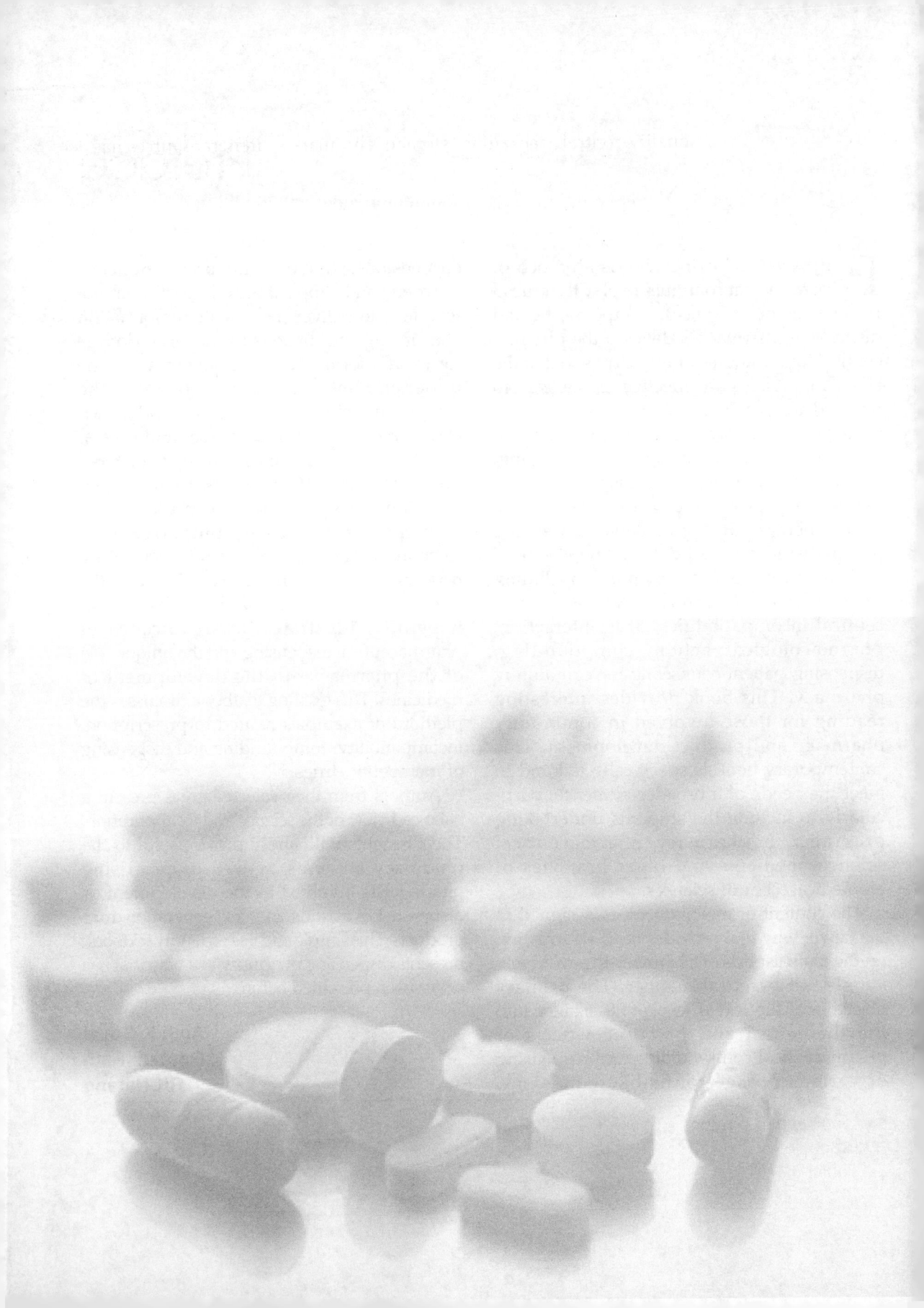

Contents

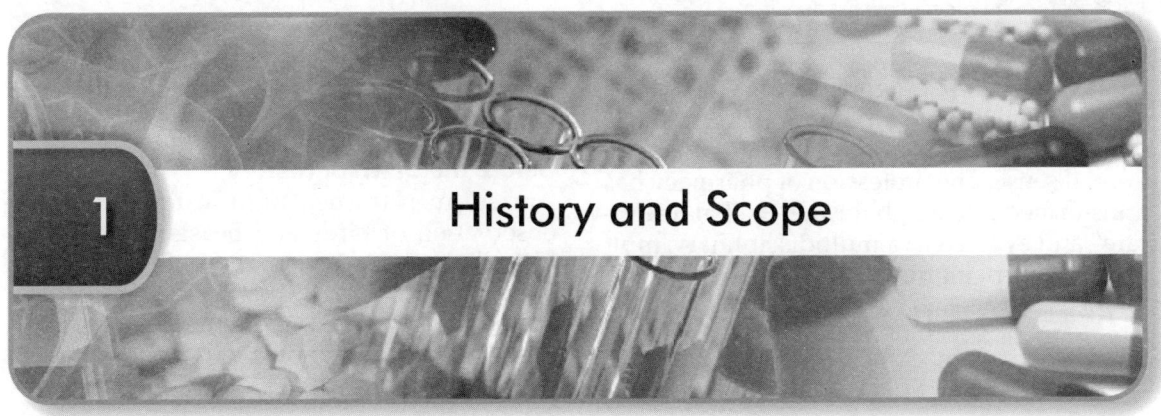

History and Scope

INTRODUCTION

The word pharmacy has been derived from the Greek word *"pharmakon"* meaning drug. Pharmacy is the art and science of compounding and dispensing drugs or preparing suitable dosage forms for the administration of drugs in men or animals. It includes all the stages related to a drug, from its discovery, collection, identification, isolation, purification, synthesis, standardization, formulation, use, quality control, packaging, storage, and marketing of medicinal substances. Thus, today's pharmacy professional is a "drug expert" in the real sense. The profession of pharmacy has transformed into a hub for the "global healthcare" and evolved as a multidisciplinary, multifaceted curriculum.

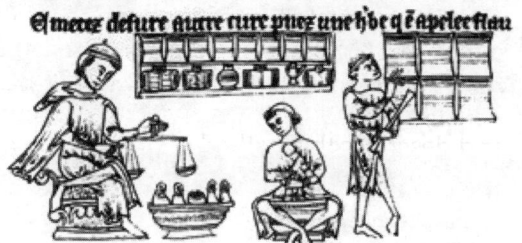

Fig. 1.1: Ancient pharmacy (middle age)

In any health system, it is essential that patients have access to reliable information and competent professional care. After physicians and nurses, pharmacists constitute the third largest group of health professionals. Pharmacists work in a wide range of settings, e.g. community, hospital, and health-system settings.

Over the past 40 years, the pharmacist's role has changed from that of compounder and dispenser to one of "drug therapy manager". This involves responsibilities to ensure that wherever medicines are provided and used, quality products are selected, procured, stored, distributed, dispensed and administered so that they contribute to the health of patients, and not to their harm. The scope of pharmacy practice now includes patient-centered care with all the cognitive functions of counseling, providing drug information and monitoring drug therapy, as well as technical aspects of pharmaceutical services, including medicines supply management.

THE HISTORY OF PHARMACEUTICAL COMPOUNDING: AN OVERVIEW

It is impossible to determine when humans first began to mix substances and create preparations that produced therapeutic effects, but it is known that the compounding of medicinal preparations from animal, vegetable and mineral sources has been practiced by a range of ancient civilizations.

Before the Dawn of History

Ancient men learned from instinct, from the observation of birds and beasts. Cold water, leaf, dirt or mud were their first soothing application. By trial, they learned more and more which served them best. Eventually, they applied their knowledge for the benefits of others.

Pharmacy in Ancient Babylonia

It provides knowledge about the earliest known practice of pharmacy known as the art of apothecary. Practitioners of healing of this era (about 2600 BC) were priests, pharmacists and physicians, all in one.

Pharmacy in Ancient China

Shengnon Bencao Jing outlined basic theory of Chinese pharmacy and investigated the medicinal value of several hundred herbs like podophyllum, ginseng, cinnamon bark, etc.

- Manuscripts on silk and bamboo describe uses of drugs of animal and plant origin.
- The text *Huangdi Neijing* listed the basic principles of pharmaceutical drug use in the third century BC.

Days of the Papyrus Ebers

Papyrus Ebers is the best known and the most important pharmaceutical records. It is a collection of 800 prescriptions mentioning 700 drugs.

Papyrus Ebers has also described contemporary materia medica, formulae, remedies and the weights and measures used in pharmaceutical compounding. Many of the vegetable-based drugs, animal products and minerals described in Papyrus Ebers are recognisable today, and indeed some remain in current use such as opium, myrrh and liquorice.

Greeks and Romans

Just as the Egyptians honored Imhotep as the god–physician, the Greeks worshipped Asklepios as their god of healing.

- Theophrastus, the greatest early Greek philosopher and natural scientist, is called "Father of botany". His observations and writings dealing with medicinal properties of herbs are usually accurate, even in the light of present knowledge.

Later on, the use of medicines was carried out by the *rhizotomoi* (experts in medicinal plants), and the *pharmakopoloi* (preparers and sellers of drugs).

Terra Sigillatan: Early Trademark Drug

Man learned the prestigious advantage of trademarks as a means of identification of source and of gaining customers confidence. One of the first therapeutic agents to bear such a mark was Terra sigillatan, a clay tablet originating on the Mediterranean islands of lemons before 500 BC.

Pharmacy in Ancient India (Vedic Evolution)

- Ayurvedic medicine was first described around 800 BC. Documents list the use of drugs together with charms for expelling demons and make reference to the god of medicine, Dhanvantari.

- The **Charaka Samhita** includes reference to drugs of animal, plant and mineral origin used until the first century AD.

Hippocrates

- Considered to be the father of medicine.

- He is associated with a number of documents collectively known as the *Hippocratic Corpus* dating to 420–370 BC, which lists 200–400 drugs of vegetable origin and describes the method of preparation of gargles, ointment and pessaries.

- His works placed emphasis on treating the patient with minimal reference to magical and religious powers.

Dioscorides: A Scientist Look at Drugs

- Prepared the document *De Materia Medica* around AD 60–78. This document provides details about medicinal herbs including side effects associated with their administration.

- His text was considered as reference source for medicine formulation, as late as the sixteenth century.

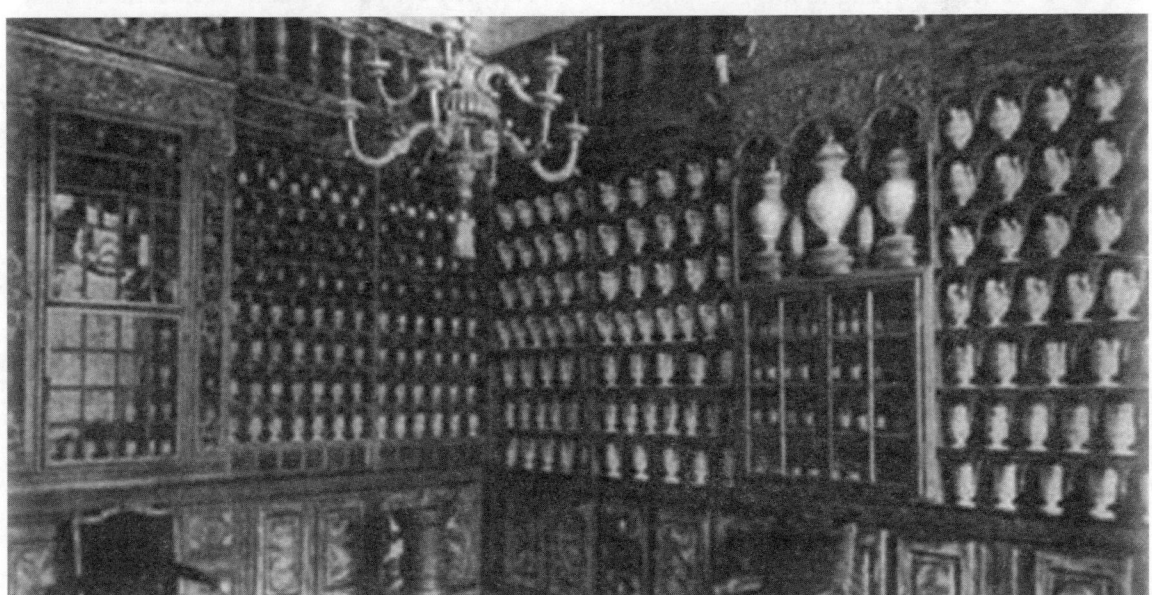

Fig. 1.2: The typical pharmacy in 17th century

Galen: Experimenter in Drug Compounding

- A physician around AD 160. He compiled medical knowledge specified by Hippocrates and Dioscorides.
- He described the use of formulations made up of numerous plants which were referred to as 'galenicals'.
- He was the originator of the formula for a cold cream.

The Arabs

- In the Arab world, a large number of texts including documents related to medicine and works by Galen were translated into Arabic and that is how these documents have been transferred along history. Documents that were prepared included formularies, herbals and books on materia medica and toxicology.
- The use of medications consisting of formulations from galenic medicine was continued.
- This required skilled preparation which laid the beginning of apothecaries in the ninth century in Baghdad. The practice of the apothecaries was inspected by the state.
- Avicenna, a Persian philosopher, compiled the book *Canon of Medicine,* in which he merged the Greek and Arab works. The book describes the use of around 760 drugs.

Evolution of Modern Pharmacy

Separation of Pharmacy and Medicine

In European countries, community pharmacy began to appear in the 17th century. In Sicily and southern Italy, pharmacy was separated from medicine.

The First Official Pharmacopoeia

The **Nuova receptario** originally written in Italian was published and became the legal standard in 1498. The idea of pharmacopoeia

with official status to be followed by all apothecary shops in Florence.

The Society of Apothecary in London

In 1617, Francis Bacon formed the society of the art and mystery of apothecary in London. This was first organization of the pharmacist in the world.

Craige: America's First Apothecary General

Craige is the first man to hold the rank of commissioned pharmaceutical officer in American army. His duties included procurement, storage, manufacture and distribution of the army's drug requirement. He also developed early whole selling and manufacturing drug business.

The Father of American Pharmacy

William Proctor, graduate from the Philadelphia College of Pharmacy in 1837 was a leader in founding the American Pharmaceutical Association, served that organization as first secretary and later as president.

Pharmacy Enters in Modern Era

Today modern pharmacist deals with complex pharmaceutical remedies far different from the elixirs, spirits, and powders described in the **Pharmacopoeia of London** (1618) and the **Pharmacopoeia of Paris** (1639). In the US today, major medicines, those regarded as having the greatest therapeutic value, are selected for inclusion in the Pharmacopoeia of the United States, first published in 1820. Similarly, the **National Formulary** was published by the American Pharmaceutical Association (founded 1852) since 1888. Any significant variation from pharmacopoeia and formulary standards may be prosecuted by the Food and Drug Administration under the Pure Food and Drug Acts.

Modern pharmaceutical practice includes the dispensing, identification, selection, and analysis of drugs. Pharmacy began to develop as a profession separate from medicine in the

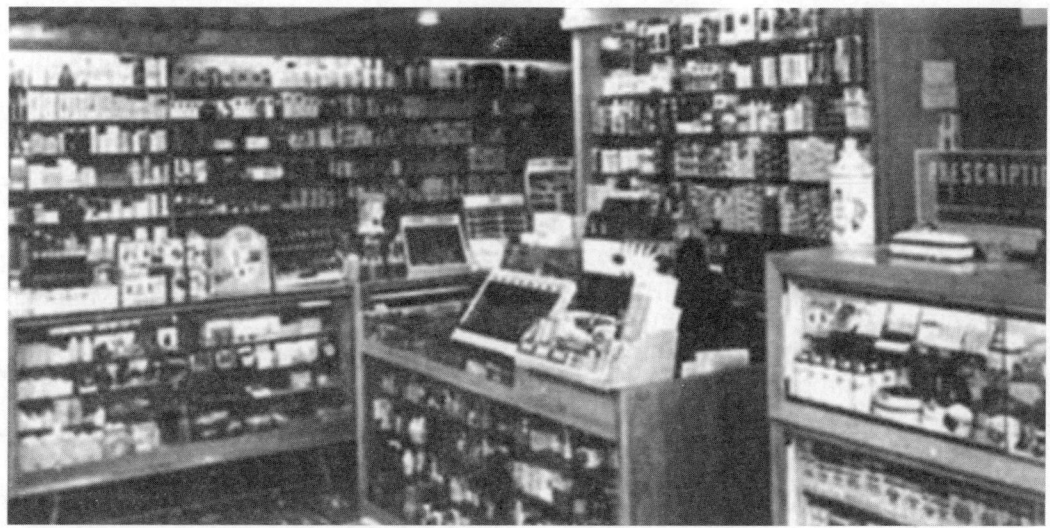

Fig. 1.3: The typical pharmacy of the 1950 – 1960

18th century, and in 1821 the first US school of pharmacy was established in Philadelphia.

The Industrial Revolution

The rapid change from hand methods to machine methods of production that characterized the industrial revolution in pharmacy, especially under the impact of the scientific developments of the nineteenth century. Phytochemistry and synthetic chemistry created new derivatives of old drugs and new chemical entities of medicinal value that strained the capacity of the individual pharmacy. Large scale drug manufacturing had its strong hold on society with the advent of machines and patents.

The Declining Art of the Apothecary

Industrialization had an impact on every aspect of the activity of the pharmacist.

First, it led to the creation of new drugs, drugs that the individual pharmacist's own resources could not produce.

Second, many drugs that the individual pharmacist was able to produce could be manufactured more economically, and in superior quality, by industry.

Third, industry assumed responsibility, traditionally vested in the pharmacist for the quality of the medication.

The Community Pharmacy

The nineteenth century did not see the end of the art of compounding, but the art did give way, to new technology. It has been estimated that a "broad knowledge of compounding" was still essential for 80% of the prescriptions dispensed in the 1920s. Although pharmacists increasingly relied on chemicals purchased from the manufacturer to make up the prescriptions. Further more, they were often called upon to provide first aid and medicines for such common ailments as burns, colic, flesh wounds, poisoning, constipation, and diarrhoea.

The Twentieth Century Pharmacist

The most notable change in pharmacy in modern times has been the virtual disappearance of the preparation and compounding of medicines. Whereas in the 1920s, 80% of the prescriptions filled in American pharmacies required knowledge of compounding, by the 1940s the number of prescriptions requiring compounding had declined to 26%. As far back as 1971, only 1%, or less, of all prescriptions combined two or more active ingredients.

All this meant that the pharmacist's education and activities had to undergo change. At the same time, the scientific education of pharmacists was steadily becoming more demanding, their role in the provision of health care was becoming more and more limited. The reaction to these conditions was apparent in the drop in the production of pharmacy graduates who were planning to go into the field of community pharmacy. In 1947, about 90% of graduates planned to go into some aspect of community pharmacy; in 1973, that figure had dropped to 76.6%; in 1988, it stood at 57.1%.

A FLASHBACK: GERMINATION OF PHARMACY EDUCATION IN INDIA

The Indian traditional systems of medicine have been Ayurveda, Siddha and Unani. Ayurveda and Siddha originated in India itself. Unani, the Greco-Arabic medical system, came from west Asia. The European colonizers brought the western system of medicine to the country. During the colonial period, the new system, commonly referred to as Allopathy, got firmly established.

The pharmacy education in India was going to pass through a mutation when the founder of Banaras Hindu University, Mahamana Pt. Madan Mohan Malviya met Prof. ML Schroff and Mahamana offered him to join BHU. By the non-tiring efforts of Prof. Schroff in July 1937 "pharmaceutical chemistry" and "pharmacognosy" were introduced as the subjects for B.Sc. degree. Since then there has been no looking back. Pharmacy came to be recognized as a well-established course with fruitful outcomes. The pharmacy education in India has a long history characterized by slow growth between 1842 and 1932.

Important events

- 1842 - First recognized pharmacy course in India (Certificate course)
- 1860 - Madras Medical College (Certificate course in pharmacy)
- 1860–1920 - Certificate courses in pharmacy at Medical Colleges of Vishakhapatnam, Kolkata, Cuttack, Dhaka, Allahabad, Banaras, Lucknow, Meerut, Mumbai and Nagpur.
- 1930 - The drugs enquiry committee under the Chairmanship of Lt. Col. Dr. Ramnath Chopra — a great leap for the profession of Pharmacy in India.

Prof. ML Schroff on the call of Pandit Madan Mohan Malviya Ji the Vice-Chancellor of Banaras Hindu University started a regular B.Pharm course of 3 years in July, 1937. Since then Pharmacy education is making rapid strides in India. Later several other Universities started B.Pharm programme. Some of the important milestones are:

- 1945 - University of Bombay
- 1947 - Department of Pharmacy, Punjab University.
- 1947 - LMCP, Ahmedabad.
- 1950 - BITS, Pilani.
- 1951 - Andhra University, Vishakhapatnam.
- 1956 - Saugar University, Saugar.
- 1956 - Department of Pharmaceutical Sciences, Nagpur University, Nagpur.

CURRENT SCENARIO

Pharmaceutical education plays a very prominent role in attaining sustainable and equitable development of a country. The curriculum of the degree in some developed countries (B. Pharm.) usually requires 5 academic years of study. In most of the European countries, successful completion of a university degree leads to a one-year internship. In India, pharmacy education is a two-tier system. After

12th with science subjects of state board, one can opt for any of the two courses, namely Diploma (D.Pharm.) and Degree (B.Pharm). However, the Diploma students can also be included in Degree course directly in second year B.Pharm. However, in the coming years, the Government and Pharmacy Council of India is planning to abolish the D.Pharm course and make B.Pharm the minimum qualification for any individual to become a pharmacy professional.

The regulatory bodies for pharmacy colleges are namely, All India Council of Technical Education (AICTE), Pharmacy Council of India (PCI) and the respective university to which the college is affiliated to. Today pharmacy education like the pharmaceutical industry is also in the process of globalization. In order to have uniformity in course contents, requisite standards of education, technical faculty, facilities and infrastructure at international levels, colleges are going for accreditation and certifications from internationally approved regulating agencies. As per PCI 2005 diary calendar, the total numbers of recognized degree institutions are 220 with intake of 12,506 students and as per AICTE, the total numbers of degree colleges are 445 with the intake of 24,672 students as well 30 institutions for the postgraduation in various fields.

The PCI controls and regulates the standards for a better pharmacy education in India. The main aims of PCI are:

- To prescribe minimum standard of education required for qualifying as a pharmacist, i.e. framing of education regulations prescribing the conditions to be fulfilled by the institutions seeking approval of the PCI for imparting education in pharmacy.
- To ensure uniform implementation of the educational standards throughout the country.
- To approve the courses of study and examination for pharmacists, i.e. approval of the academic training institutions providing pharmacy courses.

The curriculum of pharmacy education has been designed to produce the following professional categories of pharmacists:

- Community and hospital pharmacists who will work as an important link between doctor and patient and will counsel the patient on various facets of drugs like usage, side effects, indication, contraindications, compatibilities, incompatibilities, storage, dosage, etc.
- Specialist in research and development, i.e. research of new drug molecules, biotechnical research, etc.
- Occupational specialist (industrial pharmacist engaged in pharmaceutical technology), i.e. manufacture of various dosage forms, analysis and quality control, clinical trials, post-marketing surveillance, patent application and drug registration, sales and marketing.
- Academicians, i.e. teachers of pharmacy education.
- Manager and administrators of pharmaceutical services working for various regulatory authorities and pharmaceutical systems.
- Chemists and druggists engaged in selling of medicines.

The Pharmacy Council of India has now decided to start Pharm.D course from this academic year and has approved 22 colleges in the country to run Pharm.D and Pharm.D Baclaureate course (3 years after B.Pharm). The Pharm.D course will be the harbinger for the beginning of a new era in the pharmacy practice in India. Since this programme is similar to the programmes being offered in USA and UK, Indian students perusing this programme will have ample opportunities to work as pharmacists in these countries with a handsome salary. Secondly, this course gives a new dimension to pharmaceutical healthcare by giving more emphasis to patient-centered approach.

FUTURE: AN OVERVIEW

In the future, drug treatment will be increasingly and confidently tailored to the individual's need through the help of specific diagnostics. Many new drugs will be given parenterally and targeted for specific diseases. The pharmacists will need to adapt to this changing pattern in order to be seen by the patient as part of health care team. However, in spite of many lacunae in pharmacy education system, the fact cannot be overlooked that tremendous development in the field of new drug discovery and research activities, has taken place. The government expenditure alone was of the order of 150 million in 2005–06 and in subsequent years the figure has raised even higher.

The most important objectives are:

- To provide the right kind of pharmaceutical leadership by helping the individuals develop their potential.
- To provide the country with competent men and women trained in pharmacy profession.
- To bring the pharmacy colleges closer to the community through extension of pharmaceutical knowledge and its applications for problem-solving.
- Address the pharmaceutical problems for national development, particularly issues concerning self-reliance, economic growth, employment and national integration.
- Relate to the life needs and aspirations of the people.
- To improve pharmaceutical productivity by emphasizing improvement in pharmaceutical education and research.
- Inculcate social, moral and rational values in the people.

CAREER OPPORTUNITIES OF PHARMACY PROFESSIONALS

A career in pharmacy, unfolds a vista full of opportunities leading to a golden future for a young career aspirant.

Pharmaceutical industries usually employ pharmacy graduates and postgraduates for most of the operations. The various activities include manufacturing, quality control (including quality assurance), and distribution (marketing). The available career opportunities for pharmacy graduates in pharmaceutical industries and government/private sector include the following:

Production and Manufacturing

As manufacturing chemist, under whose active direction and personal supervision manufacturing of medicines takes place. The pharmaceutical production companies need such persons to obtain license for manufacturing. Graduates of pharmacy with 18 months of experience in manufacturing are treated as competent technical staff under Drugs and Cosmetics Act, which regulates the drug industries.

A pharmacy professional can work as a production person (chemist, officer, executive, manager, vice-president), involved in the production of bulk drug and intermediates or formulations and dosage forms.

Industries in the cosmetics, soaps, toiletries segment also hire pharmacy professionals. Other segments where opportunities exist are the field of dental products, biotechnological products, surgical dressings, medical devices and equipment, ayurvedic/homoeopathic/Unani medicines also involve the presence of pharmacy professionals in its production.

Research and Development

This forms the heart of any industry, as it is the key to growth and sustenance. Mainly M. Pharms and PhDs are in great demand in the various areas of Pharmaceutical R&D. Other areas where professionals are required are:

- **New drug discovery research (NDDR):** Discovering a new drug has assumed prime importance in the post-GATT era.
- **Process and development (P&D):** One of the important areas in bulk drugs indus-

try is developing viable processes for the manufacture of drugs and intermediates for their commercial production.

- **Formulation and development (F&D):** The success of any pharma company lies in the quality of its products, i.e. its formulations and dosage forms.

- **Clinical trials, bioequivalence studies, toxicological studies:** These are some of the areas of clinical research which are in high demand as they are involved in the systematic evaluation of potential drug substances prior to getting them approved by the authorities.

Analysis and Testing

The medicines that have been sampled either from manufacturing units or from retail drug stores are tested in government drug testing laboratories. The graduate pharmacists can join these government laboratories as government analyst. But the graduate pharmacists do need to undergo training on testing of drugs under a government analyst or in approved laboratories.

Quality Control/Quality Assurance

Quality assurance is a total process for assuring the quality of pharmaceutical products as per standard specified in national or other approved pharmacopoeias. Quality control is a component of quality assurance programme which deals with checking of representative samples of production to find out their compliance with standards. The graduates with aptitude in analysis of pharmaceuticals and handling of sophisticated instruments find the job interesting. There are promotional scopes too from quality control chemists to quality assurance manager.

Marketing

Pharmaceutical marketing is different from marketing of other consumer goods. Here, real consumer, the patient, has little or no choice.

The marketing takes place through doctors and chemists. Thus the job is more challenging and requires special skill and training as they deal with highly qualified doctors in one hand and the professional businessman (often called drug trader in common terminology). This is a never saturating professional area and jobs are always available. The sales personell are called as medical representatives or business executives. They can grow from medical representatives to general manager.

Hospital Pharmacy

The pharmacists in hospitals do wide range of functions ranging from procurement of medicines to dispensing to the patients. In short, they are responsible for medicine management in the hospitals. Though legally diploma in pharmacy qualification is sufficient for medicine dispensing, the degree pharmacists are preferred in procurement system in government sector and service sector in corporate hospitals. The promotional scope in this sector is limited.

Clinical Pharmacy

B.Pharm/M.Pharm degree holders can take up career in clinical research. The human testing phase is called the clinical trial. A pharmacist can work as clinical research associate or clinical pharmacist and can rise to the position of project manager. The clinical research associate plays an important role of monitoring and overseeing the conducts of clinical trials, which are conducted on healthy human volunteers. They have to see that the trials meet the international guidelines and the national regulatory requirements.

Community Pharmacy

Community pharmacies usually consist of a retail store-front with a dispensary where medications are stored and dispensed. The dispensary is subject to pharmacy legislation; with requirements for storage conditions, compulsory texts, equipment, etc. specified in legislation. Self-owned pharmacy in a good location not only gives good revenues but also provides ample opportunities to provide professional pharmaceutical services to the consumers. A license from the state drugs control authority is necessary to start a retail pharmacy business.

Through the services of community pharmacy, a pharmacist becomes a vital link between the patients and the products, i.e. drugs. The pharmacist also serves a vital link between the patients and other health care professionals, especially the medical experts. In community pharmacy a pharmacist has to play fallowing roles:

- Counseling the patients regarding the use of the drugs and dosage forms.
- Providing up-to-date infomation on drugs/ dosage forms to the patients, as well as medical staff.
- Maintaining patient records and history.
- Involved in the usage of self-diagnostic kits by the patients for disorders like diabetes, hypertension, etc.
- Providing supply of home care dosage forms. Like dosage form including home parenteral therapy and dosage form for veterinany therapy.

Medical Transcription

The B.Pharm graduate can work with medical practitioners to maintain the patient treatment history, the drug to which he/she is allergic, etc.

Academics

Excellent opportunities for the professionals are available in teaching profession also. As per the AICTE norms the minimum entry-level qualification as lecturer is M.Pharm. This is a profession associated with job satisfaction and social status, as teaching is considered to be a noble profession. The higher posts in academics are senior lecturer, reader, asst. professor, professor, principal, etc. The emoluments are satisfactory. Besides teaching, academic-related opportunities involve positions in research posts and training programs.

Regulatory Affairs

The medicines are not only required to be effective but must be safe and of assured quality. In order to assure efficacy, safety and quality, the entire pharmaceutical scenario, from manufacturing to sale of medicines, is regulated by the central and state government through a process of licensing and inspecting. The pharmaceutical graduates can join the government services usually through public service commission as drugs inspectors. They have promotional scopes to grow up to the rank of drugs controller.

With globalization process reaching out to India, the geographical barriers have become obsolete. Any country will have to compete and trade globally in order to progress and survive in the years to come. Companies have realized this fact and have stepped into the global area of competitive trade. If an Indian manufacturer wants to sell his drug or formulation to a foreign country, in order to enter into trade with the foreign countries it is mandatory to get the necessary approvals and sanctions as per the formats given by local regulatory authorities. For example, approvals to be obtained from USFDA (United States Food and Drug Administration) for USA, TGA (Therapeutic Goods Administration) for Australia and New Zealand, MCA and MHRA (Medicines and healthcare products regulatory agency) for UK and European countries and ICH guidelines going to be uniform for international levels.

Since, the business involved, worthing multibillion dollars; this branch has assumed tremendous significance and is bound to grow enormously, in the post-GATT (General agreement on tariffs and trade) era. Many big players in the drugs and pharma field have already established separate Regulatory Affairs Departments in their companies. Regulatory experts are thus in great demand.

Since, the field is highly technical, pharmacy professionals again fit in these positions.

Similarly, patents and trademarks, IPR, experts are also in high demand as far as the pharma industry is concerned.

Documentation, Library Information Services and Pharma Journalism

The regulatory affairs as well as, patenting processes and issues involve a lot of documentation work to be done and submitted to the concerned regulatory authorities, in a highly specialized and technical manner. Pharmacy professionals are again fitting in the bill. Most of the major Indian pharma companies have established separate documentation departments with a highly technical and skilled staff for this purpose. Similarly, the R&D and QC departments of the pharma companies need a wealth of technical information, which needs to be updated regularly, in order to match the pace of global competition. Therefore, library information services are another field in much demand as far as the pharma industry is concerned. Furthermore, with the advent and boom of the information technology, bio-informatics and electronic data retrieval systems, this field is already scaling new heights.

Pharma journalism is another area filled with great potentialities. This requires specialist technical personnel like pharmacy graduates on the editorial staff to cover the various aspects. There is already a very lucrative business in this field.

Consultancy

This is an ideal opportunity for highly technical and experienced pharmacy professionals to earn handsomely as self-employed entrepreneurs, even after the age of retirement. Consultancy services in pharmacy are offered in various fields against very attractive financial fees:

- Regulatory affairs
- Documentation
- Approvals
- Manufacturing processes
- Analytical series
- Research
- Market surveys and sales promotion
- Information retrieval
- Data management
- Turn key projects, etc.

Internet Pharmacy

Since about the year 2000, a growing number of internet pharmacies have been established worldwide. Many of these pharmacies are similar to community pharmacies, and in fact, many of them are actually operated as community pharmacies that serve consumers online and those that walk in their door. The primary difference is the method by which the medications are requested and received. Some customers consider this to be more convenient and private method rather than traveling to a community drugstore. Internet pharmacies (also known as online pharmacies) are also recommended to some patients by their physicians, if they are homebound.

While most internet pharmacies sell prescription drugs and require a valid prescription, some internet pharmacies sell prescription drugs without requiring a prescription. Many customers order drugs from such pharmacies to avoid the "inconvenience" of visiting a doctor or to obtain medications which their doctors were unwilling to prescribe.

Canada is home to dozens of licensed internet pharmacies, many of which sell their lower-cost prescription drugs to US consumers, who pay one of the world's highest drug prices. In recent years, many consumers in the US and in other countries with high drug costs have turned to licensed internet pharmacies in India, Israel and the UK, which often have even lower prices than in Canada.

Veterinary Pharmacy

Veterinary pharmacies, sometimes called *animal pharmacies* may fall in the category of hospital pharmacy, retail pharmacy or mail-order pharmacy. Veterinary pharmacies stock different varieties and different strengths of medications to fulfill the pharmaceutical needs of animals. Because, the needs of animals as well as the regulations on veterinary medicine are often very different from those related to people; veterinary pharmacy is often kept separate from regular pharmacies.

Nuclear Pharmacy

Nuclear pharmacy focuses on preparing radioactive materials for diagnostic tests and for treating certain diseases. Nuclear pharmacists undergo additional training specific to handling radioactive materials, and unlike in community and hospital pharmacies, nuclear pharmacists typically do not interact directly with patients.

Military Pharmacy

Military pharmacy is an entirely different working environment due to the fact that technicians perform most duties that in a civilian sector would be illegal. State laws of technician patient counseling and medication checking by a pharmacist do not apply.

Pharmacy Informatics

Pharmacy informatics is the combination of pharmacy practice science and applied information science. Pharmacy informaticists work in many practice areas of pharmacy; however, they may also work in information technology departments or for health care information technology. As a practice area and specialist domain, pharmacy informatics is growing quickly to meet the needs of major national and international patient information projects and health system interoperability goals. Pharmacists are well trained to participate in medication management system development, deployment and optimization.

Pediatric Pharmacy Practice

The pediatric patients present a unique challenge with regard to drug therapy admin- istration and monitoring. Unlike adults, dosing is most commonly based on body weight, and pharmacokinetic variables are standardized relative to weight and/or body surface area. Most commercially available drugs are not formulated for use in infants and children. In addition, the pediatric patient population poses a higher risk for medication errors. Pediatric patients are three times more likely to suffer from a medication error; and a rela- tively small magnitude of error, as compared to adults, may result in more serious conse- quences, especially in the youngest, most vul- nerable patients. Pediatric patients frequently experience adverse drug reactions similar to adults, but adverse reactions in the pediatric population may be harder to recognize or be of greater or lesser intensity. Pediatric phar- macists have specialized knowledge of the age-related differences that impact on medica- tion regimens, are able to recognize the need of the individual patient, and then make the necessary adjustments to ensure safe and effective medication use in infants, children and adolescents.

Geriatric Pharmacy Practice

Elderly patients are unique in the way that they possess an altered metabolic capacity for medications due to increased body fat, decreased muscle mass, decreased cardiac output and perfusion, decreased protein binding, reduced liver function, and reduced physiologic reserve—all of which lead to unique medication selection and dosing requirements compared to younger adults. They also often require additional assistance to understand how to take their medications to avoid possible adverse drug effects. There is a shortage of healthcare professionals trained in geriatric pharmacotherapy. As the number of elderly patients continues to increase, the contribution of the pharmacist to quality, long-term medication management will require dramatic expansion.

Nutrition Support Pharmacy

Addresses the care of patients who receive specialized nutrition support, including parenteral and enteral nutrition. Nutrition support pharmacists have responsibility for promoting maintenance and/or restoration of optimal nutritional status and designing and modifying treatment according to the needs of the individual patient. Nutrition support pharmacists have responsibility for direct patient care and often function as members of an interprofessional nutrition support team.

Oncology Pharmacy

Care to patients with cancer is called oncology. Specialists recommend for proper design, monitor and modify pharmacotherapeutic plans to optimize outcomes in patients with malignant diseases. This includes the supportive care needed to minimize side effects from the oncology treatments and the disease. Chemotherapy require specialized handling and preparation, and the patients require frequent monitoring to achieve the desired outcome. Oncology pharmacists play a key role in assuring the safety and optimum care of these patients. Oncology pharmacists may practice in hospitals or ambulatory oncology clinics, or a combination of both.

Psychiatric Pharmacy

Addresses the care of patients with psychiatric-related illnesses. As a member of an interprofessional treatment team, the psychiatric pharmacy specialist is often responsible for optimizing drug treatment and patient care by conducting such activities as monitoring patient response, patient assessment, recognizing drug-induced problems, and recommending appropriate treatment plans.

Managed Care Organizations

A pharmacist in a managed care practice provides a markedly different type of professional activity, and as a result, additional competencies are required. For a pharmacist working in this environment, patients are monitored as a population database and pharmacist care is directed through database review and querying. Economic and clinical outcomes are weighed against, and with each other, to make appropriate decisions for a "population" of patients.

Patient Care Call Centers

Call center pharmacists provide patient and prescriber education, patient counseling, drug information, and customer service, as well as drug utilization review, health management and formulary management. Pharmacists in call centers interact with patients telephonically to promote effective drug therapy. Call center pharmacists are primarily employed in health maintenance organizations (HMOs), and health plans. Some call center pharmacists focus on specific disease states.

Hospice

Hospices range from small rural organizations to very large hospices. Pharmacists practicing in this setting help to ensure that medications are appropriately selected and that management of symptoms is balanced with cost-effectiveness.

Drug and Poison

Drug and poison information services have had a long-standing role in the emergence of clinical roles for pharmacists that were built on "drug expert" contributions. Pharmacy drug information services have expanded in recent years to include hospital drug information service to community practice-based pharmacies. Easier access to information via the Internet, CD or DVD-based drug information databases, and electronic journals has contributed to this development.

Opportunities Abroad

Golden opportunities for qualified Pharmacy professionals in various courtiers including the USA, Canada; European countries like UK, France, Germany; African countries like S. Africa, Nigeria, Yemen; Gulf countries like Saudi Arabia, Kuwait; South East Asian countries like Singapore, Korea, Japan, etc.; and the Australian continent including New Zealand. There are plenty of higher education and research opportunities in the developed countries along with excellent job openings. The pharmaceutical career is one of the highest rewarding careers in these countries.

Further Studies Abroad

One may even consider venturing into pursuing higher studies abroad in order to make his career even more lucrative and challenging.

USA: One may consider opting for pursuing higher studies abroad. After graduation from a recognised university, the students can appear for their GRE (graduate record examination) and TOEFL (test of English as a foreign language) for entry into foreign universities. In USA, they can give "pharmacy equivalent examinations." For example, FPGEE (foreign pharmacist licensure examination) followed by internship and then finally NAPLEX (North American pharmacist licensure examination) both these examinations can be cleared in about one year and there one can practice retail pharmacies, which are expanding very fast in USA. In USA, M.Pharm and Ph.D. is essential to enter industry or academic institution.

Australia: Indian students know most of the universities in USA but very few know about the postgraduate studies in Australia. University of the South Australia (SA) is the largest university in the South Australia. There are about 300 programs and about 10,000 international students are studying in university SA. It offers degree in medical radiation, occupational therapy, pharmacy, physiotherapy, environmental toxicology, etc. It is top ranking university for innovative research linked to industry.

Forecasting the Demand of Pharmacy Professionals

From ancient times, pharmacy was known as a branch associated with health care services.

Times have changed now and so has the profession of pharmacy. Today, the discipline of pharmacy has made enormous progress and has matured as a distinctly independent branch of science. Of late there has been a great upgrading in the status of the pharmacy profession and now qualified pharmacists have unlimited opportunities to look forward. Going by the current trend, it has been estimated that there will be an ever-increasing demand for pharmacists in the coming years in both developed and developing countries. One might wonder why the number of people needed to work in the field of pharmacy is increasing. To answer this question, a number of factors must be taken into account:

- India has a vast and growing pharmaceutical industry. Increasing number of hospitals, nursing homes and pharmaceutical companies all over the country is a clear indication of the growing scope in this area.
- The rise in chronic health problems worldwide has resulted in a need for more pharmacists to work as health care professionals.
- The expanding pharmaceutical industry, fuelled by more lenient regulatory and patent laws, has led to a demand for more trained industrial pharmacists.
- The advent of new drug technologies has led to an increased demand for pharmacy researchers. The current boom in the biotechnology industry is creating new positions for research pharmacists as well.
- Outsourcing of clinical research by pharmaceutical companies to contract research organizations has led to increased demand for trained professional.
- There is a feeling among the pharmacy community, that the field of personalized medicines based on pharmacogenomics will affect the way drugs are prescribed in the future. This will result in greater

involvement of pharmacists in community settings and clinical care areas.

Apart from this, there are ample opportunities for carrying out further education including PhD programs, research fellowships, and postdoctorate openings.

No matter what venue is selected, pharmacy offers excellent working conditions, job satisfaction, and financial rewards in a job that can positively impact people's lives. Pharmacy offers reasonably good career opportunities both by way of jobs and in terms of starting one's own business.

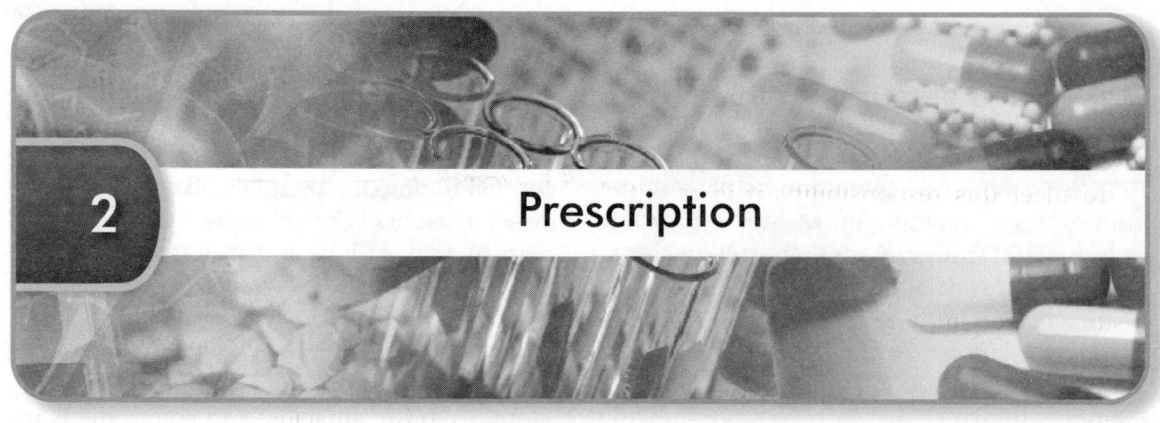

2 Prescription

INTRODUCTION

A prescription is an order issued by a physician, dentist, or other properly licensed medical practitioner to a pharmacist giving instructions regarding the dispensing of prescribed medicaments. Prescription designates a specific medication and dosage to be administered to a particular patient at a specified time. Prescriptions usually are written on printed forms that contain blank spaces for the required information. These forms are called prescription blanks and are supplied in the form of a pad. Most prescription blanks are imprinted with the name, address, telephone number and other pertinent information of the physician or his practice site, e.g. hospital or clinic.

R_X a symbol meaning "prescription". It may be intended as an abbreviation of the Latin "recipe", means "to take or take thou". The prescription order is a part of the professional relationship among the prescriber, the pharmacist and the patient. It is the pharmacist's responsibility in this relationship to provide quality pharmaceutical care that meets the medication needs of the patient.

It is also the pharmacist responsibility to advice the prescriber about the drug sensitivities the patient may have, previous adverse drug reaction (ADRs), and/or other medications that the patient may be taking that may alter the effectiveness or safety of the newly or previously prescribed medications.

To meet this responsibility, it is essential that the pharmacist maintains a high level of practice competence, keeps appropriate records on the health status and medication history of patient, and develops professional working relationship with other health professionals. Pharmacist must establish and maintain the trust of the prescriber and the patient.

TYPES OF PRESCRIPTIONS

There are two broad legal classifications of medications— those that can be obtained only by prescription and those that may be purchased without a prescription. The latter are termed nonprescription drug or over-the-counter (OTC) drugs. Medication that may be dispensed legally only on prescription are referred to as prescription drugs or legend drugs.

Over-the-counter Drugs (OTC Drugs)

OTC drugs are legal drugs that anyone can buy at places like the supermarket or the drugstore. Aspirin, antacids, and cough medicine are some kinds of OsssssTC drugs. Labels on OTC drugs give important information like dose, storage condition, contraindications, etc. Table 2.1 enlists some examples of OTC drugs.

Types of drug	Example
Allergy prevention and treatment	Benadryl, Sudafed, Actifed, Claritin, Chlora Trimaton, and Nasalcrom
Antacids and acid reducers	Tums, AXID AR, Pepcid AC, Prilosec OTC, AR, Prilosec OTC, Tagamet HB, and Zantac 75.
Anticandidal	Femstat 3, Gyne-Lotrimin, and Vagistat-1
Antihistamines	Actidil Syrup and Capsules, Actifed, Allerest, Benadryl, Claritin, Drixoral, and Triaminic
Antidiarrheal and laxatives	Ex-Lax, Pepto-Bismol, and Kaopectate
Anti fungal	Lamisil AT, Lotramin AF, and Micatin
Asthma	Primatene Mist
Cold sore/fever blister	Abreva Cream, Carmex
Condoms and other contraceptive devices	Trojans, Magnum, VGF Film and Delfen and Contraceptive Foam.
Contact lenses solutions	Bausch and Lomb, Renu, Aosept, Allergan, Boston and Opti-Free
Cough suppressants	Robitussin, Vicks 44, Chloraseptic
Decongestant	Advil Cold and Sinus, Afrin, Afrinol, Aleve Cold, Orrivin, Sudafed, Tavist-D and Tylenol
Cold and flue	Thera-flu, Alka Seltzer Cold and flu, Actidil Actifed, Allerest, Benadryl, Dimetane, Drixoral, Sudafed, and Triaminic
Diaper rash	Balmax and Desitin Ointments
Eyedrops for allergy	Ocu Hist
First-aid supplies	Ace Bandages, Band-Aids, Bandage Tape, Thermometers, Medical Gloves, Gauze, Neosporin, Rubbing Alcohol and Visine
Hemorrhoid treatments	Preparation H, Hemorid, and Tronolane

Prescription Drugs

Prescription drugs are legal drugs that can only be ordered by a doctor or a registered practitioner. Only a licensed pharmacist can sell prescription drugs. Prescription drugs are further divided into following categories:

1. Brand name prescription drugs
2. Generic prescription drugs

Brand Name Prescription Drugs

Brand name prescription drugs are those new medical agents which are patented and possess marketing exclusivity during the time period when the patents are in effect (about 20 years from discovery and 7–13 years from commercialization). Companies that develop successful patented drugs are usually rewarded very well during the patent protection period. However, these companies also incur very high research and development and marketing costs as well as the associated risk of failure. Table 2.2 enlists some branded prescription drugs.

Table 2.2: Brand name prescription drugs

Product name	Primary disease
Lipitor	Cholesterol
Nexium	Gastrointestinal disorders
Plavix	Thrombotic events
Advair Diskus	Asthma
Seroquel	Schizophrenia
Singulair	Asthma
Enbrel	Rheumatoid arthritis
Prevacid	Gastrointestinal disorders
Actos	Diabetes
Effexor Xr	Depression
Risperdal	Schizophrenia
Lexapro	Depression and anxiety
Abilify	Schizophrenia and bipolar disorder
Zyprexa	Schizophrenia
Aranesp	Anemia
Lamictal	Epilesy
Vytorin	Cholesterol
Topamax	Seizures
Cymbalta	Depression

Generic Prescription Drugs

When the patents of branded drugs expire, companies that specialize in dosage form development are allowed to manufacture and market a bioequivalent version of the branded drugs at a lower cost. This type of product is often referred to as a generic drug. The cost is lower because there are no basic research and clinical trials needed to make generics. Table 2.3 enlists example of some generic drugs.

Table 2.3: Examples of commonly prescribed generic drugs

Product name	Primary disease
Simvastatin	Cholesterol
Bupropion	Depression
Levothyroxine	Hypothyroidism
Hydrocodone	Cough
Amoxicillin	Infection
Azithromycin	Infection
Lisinopril	Hypertension
Alprazolam	Anxiety
Cyanocobalamin	Vitamin B_{12} deficiency
Hydromorphone	Pain
Atenolol	Myocardial infarction
Polymyxin B	Infection
Furosemide	Edema and hypertension
Imipramine	Depression
Metolazone	Diuretic, saluretic and hypertension
Cilostazol	Intermittent claudication
Tamoxifen	Cancer
Clorazepate	Anxiety
Indapamide	Hypertension

PARTS OF A PRESCRIPTION

A complete prescription must have following components:

• Date
• Name and address of the patient
• R_x symbol or superscription
• Medication prescribed or inscription
• Dispensing directions to pharmacist or subscription

- Directions for patient or signatura
- Refill information, special labeling or other instructions.
- Name, signature, address and registration no. of prescriber.

Figure 2.1 showing a model prescription and its various parts.

Date

Prescriptions are dated at the same time as they are written or ordered by the physician and also when they are received and filled in the pharmacy. The date is important for:

- Establishing the medication record of the patient.
- This help the pharmacist to find the cases where old prescriptions are to be repeated for a long time as in case of asthma, diabetic, hypertension, etc.
- The date prescribed is also important to a pharmacist in filling prescription for controlled substances. The drug abuse control amendment specifies that no prescription order for controlled substances may be dispensed or renewed more than 6 months after the date of prescription.

Name and Address of Patient

- It is important to identify the patient correctly.
- All names should be correctly spelled.
- An address and telephone number are important in case it becomes necessary to contact the patient at a later time.
- Age and gender of the patients become more important in case of children to check the dose of the medication.

Superscription

The "R$_X$" symbol is the superscription that heads the introduction to the prescribed medication.

R$_X$ is a Latin verb "recipe." Meaning "take thou" or "you take".

It is supposed to be the god of healing "Jupiter" for quick recovery from illness.

Inscription

This part of the prescription contains the name, strength, and quantity of medication to be prepared.

In case of complex prescription, inscription can be divided into four parts like the active ingredients, additives, vehicles and any other corrective measure to avoid possible incompatibilities.

Subscription

This section may include any special instructions or directions to the pharmacist about the method of preparation and dispensing.

Signatura

This section of the prescription is usually shortened "Sig." In Latin, the signatura means "take." The Sig is the directions to be typed on the label of the prescription container.

- It provides directions regarding the administration of the medication, i.e. how and when the dosage forms are to be administered or applied.
- Other information added to the label may be the medication's lot number and expiration date.

Refill Information

It is important for patients to know if their medication can be refilled without returning to the prescriber. If there is no refill, it is better to put this on the label than to put nothing.

Signature, Address and Registry Number of the Prescriber

The prescription must be signed by the prescriber. This is important because:

- The signature and address of the prescriber authenticates the prescription.
- If the prescription is a narcotic or controlled substance, the physician's registration number needs to be added. An example of a sample prescription is given in Table 2.4.

Name of patient:	M. Rajesh
Date:	10/10/2010
Age:	32 yrs
Address of patient:	Baba Farid Complex, Moga
Sex:	Male
R$_x$ (superscription)	
Inscription	
Calcium carbonate	15 g
Talc	15 g
Calcium phosphate	100 g
Prepare powder **(Subscription)**	
Signatura:	Tablespoonful to be taken at every morning and night
Name of prescriber:	Dr. A.K.Goyal
Regd. no:	LM-3446
Address of prescriber:	Chakki Wali Gali, Moga
Signature of prescriber	

Fig. 2.1: Model prescription and its various parts

Table 2.4: Sample prescription	
AG PHARMACY PH 9188206383 Kunal (18 yrs) 1234 Bhopal, Surendra Place, M.P 27501. **R**$_x$ Ibuprofen 800 mg Take 1 tablet by mouth 3 times a day No Refills Qty 50 R.Ph. Rajesh Verma Regd. No. MCI-123456 Date filled 20-10-2009 Discard After 20-10-2011 *Rajesh*	**AG PHARMACY** PH 9188206383 Kamal (20 yrs) 1234 Bhopal, Surendra Place, M.P 27501 **R**$_x$ Activella tablets UPS Take 1 tablet by mouth every day 11 Refills Qty 30 R.Ph. Smith Regd. No. MCI-32459 Date filled 20-1-2011 Discard After 20-10-2012 *Smit*

Table 2.4: Sample prescription (*contd.*)

AG PHARMACY PH 9188206383	**AG PHARMACY** PH 9188206383
Manish (35 yrs)	Satish (30 yrs)
1234 Bhopal, Surendra Place, M.P 27501	1234 Bhopal, Surendra Place, M.P 27501
R_x	R_x
Doxycycline mono 100 mg	Allegra-D 500 mg
Take 1 capsule twice a day after meals for 2 weeks. Take 1 capsule daily thereafter.	Take 1/2 tablet by mouth every 12 hours
No Refills Qty 100	3 Refills before 4-12-2012 Qty 30
R.Ph. Amit Awasthi	R.Ph. Katharan Dey
Regd. No. MCI-34670	Regd. No. MCI-09751
Date filled 20-10-2010 Discard After 20-10-2012	Date filled 09-08-2010 Discard After 9-8-2012

NEETU PHARMACY PH 9188206383	**NEETU PHARMACY** PH 9188206383
Manoj (40 yrs)	Ravi (35 yrs)
1234 Bhopal, Surendra Place, M.P 27501	1234 Bhopal, Surendra Place, M.P 27501
R_x	R_x
Viagra	Lodine
Take 1 capsule by mouth as needed	Take 1 tablet by mouth 2 times a day
No Refills Qty 20	6 Refills before 20-10-2010 Qty 60
R.Ph. Sperash Sharma	R.Ph. Mickal Lee
Regd. No. MCI-65195	Regd. No. MCI-45601
Date filled 20-10-2010 Discard After 20-10-2012	Date filled 20-10-2010 Discard After 20-10-2012

MEDICATION ORDER

While prescriptions are written in an outpatient setting, medication orders (Table 2.5) are written in an institutional setting. A medication order is also known as a drug order or a physician's order. These orders generally contain the name, age or date of birth, hospital ID number, room number, the date of admission to hospital, and any patient allergies. Sometimes the patient's diagnosis is included. Besides patient information, the following information about the medication is included:

- Date and time of the medication order
- Name of the drug (brand or generic)
- Dosage form

- Route of administration, e.g. oral, sublingual, intramuscular, intravenous, rectal.
- Administration schedule, e.g. times per day, milliliters per hour, at bedtime.
- Other information such as some restrictions or specifications
- Prescriber's signature
- Provision for the pharmacist's or nurse's notes

Practically, prescriptions must be difficult to understand by a layman to avoid any chance of self-medication. It is sometimes even difficult for a pharmacist to understand the prescription but after a considerable experience about the terminology, abbreviations and handwriting used on the prescription by physicians, it become easy for him to read and understand the prescription. The Latin terms which have been used in the prescription are still frequently used by some of the physicians.

Table 2.5: Sample medication order

Rajaram Health Care Hospital
Gandhi Chowk, Kotma, Dist. Anuppur, Pin. 484334, M.P. (India)

Physician's Order Sheet			Rajnagar, 42-11/A, , Dist. Anuppur, Pin. 484334 MP (India)	Admit 2/26/09 DOB 7/7/77 Dr. S. K. Agrawal Room 107
Please use Ball point pen and press firmly. You are making more than copy			Nurse Notes	
			Hour	Name
Ordered		Physician orders		
Date	Time	Start a new section with each set orders		
2/26	0900	Dynapen 259 mg. PO q6h		
2/26	0900	Datvon Compound 65 PO q4h prn pain		
2/26	0900	Vibramycin 0.2 g PO stat	0940	L, Ito
		Anshul (M.D.)		

Some of the common Latin abbreviations are given in Table 2.6.

Table 2.6: Latin terms and common abbreviations

Latin term	Common abbreviation	Translation
ad	ad	to, up to
ad lib.	ad lib.	at pleasure
adde	add	add (thou)
agita	agit	shake, stir

contd...

Table 2.6: Latin terms and common abbreviations (*contd.*)		
Latin term	**Common abbreviation**	**Translation**
alternis horis	alt. h.	every other hour
ana	a.a. or aa	of each
ante	a.	before
ante cibum	a.c.	before food, before meals
ante meridiem	a.m.	morning
amp.	amp.	ampule
aqua	aq.	water
aqua ad	aq. ad.	water up to
ag. dest; aqua dist	ag. dest; aqua dist.	distilled water
auris	aur.; a	ear
auris dexter	a.d.	right ear
aurix laevus	a.l.	left ear
auris sinister	a.s.	left ear
auris utro	a.u.	each ear
auristillae	aurist	ear-drops
a.t.c.	a.t.c.	around the clock
bis	b.	twice
bis in die	b.i.d.	twice a day
brachium	brach.	the arm
bsa	BSA	body surface area
capsula	caps	a capsule
c.c.	c.c.	cubic centimeter
chartulae	charts	powder papers; divided powders
cibus	cib.; c.	food
collunarium	collun	a nose wash
collutorium	collut.	a mouthwash
collyrium	collyr.	an eyewash
compositus	comp.	compound
congius	cong.; C.	gallon
cum	c or c.	with
cum cibus	c.c.	with food; with meals
dentur	d.	give (thou); let be given
dentur tales doses	d.t.d.	give of such doses
dexter	d.	right

contd...

Latin term	Common abbreviation	Translation
diebus alternis	dieb. alt.	every other day
dilutus	dil.	dilute, diluted
disp.	disp.	dispense
div.	div.	divide
DW	DW	distilled water
elix.	elix.	elixir
emulsum	emuls.	emulsion
et	et	and
ex modo prescripto	e.m.p.	in the manner prescribed; as directed
fac, fiat, fiant	f.; ft.	let it be made; make
f.; fl.	f.; fl.	fluid
g.; G.; gm.	g.; G.; gm.	gram
granum	gr.	grain
guttae	gtt.	a drop
hora	h	at the hour of
hora somni	h.s.	at bedtime
injectio	i.m.	intramuscular
	inj.	injection
	i.v.; IV	intravenous
	i.v.p.; IVP	intravenous push
	IVPB	intravenous piggyback
laevus	l.	left
linimentum	lin.	liniment
liquor	liq.	a solution
lot.	lot.	lotion
minimum	min; Mx	minum
misce	m.; M	mix
mcg.	mcg.	microgram
mEq.	mEq.	milliequivalent
mg.	mg.	milligram
ml.	ml.	milliliter
nocte	n.	at night
naristillae	narist.	nasal drops
nebule	neb.	a spray

Table 2.6: Latin terms and common abbreviations (contd.)

contd...

Latin term	Common abbreviation	Translation
	N.F.	National Formulary
non repetatur	non.rep.	do not repeat
	NS	normal saline
octarius	O.	pint
oculentum	occulent.	eye ointment
oculus	o.	eye
oculus dexter	o.d.	right eye
oculus laevus	o.l.	left eye
oculus sinister	o.s.	left eye
oculus utro	o.u.	both eyes, each eye
omni mane	o.m.	every morning
parti affectae applicandus	p.a.a.	to be applied to affected part
per os	p.o.	by mouth
post cibum	p.c.	after meals
	p.r.	per rectum
pro re nata	p.r.n.	as needed
pulvis	pulv.	powder
quater in die	q.i.d.	four times a day
quaque	q.	each, every
quaque die	q.d.	every day
quaque hora	q.h.	every hour
quantum sufficiat	q.s.	a sufficient quantity
quantum sufficiat ad	q.s. ad	a sufficient quantity to make
secundum artem	s.a.	according to the art
	S.C.; subc; subq	subcutaneously
semis	ss	one-half
signa	Sig.	write, label
sine	s	without
si opus sit	s.o.s.	if necessary
	sol.	solution
statim	stat.	immediately
suppositorum	supp.	suppository
syrupus	syr.	syrup
tabella	tab.	tablet

Table 2.6: Latin terms and common abbreviations (*contd.*)

contd...

Table 2.6: Latin terms and common abbreviations (*contd.*)

Latin term	Common abbreviation	Translation
	tbsp.	tablespoonful
ter in die	t.i.d.	three times a day
	tinc.; tr.	tincture
trochiscus	troche	lozenge
tussis	tuss.	a cough
ungentum	ung.	an ointment
ut dictum	ut dict.; u.d.	as directed

PROCESSING OF PRESCRIPTION ORDER

The manner in which a pharmacist processes a prescription order is important in fulfilling his/her responsibilities and can enhance his/her image with the physician and the patient. Proper procedure of dispensing and compounding consists of various steps:

1. Receiving the prescription.
2. Reading and checking the prescription.
3. Numbering and dating the prescription.
4. Preparing or compounding and labeling the prescription, packaging.
5. Rechecking, delivering and counseling, recording and filing.
6. Pricing the prescription.

Receiving the Prescription

It is desirable that the patient present the prescription order directly to the pharmacist.

- This improves the pharmacist-patient relationship.
- This helps pharmacist to collect complete data of health and medication history of the patient.
- If the pharmacist is unable to receive the prescription order personally, he/she should be available to provide information regarding refilling of prescription and to price it, if required by the patient.

- A pharmacist should not give such face expression to the patient that he/she is surprised or confused after seeing the prescription.

Reading and Checking the Prescription

The prescription order first should be read completely and carefully. This step is essential because:

- There should be no doubt as to the ingredients or quantities prescribed, units of weights and measures, quantity to be supplied and direction for use.
- The pharmacist should determine the compatibility of the prescribed medication with other drugs and also consider if any drugfood or drug-drug interactions may exist.
- In case of any prescription incompatibilities, the pharmacist should first consider alternative drug products that might be used and then consult with the prescriber to determine best therapeutic alternative for the patient.
- If something is illegible or if it appears that an error has been made, the pharmacist should consult another pharmacist or the prescriber.
- A pharmacist should never guess at the meaning of an indistinct word or unrecognized abbreviation.

- Unfamiliar or unclear abbreviations represent a source of error in interpreting and dispensing prescriptions. No official or standard list of prescription abbreviations exists. Many of those in use are derived from the Latin and generally are recognized.

- Pharmacists are frequently confronted in their interpretation of the prescription order with the names of drugs that look alike or sound alike. These similar names are a potential source for errors.

- Omissions, such as the failure to specify the desired strength of a medication or its dosage form, must be corrected, in such a case, the pharmacist should never elect to dispense the usual dose or dosage form but instead should consult the prescriber.

- The amount and frequency of a dose must be noted carefully and checked. In determining the safety of the dose of a medicinal agent, the age, weight, and condition of the patient (e.g. liver function, kidney function), dosage form prescribed, possible influence of other concomitant drugs being taken, and the frequency of administration, all must be considered.

- Several guides are available to the pharmacist in evaluating the safety of a prescribed dose. Manufacturers' catalogs, file cards, and package inserts provide dosage information on their products. References such as **Physicians' Desk Reference, Drug Today, CIMS, AMA Drug Evaluations, American Hospital Formulary Service, Drug information, Drug Facts and Comparisons, Handbook of Clinical Drug Data, Pharmacist Drug Handbook, www.drug.com** and **Pediatric Dosage Handbook** are useful general sources of such information. Some computer software programs now can check doses for pediatric patients when the child's weight is entered.

- Measurement of liquid medication may lead to dosage variation caused by differences in the capacity of household spoons and interpretation of which measuring device to use by the patient. To avoid errors in liquid dosing, pharmacists often dispense calibrated measuring devices with liquid medication.

Numbering and Dating

It is a legal requirement to number the prescription order and to place the same number on the label. This serves:

- To identify the bottle or package and to connect it with the original order for reference or to renew the prescription.

- Consecutive numbers are assigned by prescription computers or manually by use of numbering machine.

- Dating of the prescription on the date filled is also a legal requirement.

- This information is important in determining the appropriate refill frequency, patient compliance, and as an alternate means of locating the prescription order, if lost by the patient.

Weighing and Measuring Procedure

During weighing and measuring, unless strict guidelines are followed, it can be very easy to mix up different pharmaceutical ingredients. It is preferable to incorporate a weighed or measured ingredient into a product as soon as possible to prevent any accidental switching. If this is not possible, when weighing or measuring more than one ingredient, place each on a piece of labeled paper as soon as it has been weighed or measured. This will avoid any accidental cross-over of ingredients. Table 2.7 enlists some commonly used tools used to weigh and measure ingredients in compounding of pharmaceuticals.

Table 2.7: Commonly used tools to weight and measure ingredients in compounding of pharmaceuticals

Measuring device	Description
	Chemicals or small objects from 15 mg to 100 gm can be weighed with this model. This type of balance also know as despensing or prescription balance.
	The weight is measured by means of one or more bars (levers) with sliding weights that are marked with the exact weight that balances the contents in the pan. So the principle is a simple lever with weights on one side of the fulcrum that balance the weight of the unknown object in the pan. This type of balance is also known as a single beam or tarson balance.
	An analytical balance is used to measure mass to a very high degree of precision and accuracy. The measuring pan(s) of a high precision (0.1 mg or better) analytical balance are inside a transparent enclosure with doors so that dust does not collect and so any air currents in the room do not affect the balance's operation.
	A measuring cup is used primarily to measure the volume of liquid or bulk solid ingredients especially for volumes from about 50 ml (2 fl oz) upwards. The cup will usually have a scale marked in cup and fractions of a cup, and often with fluid measure and weight of a selection of dry foodstuffs. Measuring cups may be made of plastic, glass, or metal. Maximum capacity usually ranges from 0.2 to 1 litre, though larger sizes are also available (for commercial use). Smaller measuring spoons lack a scale and are filled and leveled to maximum capacity.
	A graduated cylinder, also known as a measuring cylinder, is a piece of laboratory equipment used to accurately measure the volume of an object.

contd...

Measuring device	Description
Table 2.7: Commonly used tools to weight and measure ingredients in compounding of pharmaceuticals (*contd.*)	
	A volumetric flask is used to make up a solution of fixed volume very accurately.
	Teaspoons with longer handles, such as iced tea spoons, are commonly used also for liquid formulation. Similar spoons include the table-spoon and the dessert spoon, the latter intermediate in size between a teaspoon and a tablespoon.
	Pipettes are devices that allow the users to extract or deliver small amounts of a liquid. Pipettes come in a variety of designs. Some are graduated to deliver exact quantities, but most allow for a "drop at a time" of delivery. Pipettes that dispense between 1 and 1000 µl are termed micropipettes, while macropipettes dispense a greater volume of liquid. Two types of micropipettes are generally used— air-displacement pipettes and positive-displacement pipettes.

Preparing the Prescriptions

After reading and checking the prescription order, the pharmacist should decide on the exact procedure to be followed in dispensing or compounding the medications. Most prescription call for dispensing medications already prefabricated into dosage forms by pharmaceutical manufacturer. In filling prescription with preferred products, the pharmacist should check the manufacturer's label, comparing it to the prescription order, before and after filling the order, to make certain of its correctness. When a prescription requiring compounding is received the pharmacist should take following considerations:

- The chemical and physical compatibility of the ingredients.
- The proper order of mixing
- Need for special adjuvants or techniques
- Mathematical calculation required.

Once the procedure has been decided, the pharmacist assembles the necessary materials in a single location on the prescription counter. As each ingredient is used, it is transferred to another location away from the work station. The use of this technique provides the pharmacist with a mechanical check on the introduction of each ingredient. When the pharmacist has finished, all the ingredients are returned to their storage places. Through this process, the pharmacist has the opportunity to read the label of each ingredient three times; once when the container is removed from the storage shelf, again when the contents are weighed and measured and, finally when the container is returned to the shelf.

Any calculation or compounding information that would be useful in refilling the prescription at later date should be noted either on the face or on the back of the prescription order.

Adjuvant used, order of mixing, amount of each ingredient, capsule size used, type and size of container, name and product identification number of manufacturer, auxiliary labels used, clarification of illegible words or numbers, price charged and any special notations should be recorded. The failure to do this may result in differences in the appearance of the prescription when refilled and possibly create doubt and apprehension in the mind of the patient.

Labeling

It is a legal requirement to affix a prescription label on the immediate container of prescription medications. The pharmacist is responsible for the accuracy of the label. It should bear the name, address, and the telephone number of the pharmacy, the date of dispensing, the prescription number, the prescriber's name, the name and address of the patient, and the directions for use of the medication. The label for a sample prescription is given in Table 2.4. All labels must be type written or computer generated. The details, which must appear on the label of a dispensed medicine are:

- **Identification of product:** Name of product, statement of active ingredients, pharmaceutical form like solution, syrup, ointment, powder, tablet, etc.

- **A batch number:** Batch number should be awarded to each product at the time of preparation and it should be incorporated into the label also.

- **Patient information:** Patient's name, gender, height and weight information, address and age.

- **Therapeutic indications:** Information needed for taking the product. Contraindications, precautions for use, inter actions, special warnings, including use in pregnancy, elderly, effect on ability to drive vehicles and details of any excipients which may be important for safe and effective use of the product.

- **Instructions for use:** Dosage, method and route of administration, frequency of administration, duration of treatment where limited, action to be taken in the case of an overdose or lack of dosing and risk of withdrawal effects where possible.

- **Date of dispensing and pharmacist details:** Date of dispensing and refill date (if necessary). Name, address, registration and contact number of pharmacist.

- **Storage:** Some formulations require special storage to prevent degradation and this information should be attached to the label. The pharmacists while stating the storage conditions on the label may follow the following guidelines.

  ❖ **Temperature:** A large number of products need to be stored in a cool place preferably below 15°C. For example, pessaries and suppositories, which are intended to melt at body temperature, may be spoiled, if placed near heat source. Immunological products and insulin injections are usually required to be stored between 2 and 8°C.

  ❖ **Humidity:** Dosage forms containing hygroscopic and deliquescent drugs should be protected from moisture. Such products should be supplied in air and moisture proof container and patient should be guided to replace the cap after use. In case of powders, double wrapping is must, i.e. first with wax paper and then with simple paper.

❖ **Light:** The light sensitive product like vitamins, etc. should be stored in amber color containers to avoid photodegradation. A few substances such as paraldehyde must be stored in complete darkness.

• **Instruction to the patient:** There should be clear and complete instructions to the patient on how to take or use the preparation.

❖ **Direction:** The phrases such as 'to be taken' 'to be given' or 'to be used' are preferred to 'take' 'give' 'use'. The direction written on the label of a dispensed medicine should be simple and without any confusion.

❖ **Shake the bottle before use:** Biphasic dosage forms like emulsion, suspension and aerosols need to be shaken immediately before its use, in order to ensure the homogeneous dispersion and to get equal contents of medicament in each dose so this instruction must appear on the label of such preparation.

❖ **Take with water:** Some medicaments cause gastrointestinal irritation in concentrated form so these should be diluted before administration so it should be written on the label at the time of dispense.

Table 2.8: Drug needing cautionary labeling.

Sr. No.	Drug	Particulars
1	Schedule G drugs	"Caution: It is dangerous to take this preparation except under medical supervision"
2	Schedule H drugs	I. "Schedule H drugs Warning: To be sold on the prescription of a Registered Medical Practitioner"
		II. Symbol R_x prominently on left hand top corner of the label.
		III. Symbol $N\ R_x$ prominently on the left hand top corner if drug is covered under Narcotic Drugs and Psychotropic substance Act.
3	Schedule X drugs	I. Warning: To be sold on the prescription of RMPs only.
		II. Symbol $X\ R_x$ in red on left hand top corner.
4	Schedule C drugs	I. When the test for maximum toxicity is prescribed a statement that it has passed that test.
		II. Nature and percentage of antiseptic, if any.
5	Ophthalmic solutions/ suspensions/ointments	I. Use within one month of opening. Not for injection.
		II. Name and concentration of preservative.
		III. Do not touch the dropper tip/other dispensing tip to any surface since this may contaminate.

Drugs needing cautionary labeling

• Tables 2.8 and 2.10 contain special labeling instructions of the dispensed medication, including its proper use, handling, storage, and necessary warning and precautions.

Special method of administration

In case of special method of administration, following wording may be written on the label as given in Table 2.9.

• *Cautions in use:* The wording enlisted in Table 2.10 may be written on the label in order to caution a patient about certain unusual happenings after taking the medicine.

- Special labeling instructions for particular type of dosage form. Table 2.11 enlists special labeling instructions for different dispensed medication.

Warning

Patients especially drivers should be warned if their medicine is likely to cause drowsiness, dizziness, and blurred vision. The following wording may be written on the label.

- May cause drowsiness, if affected do not drive or operate machinery, avoid alcoholic drink.
- To be taken an hour before food or empty stomach.
- Drug which causes GI irritation
- To be taken with or after food
- Some drugs cause interaction with alcohol and may provoke a reaction such as flushing when taken together such as metronidazole.

Potential interaction with food or drink

The following type of wording may be written on the label under different conditions:
- Drug in which absorption is improved, if taken before meal
- Avoid alcoholic drink.

Table 2.9: Special method of administration

Type of formulation	Warning
Mouth dissolving formulations	To be sucked or chewed
Formulations where sublingual absorption is required	To be dissolved under toung
Formulations with water soluble drugs	Dissolve or mix with water before taking
Drugs which cause gastric irritation in concentrated form	To be taken with plenty of water
Enteric coated and sustained release formulations	To be swallowed whole, not to be chewed

Table 2.10: Cautions in use

Cause	Precaution
The preparation, which may induce photosensitization	Avoid exposure of skin to direct sunlight
The preparation, which may produce unusual effect	The preparation may color the urine or stool
The preparation, which contain high proportion of flammable solvent	Keep away from naked flame

Table 2.11: Special labeling instructions for dispensed medication

Name of preparation	Labeling instructions
Aerosol inhalations	Pressurized containers, keep away from heat source. Shake before use. Do not exceed the prescribed dose, follow the instructions.
Applications	For external use only.
Capsules	Swallow with a draught of water.
Creams	For external use only. Store in a cool place.
Dusting powders	For external use only. Not to be applied on open wound or to raw or weeping surface.
Eardrops	For external use only.
Emulsions	Shake the bottle before use.

contd...

Table 2.11: Special labeling instructions for dispensed medication (*contd.*)	
Name of preparation	**Labeling instructions**
Enemas	For rectal use only. Shake well before use. Warm to body temperature before use.
Eyedrops	To be used in 30 days after first opening
Eye lotions	To be used within 24 hrs after first opening.
Gargles and mouthwashes	Not to be swallowed in large amounts. Dilute with water before use
Effervescent granules	To be dissolved or dispersed in water before taking.
Inhalations	Not to be taken. Shake the bottle before use.
Insufflations	Not to be swallowed.
Linctuses	To be slipped and swallowed slowly without the addition of water.
Liniments and lotions	For external use only. Shake the bottle before use. Do not apply on broken skin.
Mixtures	Shake the bottle before use. To be taken only after diluting with water.
Nasal drops	For nasal use only.
Ointments	For external use only. Sterile not to be used for injection.
Paints	For external use only.
Passaries	For vaginal use only. Store in cool place. For external use only.
Pastes	For external use only.
Solutions	For external use only. Sterile not to be used for injection. For rectal use only.
Suppositories	For rectal use only. Store in a cool place.
For soluble or dispersible tablets For chewable tablets For sustain release, enteric coated or unpleasant tasting tablets.	Dissolve or dispense in water before taking. Chew before swallowing. Do not crush or chew.

Auxiliary Labels

They are used to emphasize a number of important aspects of the dispensed medica-tion. The use of labels such as "for the ear" and "external use" is recommended because of the added safety they offer, even when the primary direction indicates their proper use. They should be placed in a conspicuous spot on the prescription container. Examples of some auxiliary labels are shown in Fig. 2.2.

A Package Insert or Prescribing Information

This is a document provided along with a prescription medication to provide additional information about that drug. Package inserts follow a standard format for every medica-

tion and include the same type of information. Different manufacturers may have different titles for their sections, however, to make them easier for the average person to read and comprehend, e.g. instead of "contraindications" the section may be headed, "Who should not take this medication?" The first thing listed is usually the brand name and generic name of the product. The other sections are as follows:

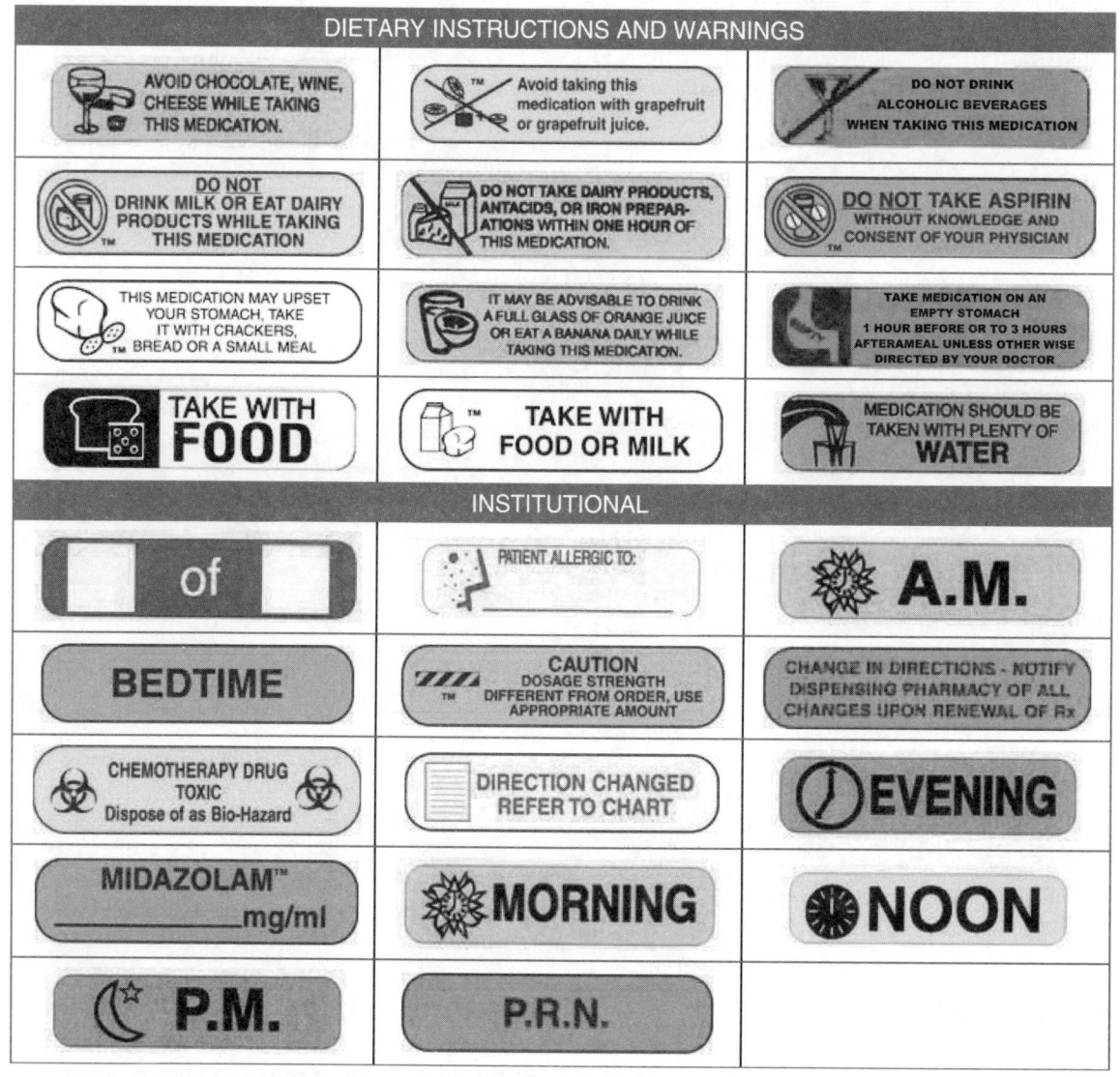

contd...

INSTRUCTIONS

 DSSOLYE UNDER THE TONGUE OR IN THE MOUTH AS DIRECTED BY YOUR DOCTOR **DO NOT CHEW OR SWALLOW WHOLE**

 DO NOT CHEW SWALLOW WHOLE

 DO NOT CRUSH

 DO NOT TAKE THIS DRUG IF YOU BECOME PREGNANT

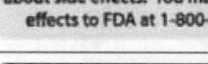 Call your doctor for medical advice about side effects. You may report side effects to FDA at 1-800-FDA-1088

 NOT TO BE TAKEN BY MOUTH

 FOR VAGINAL USE ONLY

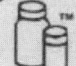 **IMPORTANT** FINISH ALL THIS MEDICATION UNLESS OTHERWISE DIRECTED BY PRESCRIBER

 OBTAIN MEDICAL ADVICE before taking non-prescription drugs, some may effect the action of this medication.

 REFRIGERATE SHAKE WELL Discard afger

 SHAKE WELL

 SHAKE WELL AND KEEP IN THE REFRIGERATOR

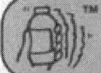 **SHAKE WELL BEFORE USING**

 SHAKE WELL STORE IN REFRIGERATOR & DISCARD UNUSED PORTION **AFTER 14 DAYS**

 This Antibiotic may decrease the effectiveness of birth control pills.

 THIS IS THE SAME MEDICATION YOU HAVE BEEN GETTING. COLOR, SIZE OR SHAPE MAY APPEAR DIFFERENT

 This item was specially compounded for you. Please contact us a day ahead to reorder.

 THIS BOTTLE IS NOT FULL BUT CONTAINS THE EXACT AMOUNT PRESCRIBED BY YOUR PHYSICIAN.

ROUTE

 DISSOLVE UNDER THE TONGUE OR IN THE MOUTH AS DIRECTED BY YOUR DOCTOR. **DO NOT CHEW OR SWALLOW WHOLE.**

 DO NOT CHEW SWALLOW WHOLE

 FOR EXTERNAL USE ONLY

 for rectal use ONLY

 FOR THE EARS

 FOR THE **eye**

 FOR THE NOSE

 FOR TOPICAL USE ONLY

 FOR VAGINAL USE ONLY

REFILL

 AVOID WAITING for your prescription refills by calling the day before you to come in. Thank you.

 PHYSICIAN'S AUTHORIZATION REQUIRED FOR REFILL, PLEASE CALL 24 HOURS IN ADVANCE

 THIS BOTTLE IS NOT FULL BUT CONTAINS THE EXACT AMOUNT PRESCRIBED BY YOUR PHYSICIAN.

 THIS IS THE LAST REFILL FOR THIS PRESCRIPTION Please contact your Physician

 THIS ITEM WAS SPECIALLY ORDERED FOR YOU. PLEASE CONTACT US A DAY AHEAD TO REORDER

This item was specially compounded for you. Please contact us a day ahead to reorder.

 Your Doctor has asked that you make an appointment.

 We OWE You

 YOU MUST see a Physician before this prescription can be refilled

contd...

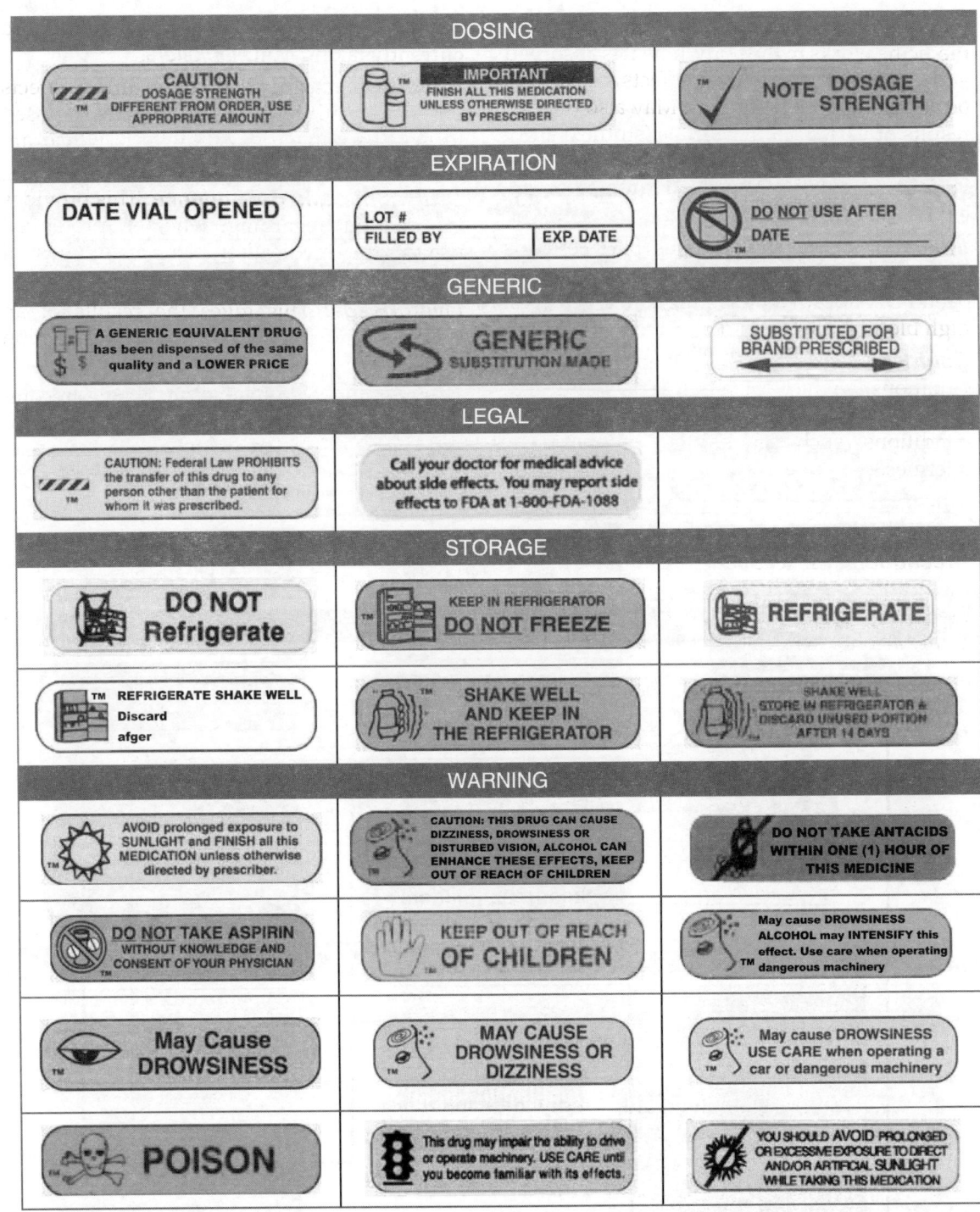

Fig. 2.2: Examples of pharmacy auxiliary labels

Clinical pharmacology: This tells how the medicine works in the body, how it is absorbed and eliminated, and what its effects are likely to be at various concentrations. May also contain results of various clinical trials (studies) and/or explanations of the medication's effect on various populations (e.g. children, women, etc.).

Indications and usage: This part contains the uses (indications) for which the drug has been FDA-approved (e.g. migraines, seizures, high blood pressure).

Contraindications: This contains the list of situations in which the medication should not be used, e.g. in patients with other medical conditions such as kidney problems or allergies.

Warnings: It covers possible serious side effects that may occur.

Precautions: It explains how to use the medication safely including physical impairments and drug interactions; e.g. "Do not drink alcohol while taking this medication"

or, "Do not take this medication, if you are currently taking *MAO inhibitors.*"

Adverse reactions: This enlists all side effects observed in all studies of the drug (as opposed to just the dangerous side effects which are separately listed in "Warnings" section).

Drug abuse and dependence: This provides information regarding whether prolonged use of the medication can cause physical dependence (only included if applicable).

Overdosage: This gives the results of an overdose and provides recommended action in such cases.

Dosage and administration: It gives recommended dosage(s); may list more than one for different conditions for different patients (e.g. lower dosages for children).

How supplied: This explains in detail the physical characteristics of the medication including color, shape, markings, etc., and storage information (e.g. "Do not store above 95°C"). Figure 2.3 gives an illustration of packaging insert.

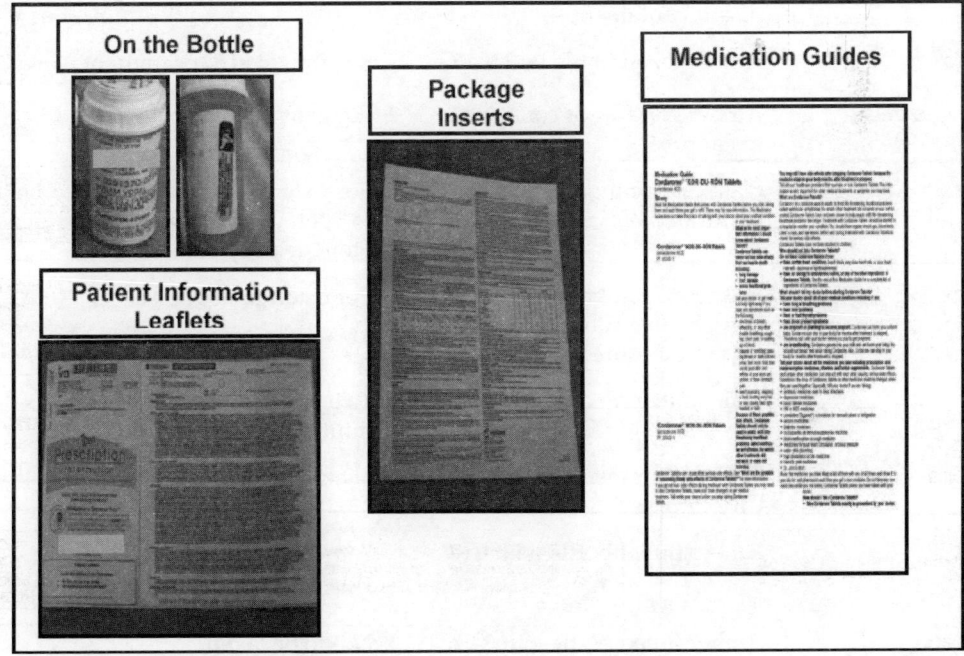

Fig. 2.3: Components of drug labeling

Packaging

In filling a prescription, pharmacists may select a container from among various shapes, sizes, mouth openings, colors and composition Selection is based primarily upon the type and quantity of medication to be dispensed and the method of its use.

Among type of containers generally used in pharmacy are round bottles, prescription bottles, wide mouth bottles, dropper bottles, applicator bottles, ointment jars and collapsible tubes, sifter top container, hinged lid or slide boxes and aerosol containers.

Most of the prescription containers usually are available in colorless or amber-colored glass or plastic. Amber-colored container is used most widely since it provides maximum protection of its contents against photochemical deterioration. In most instances, a container made of good quality amber glass will reduce light transmission sufficiently to protect light-sensitive pharmaceuticals. The closure on a prescription container is as important as the container itself. Prescription container must be moisture-proof and thus the ability of the closure to restrict entrance of moisture into the container is of prime importance. Moisture has deteriorating effect of many dosage forms, especially capsules, tablets and powders. Many pharmacies use screw cap glass or tight fitting closures to reduce moisture penetration. Here are some suggestions given in Table 2.12, to choose suitable containers and auxiliary labels for extemporaneous preparations.

Preparation	Container	Important auxiliary labels
Table 2.12: A guide to auxiliary labels and container for extemporaneous preparations		
Applications	Amber fluted bottle with CRC	For external use only.
Cachets	Colored or colorless, glass or plastic container	Swallow with a draught of water.
Capsules	Amber tablet bottle with CRC	Swallow with a draught of water.
Creams and gels	Amber glass jar or collapsible metal tube	For external use only.
Dusting powders	Plastic jar preferably with a perforated reclosable lid	For external use only. Not to be applied to open wounds or raw weeping surfaces Store in a dry place.
Ear drops	Hexagonal amber fluted glass bottle with a rubber teat and dropper closure	For external use only.
Elixirs	Plain amber medicine bottle with CRC	To be swallowed slowly without dilution.
Emulsions	Plain amber medicine bottle with CRC	Shake the bottle before use.
Enemas	Amber fluted bottle with CRC	For rectal use only. Warm to body temperature before use.
Gargles and mouthwashes	Amber fluted bottle with CRC	Not to be taken. Do not swallow in large amounts.

contd...

Table 2.12: A guide to auxiliary labels and container for extemporaneous preparations (*contd.*)

Preparation	Container	Important auxiliary labels
Granules	Colorless, plain, glass or plastic jar	Not to be swallowed in large amounts. Dilute with water before use.
Inhalations	Amber fluted bottle with CRC	Not to be taken. Shake the bottle.
Linctuses	Plain amber medicine bottle with CRC	To be slipped and swallowed slowly without the addition of water.
Liniments and lotions	Amber fluted bottle with CRC	For external use only. Shake the bottle. Avoid broken skin.
Mixtures and suspensions	Plain amber medicine bottle with CRC	Shake the bottle.
Nasal drops	Hexagonal amber fluted glass bottle with a rubber teat and dropper closure.	Not to be taken.
Ointments	Amber glass jar	For external use only.
Pastes	Amber glass jar	For external use only.
Pessaries	Wrapped in foil and packed in an amber glass jar	For vaginal use only.
Powders (individual)	Wrapped in powder papers and packed in a cardboard carton	Store in a dry place. Dissolve or mix with water before taking.
Solution	Amber fluted bottle with CRC	For external or internal use only (as directed).
Suppositories	Wrapped in foil and packed in an amber glass jar	For rectal use only. Store in a cool place.
Tablet	Amber tablet bottle with CRC	Dissolve or dispense in water before taking.

CRC–child resistant closure.

Although different pharmaceutical preparations will be packaged in different containers depending on the product type. Pharmaceutical packaging can largely be grouped into a few main types (Table 2.13).

Table 2.13: Different containers used in pharmaceutical packaging

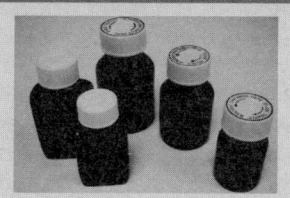

Tablet bottles

Tablet bottles come in a variety of shapes and sizes and are usually made of either glass or plastic. Generally, tablet bottles are colored amber to reduce the likelihood of the contents reacting with light. They are used for solid, single-dose preparations that are intended for oral use (i.e. tablets and capsules).

contd...

Table 2.13: Different containers used in pharmaceutical packaging (*contd.*)

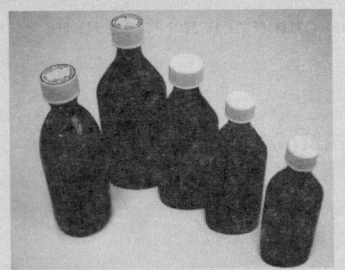

Plain amber medicine bottles

Plain amber medicine bottles can be used to package all internal liquid preparations. Traditional amber medicine bottles have two different sides— one curved and one flat. The label or labels are usually placed on the curved side of the bottle as the patient's natural action will be to pick the bottle up with the curved side of the bottle facing the inside of the palm. This will prevent the label becoming damaged by any dribbles of liquid running down the side of the bottle during pouring of a dose. Plain amber medicine bottles usually come in the following sizes— 50, 100, 150, 200, 300 and 500 ml.

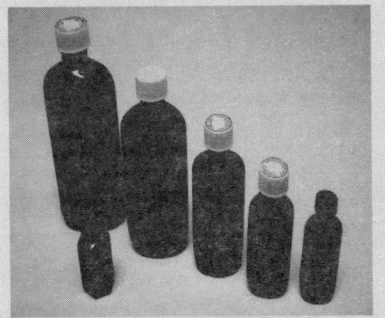

Fluted amber medicine bottles

Fluted (or ribbed) amber medicine bottles are similar to the plain amber medicine bottles but, instead of having a flat plain side, this side is curved and contains a number of ridges or grooves running from the top of the bottle down to the bottom. The ridges or grooves are intended to be both a visual and tactile warning to the patient that the contents of the bottle are not to be administered via the oral route (the tactile nature of the warning is particularly useful for blind or partially sighted patients). For this reason, these types of container are often referred to as 'external medicine bottles' or 'poison bottles'. Fluted bottles can be used with specific types of pharmaceutical preparations— embrocations, liniments, lotions, liquid antiseptics, other liquids or gels for external use.

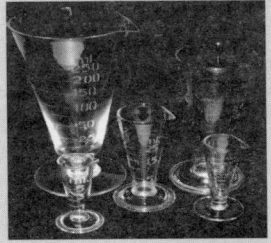

Conical measures

Liquid preparations are normally made up to volume in a conical measure. There are occasions where a tared or calibrated bottle may be used. A tared bottle is normally only employed when, because of the viscosity of the final product, the transference loss from the measure to the container would be unacceptable. For example, Kaolin Mixture BP is a very dense suspension and transference may cause problems; similarly, a thick emulsion will also prove difficult and time-consuming to transfer in its entirety because of the viscosity of the finished product.

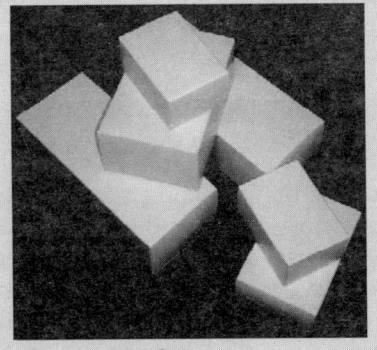

Cartons

Cardboard cartons come in a variety of differing sizes, the sizes being dependent on the manufacturer. They tend to be rectangular in shape and the label is placed on the larger side of the box. They are used to package blister strips of tablets or capsules, powder papers and other pharmaceutical products that may be of a shape that is not suitable for labeling. Although it is good dispensing practice to label the primary container of a medicinal product, in some cases this is not possible. By placing the primary container into a labeled carton, this provides the next best method for labeling the product in question (e.g. the labeling of very small eye/ear/nose dropper bottles). Additional care must be exercised in the storage of pharmaceutical products in cardboard cartons as they do not come with child-resistant closures.

contd...

Table 2.13: Different containers used in pharmaceutical packaging (*contd.*)

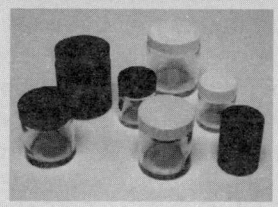 Ointment jars	Ointment jars come in a variety of different sizes and can be made of either colorless glass or amber glass. Amber ointment jars are used for preparations that are sensitive to light. They are used to package ointments and creams and can be used for individually wrapped suppositories. As with cartons, additional care must be exercised in the storage of preparations in ointment jars as they do not come with child-resistant closures.

Rechecking

Once the medication has been prepared and labeled, it needs to have a terminal check before it can be dispensed to the patient. The pharmacist must do this. Every prescription should be rechecked and the ingredients and amounts used verified by the pharmacist. All the details of the label should be rechecked against the prescription order to verify directions, patients name, prescription number, date and prescriber's name. After checking, the pharmacist's initials are added to the label and the patient's record.

Delivering and Patient Counseling

The pharmacist personally should present the prescription medication to the patient unless it is to be delivered to the patient's home or workplace. This gives the pharmacist assurance that the patient knows how to use the medication properly. When presenting the medication to the patient, the pharmacist also should call attention to any auxiliary labeling instructions and provide further information regarding the medication as may be desirable. When personal delivery of the prescription is not possible, the pharmacist should make certain that the appropriate instructions are provided to the patient and that he/she is encouraged to enquire phone, if there be any question.

The three **C**s of effective patient counseling are communication, comprehension, and compliance.

- **Communication:** To communicate effectively with patients, pharmacists need to remove any barrier to good communication, be good listener, and use open-ended questions.
- **Comprehension:** To counsel patients properly, pharmacists should select only a few key counseling points and verify that patients understand what they need to know.
- **Compliance:** Unless counseled, most patients will not take their medication exactly as prescribed. It is important to stress how often to take the medication and what may happen, if the patient does not take it as prescribed.

Recording and Filling

A record of the prescription dispensed is maintained in the pharmacy through the use of computer and hard copy prescription files.

Prescription Refilling

Instructions for refilling a prescription are provided by the prescriber on the original prescription or by verbal communication. Although prescriptions for noncontrolled substances have no limitation according to FDA. No prescription should be renewed indefinitely without the patient being re-evaluated by the prescriber to assure that the medication as originally prescribed remains the medication of choice. Renewal should be noted on the reverse side of the prescription order or in the prescription computer with the date and the quantity dispensing the medication.

STANDARDS FOR EXTEMPORANEOUS DISPENSING

Patients who visit a pharmacy with a prescription for a product needing to be extemporaneously prepared are entitled to expect the standards within a pharmacy to be comparable to those of a licensed manufacturing unit. The products produced within the pharmacy must be suitable for use, accurately prepared and prepared in such a way as to ensure that the products meet the required standard for quality assurance. So, although this is small-scale production, the same careful attention to detail is required as would be found in a manufacturing unit. The following measures must be taken into consideration when preparing a product extemporaneously.

Personal hygiene: Personal hygiene is extremely important. Hygiene standards within a pharmaceutical environment should be as high as, if not higher than, those found in food kitchens. This is because within a pharmaceutical environment, medication is being prepared for patients who may already be ill.

Personal protective equipment: A clean white coat should be worn to protect the compounder from the product and conversely the product from contamination from the compounder. During the compounding process, safety glasses should always be worn and, depending on the nature of the ingredients to be incorporated into the preparation, additional safety equipment (e.g. face masks, gloves) may also be required. It is the responsibility of the individual compounder to assess the risk posed by any pharmaceutical ingredient and to ensure that the correct safety equipment is in use. Similarly, long hair should be tied back and hands washed, ensuring any open cuts are covered.

Clean work area and equipment: The cleanliness of the work area and equipment used during the compounding procedure is of paramount importance. The risk of contaminating the final product with either dirt or microorganisms from the surroundings or from ingredients from a previous preparation can be considerable, if attention is not paid to the cleanliness of the work area and equipment. Before starting to compound a product, the work area and equipment should be cleaned with a suitable solution [e.g. industrial denatured alcohol (IDA), formerly known as industrial methylated spirits (IMS)], which must be allowed to dry fully.

Work area: In addition to the cleanliness of the work area, considerable attention needs to be given to the work area itself to ensure that it is suitable for its intended purpose. Both lighting and ventilation need to be adequate. Some pharmaceutical ingredients are highly volatile and so, if the ventilation within the work area is inadequate, this could cause problems for the compounding staff.

Label preparation: The label for any pharmaceutical product must be prepared before starting the compounding procedure. This will enable the product to be labeled as soon as it has been manufactured and packaged. This will eliminate a situation where an unlabeled product is left on the bench and would reduce the possibility of the product being mislabeled and given to the wrong patient.

ERRORS IN PRESCRIPTION

Causes of Prescription Errors

Prescription errors may result due to improper diagnosis or medical malpractice which includes:

- Ordering a medication for a patient with known allergies to that drug.
- Current medications could adversely react with the new medication.
- People with special health concerns, such as liver or kidney problems, may suffer as a result of prescription errors when an inappropriate or unsafe medicine is administered.

- Wrong medication or the wrong dose being administered altogether.
- Doctors are notorious for illegible handwriting. If a pharmacist is unable to read their handwriting or misreads the instructions, he/she may make prescription errors that could be injurious to that patient's health. When a person receives the wrong medication, he/she is most likely not receiving the necessary treatment he/she needs. A person may actually develop health symptoms as a result of prescription errors. These drug reactions may be mistaken for another condition and treated inappropriately with additional medications.

Prescribing faults and prescription errors are major problems among medication errors. They occur both in general practice and in hospital, and although they are rarely fatal they can affect patients' safety and quality of healthcare. Prescription errors encompass those related to the act of writing a prescription, whereas prescribing faults encompass irrational prescribing, inappropriate prescribing, underprescribing, overprescribing, and ineffective prescribing, arising from facility medical judgement or decisions concerning treatment or treatment monitoring. Appropriate prescribing results when errors are minimized and when the prescriber actively endeavours to achieve better prescribing— both actions are required.

All procedures related to prescribing are error-generating steps. A prescribing fault can arise from the choice of:

- The wrong drug.
- The wrong dose.
- The wrong route of administration.
- The wrong frequency or duration of treatment.
- Inaccuracy in writing.
- Poor legibility of handwriting.
- The use of abbreviations or incomplete writing of a prescription.

Inappropriate prescribing most often derives from a wrong medical decision, because of lack of knowledge or inadequate training. Junior doctors often work in stressful circumstances that are perceived as routine by experienced doctors. Inadequate staffing, lack of skills and knowledge of relevant rules, tasks outside the routine, or taking care of another doctor's patient have also been identified as conditions associated with prescribing faults.

Factors related to patient's medical history can also result in errors, leading to adverse effects, since these are associated in most cases with identifiable clinical conditions, such as reduced renal and hepatic function or a history of allergy requiring a typical or unusual dosage and frequency. Monitoring of drug action is necessarily a part of the prescribing process, to allow optimization or adjustments of doses or treatments. In ambulatory care, prescribing faults are mostly related to the use of inappropriate doses and inadequate monitoring.

Prescription Errors Involving Children

Prescription errors can be particularly dangerous when they involve children and infants. Young children are much more susceptible to injuries because of dose-related prescription errors than adults. Children do not have the immune systems or the chemical tolerance to handle, taking the wrong medicine as well as adults. Evaluating specific age and weight factors are of particular importance in pediatrics to ensure that prescription errors are avoided. It is estimated that one in every eighteen prescriptions written for children involve prescription errors related to the type of medication or dosage.

PREVENTING PRESCRIPTION ERRORS

While there is absolutely no excuse for a medical professional's negligence, there are some actions that consumers can take to avoid prescription errors. Checking all medications to ensure that the information is correct, asking the pharmacist about drug interactions and side effects, and reading available information on the drug you are given can help you catch

Textbook of Pharmaceutical Dispensing

any possible prescription errors that may have occurred.

Following strategies can be adopted to avoid or minimize prescription error:

1. Reduction of complexity in the act of prescribing by the introduction of automation.
2. Improved prescribers' knowledge by education and the use of online aids.
3. Feedback control systems and monitoring of the effects of interventions.

Computerized systems: The use of automated prescribing systems is recommended as an effective tool to reduce medication errors. They can reduce the risk of harm that arises from prescribing faults and improve the quality of medical care by reducing errors in drug dispensing and administration. Computerized advice can give significant benefits by guiding the prescription of optimal dosages.

Education and systems approaches: Education of medical students and junior doctors is highly advisable. Training and feedback control of prescribing by tutors and senior doctors should be associated with availability of online references for immediate identification and verification of potential prescribing faults. The choice of treatment should generally be in line with approved guidelines, although flexibility may be necessary in individual cases.

Constraints can minimize omissions, e.g. the introduction of check lists or strict rules in writing a prescription, and the use of well-structured medication charts. Handwritten prescriptions should not contain ambiguous abbreviations or symbols. Frequent and immediate review of prescriptions as well as monitoring of potential harms deriving from treatment should be encouraged.

MEDICATION ERROR

A medication error can be defined as 'a failure in the treatment process that leads to, harm to the patient'.

Medication errors can occur in:

- **Choosing a medicine**—irrational, inappropriate, and ineffective prescribing, underprescribing and overprescribing.
- **Writing the prescription**—prescription errors, including illegibility.
- **Manufacturing the formulation to be used**—wrong strength, contaminants or adulterants, wrong or misleading packaging.
- **Dispensing the formulation**—wrong drug, wrong formulation, wrong label.
- **Administering or taking the drug**—wrong dose, wrong route, wrong frequency, wrong duration.
- **Monitoring therapy**—failing to alter therapy when required, erroneous alteration.

Table 2.14: Enlisted some official formulas, methods of preparation and uses

Types of dosage form: Liquid dosage form (solution)		
Preparation: Strong sodium salicylate mixture BPC	Sent: 50 ml	Use: Analgesic and antipyretic
Ingredients	Official quantity	Required quantity
Sodium salicylate	10 g	0.5 g
Sodium metabisulfate	1 g	0.05 g
Double strength chloroform water	525 ml	26.25 ml
Water	1000 ml	50 ml

contd...

Table 2.14: Enlisted some official formulas, methods of preparation and uses (*contd.*)

Procedure:

Dissolve all the ingredients in chloroform water and two-thirds of water; filter if necessary and then make up the volume as desired.

Preparation: Peppermint water BP	Sent: 100 ml	Use: Carminative and flavor
Ingredients	Official quantity	Required quantity
Peppermint	2 ml	0.2 ml
Talc	15 g	1.5 g
Purified water q.s	1000 ml	100 ml

Procedure:

Weigh 1.5 g of talc and put it into a mortar.

Add 0.2 ml of peppermint and levigate to absorb the oil on to the finely talc powder to ensure dispersion.

Add water to the mortar and mix well.

Transfer to the bottle and add the remaining water and shake it for 10 min.

Filter and place it in dispersing bottle and adjust volume.

Preparation: Aqueous iodine solution	Sent: 100 ml	Use: Disinfectant
Ingredients	Official quantity	Required quantity
Iodine	50 g	5 g
Potassium iodide	100 g	10 g
Water q.s	1000 ml	100 ml

Procedure:

Potassium iodide and iodine are dissolved in small portion of purified water by stirring and shaking till dissolve completely. Sufficient water is added to make the required volume.

Preparation: Lysol	Sent: 100 ml	Use: External disinfectant
Ingredients	Official quantity	Required quantity
m-Cresol	500 ml	50 ml
Vegetable oil	180 ml	18 ml
Potassium hydroxide	42 g	4.2 g
Water q.s	1000 ml	100 ml

Procedure:

Weigh potassium hydroxide and dissolve it in small portion of water and add 18 ml of linseed oil (vegetable oil).

Heat in water bath with constant stirring.

After saponification add m-Cresol with constant agitation till clean solution results.

contd...

Table 2.14: Enlisted some official formulas, methods of preparation and uses (*contd.*)		
Types of dosage form: Liquid dosage form (syrup)		
Preparation: Syrup BP	**Sent: 100 ml**	**Use: Pharmaceutical aid**
Ingredients	Official quantity	Required quantity
Sucrose	667 g	66.7 g
Water q.s	1000 g	100 ml

Procedure:
Dissolve the sucrose in purified water in beaker by careful heating on water path. Stir frequently until dissolved and adjust volume.
Cool it and filter through gauze.
It is preferred to add 10% glycerol to prevent crystal formation during storage.

Types of dosage form: Liquid dosage form (elixir)		
Preparation: Aromatic elixir USP	**Sent: 100 ml**	**Use: Pharmaceutical aid and soothing effect**
Ingredients	Official quantity	Required quantity
Rose oil	0.6 ml	0.06 ml
Peppermint oil	0.6 ml	0.06 ml
Syrup	375 ml	37.5 ml
Talc	30 g	3 g
Alcohol	30 g	3 g
Water q.s	1000 ml	100 ml

Procedure:
Put rose oil, peppermint oil, talc and alcohol in a dispensing bottle and shake very well.
Add 20 ml of purified water and shake well.
Filter using buchner funnel.
Transfer the filtrated into a measuring cylinder and all syrup and complete volume to 100 ml by purified water.
Write label.

Types of dosage form: Liquid dosage form (eardrops)		
Preparation: Sodium bicarbonate ear-drops BP	**Sent: 50 ml**	**Use: Softening of earwax.**
Ingredients	Official quantity	Required quantity
Sodium carbonate	5 g	2.5 g
Glycerol	30 ml	15 ml
Distilled water	100 ml	50 ml

Procedure:
Dissolve sodium bicarbonate in a portion of water and shake well.
Add 15 ml of glycerol and shake and complete volume with water to 50 ml.
Write label.

contd...

Table 2.14: Enlisted some official formulas, methods of preparation and uses (*contd.*)		
Types of dosage form: Liquid dosage form (emulsion)		
Preparation: Almond oil emulsion	**Sent: 100 ml**	**Use: Demulcent and mild laxative**
Ingredients	Official quantity	Required quantity
Almond oil	50 ml	25 ml
Double strength chloroform water	100 ml	50 ml
Water	200 ml	100 ml

Procedure:

Almond oil is a fixed oil, therefore, the qualities for primary emulsion are (oil: water: gum = 4:2:1)

Almond oil	25 ml
Water	12.5 ml
Acacia	6.25 g

Use the dry gum technique for acacia emulsion as follows:

Weigh the acacia and place it in dry mortar.

Dispense the acacia powder lightly in the water.

Add 25 ml oil at once and triturate until the primary emulsion is well established.

The primary emulsion is then diluted with the remaining ingredients and transferred to measuring cylinder to adjusted volume with water.

Use amber dispensing bottle with a wide mouth.

Write label and add "shake the bottle before use" label.

Types of dosage form: Liquid dosage form (liniment)		
Preparation: White liniment BP	**Sent: 100 ml**	**Use: Counterirritant and rubefacient**
Ingredients	Official quantity	Required quantity
Ammonium chloride	12.5 g	25 g
Dilute ammonia solution	2.25 ml	4.5 ml
Oleic acid	4.25 ml	8.5 ml
Turpentine oil	12.25 ml	24.5 ml
Purified water	31.25 ml	62.5 ml

Procedure:

Make emulsifier (ammonium oleate) the reaction between dilute ammonia and oleic acid as follows. Take 8.5 ml of oleic acid and 24.5 ml of turpentine oil and 4.5 ml of dilute ammonia solution (2.5%) and 10 ml of water. Shake vigorously to form turpentine water emulsion.

Dissolve ammonium chloride in the remaining water and mix it with to produce the preparation after adjusting the volume with water to 100 ml.

Write label.

contd...

Table 2.14: Enlisted some official formulas, methods of preparation and uses (*contd.*)

Types of dosage form: Liquid dosage form (lotion)

Preparation: Calamine lotion BP	Sent: 50 ml	Use: Astringent and protective
Ingredients	Official quantity	Required quantity
Calamine	15 g	7.5 g
Zinc oxide	5 g	2.5 g
Bentonite	3 g	1.5 g
Sodium citrate	0.5 g	0.25 g
Liquid phenol	0.5 g	0.25 g
Glycerin	5 ml	2.5 ml
Purified water	100 ml	50 ml

Procedure:

Dissolve sodium citrate in 35 ml purified water

Weigh calamine, zinc oxide and bentonite and triturate them with sodium citrate solution.

Add liquid phenol, the glycerin and sufficient quantity of water to make up the required volume.

Write label.

Types of dosage form: Liquid dosage form (powder)

Preparation: Camphor powder	Sent: 20 g	Use: Counterirritant
Ingredients	Official quantity	Required quantity
Camphor	0.1 g	2 g
Starch	0.6 g	12 g
Zinc	0.3 g	6 g

Procedure:

Weigh the camphor and try to pulverize in the mortar with pestle.

Add few drops of alcohol and pulverize.

Mix starch and zinc oxide and gradually add to camphor while trituration until uniformity.

Pass through 90-mesh sieve.

Types of dosage form: Solid dosage form (granules)

Preparation: Sodium citrate tartrate granule	Sent: 30 g	Use: Antacid
Ingredients	Official quantity	Required quantity
Sodium bicarbonate	510 g	15.3 g
Tartaric acid	270 g	8.1 g
Citric acid	180 g	5.4 g

contd...

Table 2.14: Enlisted some official formulas, methods of preparation and uses (*contd.*)		
Sucrose	150 g	4.5 g

Procedure:

Thus 33.3 g is the total amount of ingredient after adding the amounts which can loose during handling and during chemical reactions.

If the amount of sodium bicarbonate is not known, calculate it as follows

Amount of sodium bicarbonate = (Amount of citric acid x Eq. wt. of sod. bicarb.) / Eq. wt. of citric acid + (amount of tartaric acid x Eq. wt. of sod. bicarb.) / Eq. wt. of tartaric acid

= ((180 x 84)/70 + (180 x 84)/75) = 519.4

In the prescription, the amount used is 510 g so the final solution will be slightly acidic.

Types of dosage form: Solid dosage form (tablet by direct comp.)		
Preparation: Aspirin tablet by direct compression	**Sent: 100 tab**	**Use: Analgesic**
Ingredients	Official quantity	Required quantity
Aspirin	90%	32.5 g
Starch	7%	2.5 g
Talc	2.4%	0.9 g
Stearic acid	0.6%	0.2 g

Procedure:

Screen aspirin on 40 mesh sieve to remove the fine particles.

Blend all the ingredients in a mortar using plastic spatula.

Compress into tablets using 9 mm standard concave punches.

Types of dosage form: Liquid dosage form (tablet by dry gran.)		
Preparation: Aspirin tablet by dry granulation.	**Sent: 100 tab**	**Use: Analgesic**
Ingredients	Official quantity	Required quantity
Aspirin	90%	32.5 g
Starch	7%	2.5 g
Talc	2.4%	0.9 g
Stearic acid	0.6%	0.2 g

Procedure:

Mix all the above ingredients (except) 50% of starch, talk and magnesium stearate.

Compress into slug using 18 mm flat face punches.

Grind the slugs using 20 mesh screens.

Transfer into cubic mixture and the reminder disintegrant and lubricant, mix for 10 minutes.

Compress to weight using 9 mm concave punches.

contd...

Table 2.14: Enlisted some official formulas, methods of preparation and uses (*contd.*)

Types of dosage form: Solid dosage form (tablet by wet gran.)

Preparation: Chewable antacid tablets	Sent: 100 Tab	Use: Antacid
Ingredients	Official quantity	Required quantity
Aluminum hydroxide	300 mg	30 g
Calcium carbonate	150 mg	15 g
Mannitol	100 mg	10 g
Gelatin	20 mg	2 g
Magnesium stearate	15 mg	1.5 g
Talc	15 mg	1.5 g
Oil of peppermint	0.2 mg	0.2 g

Procedure:

Mix the first three ingredients and moisten with a 10% gelatin solution until formation of coherent mass. Granulate by passing through 10 mesh screen.

Dry at 50°C overnight, screen the drug granules through 20/35 mesh.

Add the oil of peppermint mixed with talc and finally the magnesium stearate.

Mix for 5 minutes in a cubic mixer.

Compress using 12 mm flat face punches.

Types of dosage form: Liquid dosage form (capsule)

Preparation: Ephedrine sulfate and phenobarbital capsules	Sent: 10 cap	Use: Treatment of bronchial asthma.
Ingredients	Official quantity	Required quantity
Ephedrine sulfate	0.025 g	0.25 g
Phenobarbital	0.015 g	0.15 g

Procedure:

The powders are triturated intimately and mixed by geometric dilution.

The resting powder is placed on a powder paper and smoothed with a spatula to a height approximately half the length of capsule body.

The open end of the capsule base is repeatedly pushed into the powder until the capsule is filled.

The cap is then placed back to close the capsule.

Each filled capsule is weighed using empty capsule as counterpoise, powder is added or removed until the correct weight is obtained.

Finally, the capsule is cleaned to remove any trace of powder trapped on the surface

Calculation:

Calculate for 10 capsules using no. 0 capsules

Fill one capsule with lactose in previously described manner and determine the exact capacity of capsule by weighing suppose it is 0.5 g.

contd...

Table 2.14: Enlisted some official formulas, methods of preparation and uses (*contd.*)

Calculate the amount of drugs for 10 capsules and substrate from total amount of lactose (0.5 g × 10) to get amount of lactose which you will use, e.g. (0.5 g × 10 – (0.025 × 10 + 0.015 × 10)) = 4.6 g lactose.

Weigh the calculated amounts of lactose (4.6 g), ephedrine sulfate (0.25 g) and phenobarbital (0.15 g).

Types of dosage form: Semisolid dosage form (suppository)		
Preparation: Boroglycerin suppository	**Sent: 3 sup.**	**Use: Antiseptic**
Ingredients	Official quantity	Required quantity
Boric acid	7.5 g	0.375 g
Gelatin	15 g	0.750 g
Glycerin	62.5 g	3.125 g
Water	15 g	0.750 g

Procedure:

Calculation:

The formula gives 100 g of suppository mass.

To prepare 3 supp. Calculate for 5.

If we use mould of 1 g capacity the amounts are as follows :

Boric acid = (1 × 5 × 7.5) / 100 = 0.375 g

Gelatin   = (1 × 5 × 15) / 100 = 0.750 g

Glycerin   = (1 × 5 × 62.5) / 100 = 3.125 g

Water   = (1 × 5 × 15) / 100   = 0.750 g

Preparation:

In a porcelain dish soak gelatin in water, then transfer to dish over a water bath.

Dissolve boric acid in glycerin by the aid of gentle heat.

Add the dissolved boric acid, the gelatin solution and continue heating over a water bath until a clear solution produced and constant weight is attained.

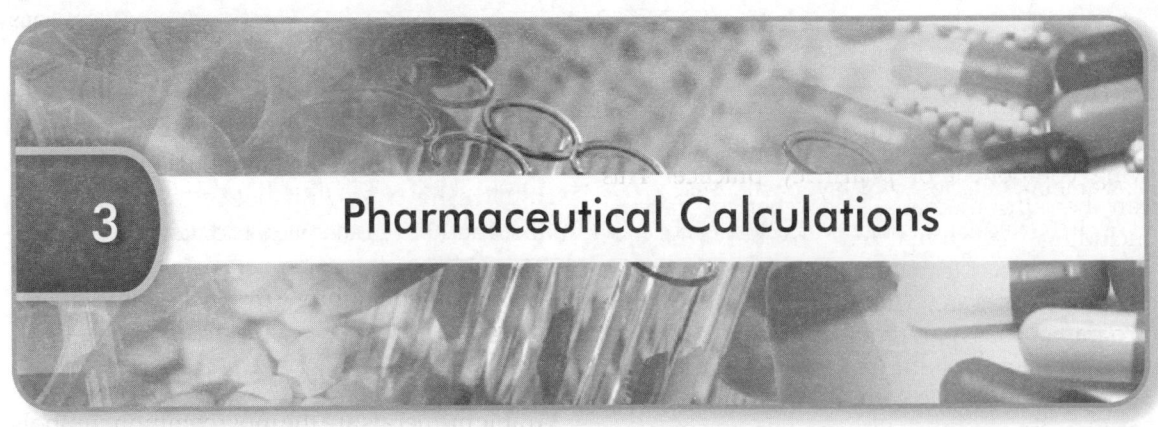

3   Pharmaceutical Calculations

INTRODUCTION

Prescription compounding is a rapidly growing component of pharmacy practice. This can be attributed to a number of factors, including individualized patient therapy, lack of commercially available products, home healthcare, intravenous admixture programs, total parenteral nutrition programs and "problem solving" for the physician and patient in enhancing compliance with a specific therapeutic regimen. Pharmacists are creative and should have the ability to formulate patient-specific preparations for providing pharmaceutical care. Most compounded prescriptions require a number of calculations as part of preparation, packaging and dispensing.

POTENTIAL FOR ERROR

One of the greatest potentials for error in prescription compounding is in the area of pharmacy math, or pharmacy calculations. Even though most of the processes are relatively simple, a misplaced decimal or "estimated" value for a medication can have serious consequences, including death. There is no excuse for ignorance in this area and, an individual unprepared to do the necessary calculations should not be involved in pharmaceutical compounding. It is of utmost importance that pharmacists be extremely well-grounded in the practice of pharmaceutical calculations as there is "zero-tolerance" allowed in these vital operations.

NUMBERS AND NUMERALS

A number is a total quantity or amount, whereas a numeral is a word, sign, or group of words and signs representing a number.

Roman Numerals

Roman numerals are a numeral system of ancient Rome based on letters of the alphabet, which are combined to signify the sum of their values. The first ten Roman numerals are: I, II, III, IV, V, VI, VII, VIII, IX, X. The Roman numeral

system is decimal but not directly positional and does not include a zero. It is a cousin of the Etruscan numerals, and the letters derive from earlier non-alphabetical symbols; over time the Romans came to identify the symbols with letters of their Latin alphabet. The system was modified slightly during the middle ages to produce the system used today.

Arabic Numerals

Arabic numerals are the most common symbols used to represent numbers. Every number can be expressed in Arabic numerals by using 10 basic symbols, alone or in combination. The basic symbols, called digits, are: 0, 1, 2, 3, 4, 5, 6, 7, 8, and 9. The position of a digit in an Arabic numeral determines its value.

The Arabic numeral for the number two hundred and thirty-seven is the sequence of digits 237. In this numeral, the digit 2 has a value of two hundred, the digit 3 has a value of thirty, and the digit 7 has a value of seven. Roman numerals are based on seven symbols: a stroke (identified with the letter I) for a unit, a chevron (identified with the letter V) for a five, a cross-stroke (identified with the letter X) for a ten, a C (identified as an abbreviation of Centum) for a hundred, etc.

Table 3.1: Common Arabic numbers	
Roman	Arabic
I	1 (one) (unus)
V	5 (five) (quinque)
X	10 (ten) (decem)
L	50 (fifty) (quinquaginta)
C	100 (one hundred) (centum)
D	500 (five hundred) (quingenti)
M	1000 (one thousand) (mille)

Symbols are iterated to produce multiples of the decimal (1, 10, 100, 1000) values, with V, L, D substituted for a multiple of five, and the iteration continuing: I "1", II "2", III

"3", V "5", VI "6", VII "7", etc., and the same for other bases: X "10", XX "20", XXX "30", L "50", LXXX "80"; CC "200", DCC "700", etc. At the fourth iteration, a subtractive principle may be employed, with the base placed before the higher base: IIII or IV "4", VIIII or IX "9", XXXX or XL "40", LXXXX or XC "90", CCCC or CD "400", DCCCC or CM "900".

Table 3.2: Roman and Arabic numbers							
Nits		Tens		Hundreds		Thousands	
Arabic	Roman	Arabic	Roman	Arabic	Roman	Arabic	Roman
1	I	10	X	100	C	1000	M
2	II	20	XX	200	CC	2000	MM
3	III	30	XXX	300	CCC	3000	MMM
4	IV	40	XL	400	CD	4000	MV
5	V	50	L	500	D	5000	V
6	VI	60	LX	600	DC	6000	VM
7	VII	70	LXX	700	DCC	7000	VMM
8	VIII	80	LXXX	800	DCCC	8000	VMMM
9	IX	90	XC	900	CM	9000	MV

Fractions

A fraction (from the Latin fractus, broken) is a number that can represent part of a whole. The earliest fractions were reciprocals of integers, symbols representing one-half, one-third, one-quarter, and so on. A much later development were the common or "vulgar" fractions which are still used today, and which consist of a numerator and a denominator, the numerator representing a number of equal parts and the denominator telling how many of those parts make up a whole. An example is 3/4, in which the numerator, 3, tells us that the fraction represents 3 equal parts, and the denominator, 4, tells us that 4 parts make up a whole. There are two types of fractions: (a) common fractions, such as 1/4 and 3/4 (referred to simply as fractions) and, (b) decimal fractions, such as 0.25 or 0.75 (usually referred as decimals).

Following are some important terms in dealing with fractions:

Example 1:

Proper fractions: A proper fraction should always be less than 1, i.e. the numerator is smaller than the denominator:

$$\frac{A}{B} \text{ where, } A < B$$

A proper fraction such as 3/5 may be read as "3 of 5 parts" or as "3 divided by 5."

Example 2: 3/4, 5/7, 2/7

Improper fractions: An improper fraction has a numerator that is greater than or equal to the denominator.

$$\frac{A}{B} \text{ where, } A \geq B$$

Example 3: 2 3/4, 1 5/8. 1 2/3

Mixed fractions: In mixed fractions, a whole number and a proper fraction are combined. The value of the mixed fraction is always greater than 1.

$$C\frac{A}{B} \text{ where C is whole number}$$

Example 4: 5/3, 19/7, 7/4

Complex fractions: In complex fractions, the numerator or the denominator, or both, may be a whole number, proper fraction, or mixed fraction. The value of complex fractions can be less than or greater than 1.

$$\frac{A}{B} \text{ where A and B are kinds of fractions}$$

> Example 5: $\dfrac{5}{8} \div \dfrac{1}{3} = \left[\dfrac{5}{8}\right] / \left[\dfrac{1}{3}\right]$

Equivalent fractions: Fractions that represent the same number are called equivalent fractions. For example, 1/2, 2/4, and 4/8 are all equivalent fractions.

$$\frac{A}{B} = \frac{A \times C}{B \times C}$$

ARITHMETIC WITH FRACTIONS

Addition

1. Add like quantities. If, in the metric system, the quantities are not alike, change them to a common unit. For the apothecary or avoirdupois systems, place in columns of like quantities arranged in descending order of magnitude toward the right.
2. In the apothecary or avoirdupois systems, add together the smaller quantities first, and then advance to the next higher units.
3. When adding decimals, keep the decimal points directly under each other.
4. When adding fractions, reduce to the lowest common denominator, add the resulting numerators, and reduce the fraction, if possible by cancelling.

The first rule of addition is that only like quantities can be added, e.g. various quantities of quarters. Unlike quantities, such as adding thirds to quarters, must first be converted to like quantities as described below: Imagine a pocket containing two quarters, and another pocket containing three quarters; in total, there are five quarters.

Since four quarters is equivalent to one (dollar), this can be represented as follows:

> Example 1:
> $$\frac{2}{4} + \frac{3}{4} = \frac{5}{4} = 1\frac{1}{4}$$

Subtraction

The process for subtracting fractions is the same as that of adding them— find a common denominator, and change each fraction to an equivalent fraction with the chosen common denominator. The resulting fraction will have that denominator, and its numerator will be the result of subtracting the numerators of the original fractions. For instance,

> Example 2:
> $$\frac{2}{3} - \frac{1}{2} = \frac{4}{6} - \frac{3}{6} = \frac{1}{6}$$

Multiplication of fractions

To multiply fractions, the following steps can be used:

1. Multiply the two numerators and the two denominators.

> Example 3:
> $$\frac{3}{4} + \frac{5}{8} = \frac{3 \times 5}{4 \times 8} = \frac{15}{24}$$

2. Reduce the answer, when possible, to lowest terms by dividing both numerator and denominator with the least common factor (LCF).

> Example 4:
> $$\frac{15}{24} = \frac{\frac{15}{3}}{\frac{24}{3}} = \frac{5}{8}$$

3. When possible, divide the numerator of any of the fractions and the denominator of any of the fractions by the same number. Then multiply the numerators and denominators.

> Example 5:
> Solve $\dfrac{3}{9} \times \dfrac{4}{12}$

In such cases, no further reduction can be made, since the fraction is already in its lowest terms.

Example 6:

First, simplification of the fractions:

First fraction: $\dfrac{\frac{3}{3}}{\frac{9}{3}} = \dfrac{1}{3}$

Second fraction: $\dfrac{\frac{4}{4}}{\frac{12}{4}} = \dfrac{1}{3}$

Multiply the products of each of the simplified terms.

$$\frac{1}{3} \times \frac{1}{3} = \frac{1 \times 1}{3 \times 3} = \frac{1}{9}$$

4. To multiply a fraction with a whole number, assume the denominator of the whole number to be 1. Then multiply the numerator and denominator in the same way as explained above in step 1. For example, 5 can be expressed as 5/1.

Example 7:

Find the product of : $30 \times 6\dfrac{2}{5}$

$$= \frac{30}{1} \times \frac{(5 \times 6 + 2)}{5} = \frac{30 \times 32}{5}$$

$$= \frac{960}{5} = \dfrac{\frac{960}{5}}{\frac{5}{5}} = 192$$

Division of fractions

Division of any number by a fraction is similar to multiplying fractions, except for one additional step.

1. Multiply the number by the reciprocal of the fraction.
2. Simplify the resulting fraction, if possible.
3. Multiply the result with the divisor. This value should be equal to the original dividend.

Note: Only non-zero fractions can be divided. In the division of fractions, the following terms should be recognized:

$$\frac{A}{B} = C = \frac{Dividend}{Divisor} = Quotient$$

Dividend (A) = the number to be divided.

Divisor (B) = the number by which the dividend is divided.

Quotient (C) = the number obtained by dividing the dividend with the devisor.

Dividend ÷ divisor = quotient; this expression may be read as "dividend is divided by divisor to obtain the quotient."

Problem 1:

Work out the answers to these additions and substraction:

(a) $\dfrac{3}{7} + \dfrac{1}{7} =$

(b) $\dfrac{1}{9} + \dfrac{7}{9} =$

(c) $\dfrac{1}{5} + \dfrac{3}{5} =$

(d) $\dfrac{2}{7} + \dfrac{4}{7} =$

(e) $\dfrac{7}{9} - \dfrac{5}{9} =$

(f) $\dfrac{8}{11} - \dfrac{3}{11} =$

(g) $\dfrac{4}{15} - \dfrac{2}{15} =$

(h) $\dfrac{6}{13} - \dfrac{3}{13} =$

(i) $\dfrac{4}{7} - \dfrac{3}{7} =$

(j) $\dfrac{6}{25} - \dfrac{2}{25} =$

Problem 2:

Work out the answers to these additions and subtractions:

(a) $\dfrac{1}{3} + \dfrac{1}{2} =$

(b) $\dfrac{3}{4} + \dfrac{2}{3} =$

(c) $\dfrac{1}{5} + \dfrac{1}{4} =$

(d) $\dfrac{3}{5} + \dfrac{2}{3} =$

(e) $\dfrac{5}{8} + \dfrac{1}{4} =$

(f) $\dfrac{4}{5} + \dfrac{2}{7} =$

(g) $\dfrac{1}{7} + \dfrac{2}{3} =$

(h) $\dfrac{6}{7} + \dfrac{2}{3} =$

(i) $\dfrac{7}{8} - \dfrac{3}{4} =$

(j) $\dfrac{8}{9} - \dfrac{3}{4} =$

(k) $\dfrac{3}{7} - \dfrac{1}{3} =$

(l) $\dfrac{4}{5} - \dfrac{3}{4} =$

Answers:

(1) a. 4/7, b. 8/9, c. 4/5, d. 6/7, e. 2/9, f. 5/11, g. 2/15, h. 3/13, i. 1/7, j. 4/25

(2) a. 5/6, b. 17/12, c. 9/20, d. 19/15, e. 7/8, f. 38/35, g. 17/21, h. 32/21, i. 1/8, j. 5/36, k. 2/21, l. 1/20

Decimals

Decimals are another means of expressing a fractional amount. A decimal is a fraction whose denominator is 10 or a multiple of 10.

Example 8:

$$0.7 = \dfrac{7}{10}$$

$$0.06 = \dfrac{6}{100}$$

$$0.006 = \dfrac{6}{1000}$$

A decimal mixed number is a whole number and a decimal fraction.

Example 9:
$$4.3 = 4(3/10)$$

Each position to the left of the decimal is ten times the previous place, and each position to the right is one-tenth the previous place. The position to the left or right of the decimal point is referred to as place value, which determines the size of the denominator.

Adding zeros to a decimal that do not change the place value of the numerals does not affect the value of the number. However, adding or subtracting zeros between the decimal point and the numeral does change the value of the number.

Example 10:

0.3, 0.30 or 0.300; all these represent two-tenths
But, 0.3   = three-tenths 3/10
     0.03 = three-hundredths 3/100
     0.003 = three-thousandths 3/1000

USING RATIOS, PROPORTIONS AND PERCENTAGES IN DOSAGE CALCULATIONS

Calculations involving ratios, proportions, and percentages are very important in the dispensing and compounding of medications. Following is a discussion on these topics, followed by a variety of practice problems highlighting some of the important applications of ratios, proportions, and percentage calculations.

Ratio

A ratio is a comparison of two numbers. We generally separate the two numbers in the ratio with a colon (:). Suppose we want to write the ratio of 8 and 12.

We can write this as 8:12 or as a fraction 8/12, and we say the ratio is eight to twelve.

Example 1:

Are the ratios 3 to 4 and 6:8 equal?

The ratios are equal if, 3/4 = 6/8.

These are equal, if their cross products are equal; that is, if 3 × 8 = 4 × 6. Since both of these products equal 24, the answer is yes, the ratios are equal.

Proportion

A proportion is an equation with a ratio on each side. It is a statement that two ratios are equal.

3/4 = 6/8 is an example of a proportion.

When one of the four numbers in a proportion is unknown, cross products may be used to find the unknown number. This is called solving the proportion. Question marks or letters are frequently used in place of the unknown number.

Example 2:

Solve for n: 1/2 = n/4.

Using cross products we see that 2 × n = 1 × 4 =4, so 2 × n = 4. Dividing both sides by 2, n = 4 ÷ 2 so that n = 2.

Example 3:

A vial of Rocephin contains 100 milligrams per milliliter. How many milliliters should be given to a patient to obtain 650 milligrams?

The expression of strength will be the first ratio of the proportion:

1 ml/100 mg = Assign the "X" value:

1 ml /100 mg = X ml

Find the other known factor:

1 ml/100 mg = X ml/650 mg

Then, cross-multiply:

100 X = 650 (1)

Solve for "X":

X = 6.5 ml (NOTE: Don't forget to add the unit of measurement.)

Basic principles - Always look for what is being asked:

*Number of doses

*Total amount of drug

*Size of dose

Given any two of the above, you can solve for the third.

General formula:

Number of doses = Total amount/size of dose

Can also be rearranged to:

Total amt = number of doses x size of dose

Size of dose = Total amount/number of doses

Example 4:

How many doses are in 120 ml of Benadryl Elixir, if one dose contains 1 dram?

X numbers of doses = 120 ml/5 ml

Divide to solve for (X):

X = 24 doses

Example 5:

How many milligrams of theophylline does a patient receive per day, if the prescription indicates 300 mg tid?

X total amt = 3 × 300 mg

Multiply to solve for (X):

X = 900 mg total

Example 6:

How much propanolol will a patient receive every 6 hours, if he is to receive 160 mg per day?

X dose = 160 mg/4 doses

Divide to solve for (X):

X = 40 mg

Problems

1. If you stock aminophylline for injection, 250 mg/10 ml, how many milliliters should be used to deliver a 200 mg dose?
2. When erythromycin lactobionate is reconstituted, it yields a concentration of 50 mg/ml. How many milliliters are required to give a 0.9 gm dose?
3. If 20 milliequivalents (mEq) of a drug is ordered daily and the drug on hand contains 40 mEq/2 ml, how many milliliters should be dispensed for a 30-day supply?
4. A 1,000,000 unit vial of penicillin G potassium contains 100,000 units/ml when reconstituted with 9.6 ml of sterile

water for injection. How many milliliters are needed to administer a dose of 600,000 units?

5. If an injectable medication is labeled 500 µg/2 ml, and the dose needed is 0.125 mg, how many milliliters would you need?

6. An IV order calls for 100 mg of hydrocortisone. The available stock is 250 mg/2 ml vials. How many milliliters would you need to fill the order?

7. How many 5 gr tablets should be dispensed to fill the following prescription?
R$_x$: 648 mg of ASA q8h × 2 weeks

8. How many tablets would be dispensed for the following prescription?
R$_x$: Take 2 grams initially then 500 mg qid for 6 days (Note: Each tablet is 250 mg).

9. How many milliliters of alcohol would be used to make 240 ml of preparation, if each teaspoonful contains 2.8 ml of alcohol?

10. In supply, you find a vial of kanamycin injection labeled 1.0 g per 3 ml. How many milliliters of this solution must be given to administer a dose of 750 mg of drug?

11. You have a vial of ephedrine injection labeled 25 mg/ml. How many milliliters must be injected in order to administer a dose of 12.5 mg?

12. How many milligrams of drug are contained in a 30 ml vial of naloxone, labeled 0.4 mg/ml ?

13. How many tablets you would you dispense for the following prescription?
R$_x$: 0.9 gm initially then 0.3 gm po tid for 14 days (Note each tablet is 300 mg)

14. How many milligrams of drug would be in one pint if each dram has 1/8th of a grain?

15. If 0.3 mg is the dose to taken daily for 30 days, how many grams will you dispense?

16. The prescription calls for the patient to take one teaspoonful four times a day for 10 days. How many milliliters will you dispense?

17. The dose is one tablespoonful every 6 hours for 1 week. How many milliliters will you dispense?

18. How many doses are in 180 ml, if each dose contains 2 tablespoonfuls?

19. How many teaspoonful doses are contained in 60 ml of a preparation?

20. The physician prescribes 8 fluid ounces of penicillin to be taken in 10 ml doses. How many doses will the patient receive?

21. The patient will take 350 mg in each dose which is to be taken six times a day for 14 days. How many total grams will this patient need?

22. Twenty doses are to be obtained from 1oz of a chemical. How many milligrams are in each dose?

23. Forty grams of a medication is to be divided into 500 doses. What is the strength of each dose in milligrams?

24. One pound of chemical will make 60 doses. How many milligrams will each dose contain?

25. Six fluid ounces are to be divided into 20 doses. How many milliliters are in each dose?

26. What is the dosage in tablespoonfuls, if 480 ml of medication is divided into 64 doses?

27. How many tablets would you dispense, if 2 tablets are to be taken every 3 hours for 15 days?

28. If a patient takes 2 and 1/2 teaspoonfuls every 8 hours for 10 days, how many milliliters of medication would you dispense?

29. If 250 mg of medication are to be taken daily for 3 weeks, how many grams would you dispense?

30. How many doses can be obtained from 450 ml of medication, if the size of each dose is 1.5 teaspoonfuls?

Answers:
(1) 8 ml (2) 18 ml (3) 30 ml (4) 6 ml (5) 0.5 ml (6) 0.8 ml (7) 84 tabs (8) 56 tabs (9) 134.4 ml (10) 2.25 ml (11) 0.5 ml (12) 12 mg (13) 45 tabs (14) 766.26 mg (15) 0.009 gm (16) 200 ml (17) 4 20 ml (18) 6 doses (19) 12 doses (20) 23.65 doses (21) 29.4 gm (22) 1,417.5 mg (23) 80 mg (24) 7,566.6 mg (25) 8.87 ml (26) ½ tablespoonsful

(27) 240 tabs (28) 375 ml (29) 5.25 gm (30) 60 doses

Rate

A rate is a ratio that expresses how long it takes to do something, such as traveling a certain distance. To walk 3 kilometers in one hour is to walk at the rate of 3 km/h. The fraction expressing a rate has units of distance in the numerator and units of time in the denominator.

Problems involving rates typically involve setting two ratios equal to each other and solving for an unknown quantity that is, solving a proportion.

Percentage

A percentage is a way of expressing a number as a fraction of 100 (percent meaning "per hundred"). It is often denoted using the percent sign, "%". For example, 45% (read as "forty-five percent") is equal to 45 / 100, or 0.45.

Percentages are used to express how large one quantity is, relative to another quantity. The first quantity usually represents a part of, or a change in, the second quantity, which should be greater than zero. For example, an increase of Rs 0.25 on a price of Rs 2.50 is an increase by a fraction of 0.25/2.50 = 0.10. Expressed as a percentage, this is therefore a 10% increase.

The fundamental concept to remember when performing calculations with percentages is that the percent symbol can be treated as being equivalent to the pure number constant 1/100 = 0.01., for an example, 35% of 300 can be written as (35/100) × 300 = 105.

To find the percentage of a single unit in a whole of N units, divide 100% by N. For instance, if you have 1250 apples, and you want to find out what percentage of these 1250 apples a single apple represents, 100%/1250 = (100/1250)% provides the answer of 0.08%.

To calculate a percentage of a percentage, convert both percentages to fractions of 100, or to decimals, and multiply them. For example, 50% of 40% is:

(50/100) × (40/100) = 0.50 × 0.40 = 0.20 = 20/100 = 20%.

It is not correct to divide by 100 and use the percent sign at the same time (e.g. 25% = 25/100 = 0.25, not 25% / 100, which actually is (25 / 100) / 100 = 0.0025.)

Percent Concentration Expressions

The concentration of a solution may be expressed in terms of the quantity of solute in a definite volume of solution or as the quantity of solute in a definite weight of solution. The quantity (or amount) is an absolute value (e.g. 10 ml, 5 g, 5 mg), whereas, concentration is the quantity of a substance in relation to a definite volume or weight of other substance (e.g. 2 g/5 g, 4 ml/5 ml, 5 mg/1 ml).

Mass percentage (fraction)

Weight-in-weight(w/w) percentage means parts of a drug in parts of a mixture by weight. Percent weight-in-weight expresses the number of grams of a drug or active ingredient in 100 grams of a mixture (g/g). For instance, if a bottle contains 40 grams of ethanol and 60 grams of water, then it contains 40% ethanol by mass or 0.4 mass fraction ethanol. In older texts and references, this is sometimes referred to as weight-weight percentage (abbreviated as w/w or wt%). In chemistry, a common term of measuring total mass percentage of dissolved solids in an aqueous medium is total dissolved solids.

Example 7:
Prepare 500 ml of phenol glycerin

Phenol 150 g
Glycerin q.s 850 g
Weight per ml of glycerin = 1.25

So preparing 500 ml of phenol glycerin, the quantity of glycerin required = 500 × 1.25 = 625 g

Quantity of phenol required = 150 × 625/850 = 110 g

For preparing 500 ml of phenol glycerin, the formula becomes:

Phenol   110 g
Glycerin   625 g

Example 8:

Prepare 500 ml of sugar solution
   Sugar 100 g
   Water q.s 900 g
   Weight per ml of water = 1g
   So preparing 500 ml of solution the quantity of water required = 500 × 1 = 500 g
   Quantity of sugar required
             = 100 × 500/900 = 55 g
   For preparing 500 ml of sugar solution the formula becomes;
   Sugar 55 g
   Water 500 g

Mass–volume percentage

Weight-in-volume (w/v) percentage is a part by weight in parts by volume expresses the number of grams of a drug or active ingredient in 100 milliliters of a mixture. Mass-volume percentage is often used for solutions made from a solid solute dissolved in a liquid. For example, a 40% w/v sugar solution contains 40 g of sugar per 100 ml of resulting solution.

Example 9:

Calculate the quantity of sodium chloride required to prepare 400 ml of 2% solution.
   1 g of sodium chloride with water produces 100 ml of 1% solution.
   1 × 2 g with water to produce 100 ml makes 2% w/v solution.
   2 × 400/100 with water to produce 400 ml makes 2% w/v solution = 8 g.
   Hence 8 g of sodium chloride is dissolved in water to produce 400 ml makes 2% w/v solution.

Example 10:

Prepare 500 ml of a 5% solution and label with a direction for preparing 2 liter quantities of a 1 in 5000 solution.

Strength of concentrate = 5%
Strength of dilute solution = 1in 5000 = 0.02%
Degree of dilution = strength of concentrate/ strength of dilute solution
   = 5/0.02 = 250 times
Volume of solution to be prepared = 2 litre
   = 2000 ml
Therefore, dilute solution is obtained by diluting 2000/250 = 8 ml of concentrated solution to 2 litre.

Example 11:

Prepare 500 ml of a 1 in 10000 solution from 1 in 5000 solution.
   Strength of concentrate 1 in 5000 = 100/5000 = 0.02%
   Strength of dilute solution = 1 in 10000 = 100/10000 = 0.01%
   Degree of dilution = strength of concentrate/ strength of dilute solution = 0.02/0.01 = 2 times
   Volume of solution to be prepared =500 ml
   Therefore, dilute solution is obtained by diluting 500/2 = 250 ml of 1 in 5000 solution to 500 ml.

Example 12:

How much of a 5% will be required to prepare 1000 ml of a 1 in 500 solution?
   Strength of concentrate = 5%
   Strength of dilute solution = 1 in 500 = 100/500 = 0.2%
   Degree of dilution = strength of concentrate/ strength of dilute solution = 5/0.2 = 25 times
   Volume of solution to be prepared = 1000 ml
   Therefore, dilute solution is obtained by diluting 1000/25 = 40 ml of 5% solution to 1000 ml.

Volume–volume percentage

Volume-in-volume (v/v) percentage is parts by volume of the total mixture. Percentage volume in volume expresses the number of milliliters of a drug or active ingredient in 100 milliliters of a mixture and is usually used for mixtures of liquidsssss in liquids. This is most useful when a liquid–liquid solution is being prepared, although it is used for mixtures of gases as well. For example, a 40% v/v ethanol solution contains 40 ml ethanol per 100 ml total volume. The percentages are only additive in the case of mixtures of ideal gases.

Example 13:

Prepare 500 ml of 5% solution of chloroform in 50% alcohol.

1 ml chloroform dissolved in 100 ml of alcohol = 1% v/v solution.

5 ml chloroform dissolved in 100 ml of alcohol = 5% v/v solution.

$5 \times 5 = 25$ ml chloroform dissolved in 500 ml of alcohol = 5% v/v solution.

Therefore dissolve 25 ml of chloroform in sufficient quantity of 50% alcohol to make 500 ml of solution.

Example 14:

Prepare 1 litre of 5% solution of water in 50% alcohol.

1 ml water dissolved in 100 ml of alcohol = 1% v/v solution.

$5 \times 10 = 50$ ml water dissolved in 1000 ml of alcohol = 5% v/v solution.

Therefore, dissolve 50 ml of water in sufficient quantity of 50% alcohol to make 1 lt solution.

Ratio strength

Ratio strength (1:N) is one part by weight or volume in N parts by weight or volume. 1:200 ratio strength can be 1 gm solid to 200 ml solid or 1 ml liquid to 200 ml liquid or 1 gm solid to 200 ml liquid.

Example 15:

If 2000 gm of ointment contain 75 gm of hydrocortisone, what is the percentage strength (w/w) of the ointment?

2000 gm of ointment contain 75 gm of hydrocortisone.

1 gm of ointment contain:

(Active ingredient) 75 gm/(total amt) 2000 gm

100 gm of ointment contain: $\dfrac{75 \times 100}{2000} = 3.75\%$

$x = 3.75\%$

Example 16:

If 8 ml of phenol were added to 480 ml of lotion, what is the percentage of phenol in the lotion?

480 ml of lotion contain 8 ml of phenol

1 ml of lotion contain: $8 / 480 = 0.0166$ ml of phenol

100 ml of lotion contain $0.0166 \times 100 = 1.6\%$ of phenol

Example 17:

If 1.2 gm of menthol is added to 480 ml of lotion, what is the percentage of menthol in the lotion?

480 ml of lotion contain 1.2 gm of menthol

1 ml of lotion contain: $1.2 / 480 = 0.0025$ gm of menthol

100 ml of lotion contain $0.0025 \times 100 = 0.25\%$ of menthol

Problems

1. How many grams of mercuric chloride are required to prepare 250 ml of a 5% solution?
2. How many grams of boric acid are there in 30 ml of a 2% solution?
3. How many grams of phenol are required to prepare 480 ml of a 1/10% solution?
4. How many grains of silver nitrate will be required to prepare 6 fl oz of a 0.25% solution?
5. If 425 gm of sucrose is dissolved in enough water to make 500 ml, what is the percentage strength of the solution?
6. If 2 liters of a solution of iodine in alcohol contains 7 grams of iodine, what is the percentage strength of the solution?

7. What are the percentages of the ingredients in the following prescription?

Zinc sulfate   2 grains _____ %

Boric acid   20 grains _____ %

Distilled water q.s 1 fl

8. How many milliliters of a 0.1% solution can be made from one gram of atropine sulfate?

9. How many fluid ounces of a 0.55% solution can be prepared from 75 grains of scopolamine hydrobromide?

10. With 43 gm of hydrocortisone powder, how many grams of a 1.5% ointment could you make?

11. How many liter of a 2% iodine tincture can be made from 123 gm of iodine?

12. If 1 gallon of a solution contains 474 gm of solute, what is the percentage strength of the solution?

13. How many grains of gentian violet should be used in preparing 2 fl oz of a 1/2% solution?

14. How many milliliters of a 6% solution can be prepared from 14 gm of neomycin sulfate?

15. What is the percentage strength of solution if 1/4 pound of chemical is dissolved in 0.25 liter?

16. How many pounds of medication are required to make 3 gallons of 7% solution?

17. How many fl oz of 16% solution can be made from 7000 grains of chemical?

18. How many quarts of 5% solution can be made from 47.3 grams of drug?

19. How many grains are needed to make 4 quarts of a 1/8% solution?

20. How many fl oz. (apothecary) of a 16% solution can be made from 9100 grains of drug?

21. If 12 grains of powder are dissolved in enough water to make one pint of solution, what is the percentage strength?

22. How many grains of NaCl are needed to make 8 fl oz of 0.9% solution?

23. How much thymol would be needed, if a prescription was written for 240 gm of 4%?

24. If 1000 ml contains 0.25 mg, what is the percentage of the solution?

25. If 10 grains are dissolved in 250 ml of solution, what is the percentage of this solution?

Answers:

(1) 12.5 gm (2) 0.6 gm (3) 0.48 gm (4) 6.83 gr (5) 85% (6) 0.35% (7) 0.43%, 4.3% (8) 1000 (9) 29.97 fl oz (10) 2866 gm (11) 6.15 L (12) 12.5% (13) 4.55 gr (14) 233.3 ml (15) 45.4% (16) 1.75 lb (17) 96.15 fl oz (18) 1 quart (19) 72.8 gr (20) 124.65 fl oz (21) 0.164% (22) 32.76 gr (23) 9.6 gm (24) 0.00002% (25) 0.25%

CONCENTRATION AND DILUTION

Stock solutions are bulk solutions of known concentration frequently prepared for convenience in dispensing. They are frequently concentrated solutions from which more dilute solutions can be quickly prepared. Although, dilute solutions are also compounded.

These solutions can be used with ratio strengths or percentage strengths.

General formula for solving:

$$V1 \times S1 = V2 \times S2$$

V1 = The quantity or amount of the original preparation.

S1 = The % strength of the original preparation expressed as a decimal or percent.

V2 = The quantity or amount of the wanted preparation.

S2 = The % strength of the wanted preparation expressed as a decimal or percent.

To solve concentration and dilution problems, you need to identify the two preparations in the equation, convert ratio or percentage strengths to decimal expressions and convert to same systems of measurement.

Example 1:

If 500 ml of a 15% solution are diluted to 1500 ml, what will be the percent strength?

$V1 \times S1 = V2 \times S2$

Step 1: Identify the two preparations in the problem and assign values to appropriate terms.

Step 2: Solve the equation by multiplying and solving for X.

500 ml (V1) × 15% (S1) = 1500 ml (V2) × (S2) X%

7500 = 1500 S2

7500/1500 = S2 = 5%

Example 2:

If 1000 ml of a 20% solution are diluted to 5000 ml, what will be the percent strength?

$V1 \times S1 = V2 \times S2$

1000 ml (V1) × 20% (S1) = 5000 ml (V2) × (S2) X%

20000 = 5000 S2

20000/5000 = S2 = 4%

Problems

1. How many milliliters of a 25% solution can be prepared from 750 ml of a 65% solution?

2. If 30 gm of a 45% powder was diluted to make a 30% powder, how many grams will the new preparation weigh?

3. If you dilute 2 pints of a 65% solution to 30%, how many fl oz will the new preparation measure?

4. How many grams of a 10% phosphoric acid can be made from 1 kg of 85% phosphoric acid?

5. If 20 ml of a 1:200 solution of a chemical is diluted to 500 ml, what is the ratio strength?

6. If 55 ml of an 18% solution is diluted to 330 ml, what will be the percentage strength?

7. How many milliliters of a 1:400 stock solution should be used to prepare 2l of a 1:2000 solution?

8. If 24 fl oz were prepared by diluting 1 pint of a 1:500 solution, what percentage strength would it be?

9. If 2 fl oz (apothecary) of a 25% solution is diluted to 5%, how many fluid ounces will the new solution measure?

10. How many pounds of a 1% cream can be made from 10,000 gm of an 8.5% cream?

11. How many milliliters of a 15% solution can be made from a quart of a 60% solution?

12. How many liters of a 1/1,000 solution can be made form 200 ml of a 0.1% solution?

13. How many milliliters of a 6% solution can be made from 2l of a 36% solution?

14. How many pints of a 6% solution can be made from 4 fl oz (apothecary) of a 15% solution?

15. How much of a 25% solution is needed to prepare 473 ml of a 10% solution?

Answers:

(1) 1950 ml (2) 45 gm (3) 69.33 fl oz (4) 8500 gm (5) 1:5000 (6) 3% (7) 400 ml (8) 0.13% (9) 10 fl oz (10) 187.22 lb (11) 3784 ml (12) 0.2 l (13) 12000 ml (14) 0.625 pts (15) 189.2 ml

MASS VERSUS VOLUME

Some units of concentration particularly the most popular one, molarity require knowledge of a substance's volume, unlike mass volume is variable depending on ambient temperature and pressure. In fact (partial) molar volume can even be a function of concentration itself. This is why volumes are not necessarily completely additive when two liquids are added and mixed. Volume-based measures for concentration are therefore not to be recommended for non-dilute solutions or problems where relatively large differences in temperature are encountered (e.g. for phase diagrams).

The volume of a liquid is usually determined by calibrated glassware such as burettes and volumetric flasks. For very small volumes precision syringes, pipettes and micropipettes are available. The use of graduated beakers and cylinders is not recommended as their indication of volume is mostly for decorative rather than quantitative purposes. The volume of solids, particularly of powders, is often difficult to measure. For gases, the opposite is true: the volume of a gas can be measured in a gas burette, if care is taken to control the pressure, but the mass is not easy to measure due to buoyancy effects.

Molarity

Molarity (in units of mol/L, molar, or M) or molar concentration denotes the number of moles of a given substance per liter of solution. A capital letter M is used to abbreviate units of mol/L. For instance:

$$\text{Moles of solute} = \frac{\text{Molarity of solution}}{\text{Liters of solution}}$$

Example 1:

2.0 moles of dissolved solute/4.0 liters of solution = Solution of 0.5 mol/L.

Such a solution may be described as "0.50 molar." It must be emphasized a 0.5 molar solution contains 0.5 mole of solute in 1.0 liter of solution. This is not equivalent to 1.0 liter of solvent. A 0.5 mol/L solution will contain either slightly more or slightly less than 1 liter of solvent because the process of dissolution causes volume of liquid to increase or decrease.

When discussing molarity of minute concentrations, such as in pharmacological research, molarity is expressed in units of millimolar (mmol/L, mM, 1 thousandth of a molar), micromolar (µmol/L, µM, 1 millionth of a molar) or nanomolar (nmol/L, nM, 1 billionth of a molar).

Example 2:

Prepare 1000 ml of one molar solution of sodium chloride

Molecular weight of sodium chloride = 60

That means if 60 grams of sodium chloride is dissolved in 1 litre water that will produce 1 litre of 1 molar solution of sodium chloride.

Example 3:

Prepare 10 litres of 5 molar solution of sodium chloride.

Molecular weight of sodium chloride = 60.

60 gm of sodium chloride is required for 1 M solution.

For 5 M solution 60 × 5 = 300 g sodium chloride require to produce 1 litre of 5 M solution.

For 10 litres solution 300 × 10 = 3000 g of sodium chloride.

That means if 3000 grams of sodium chloride are dissolved in 10 litres water that will produce 10 litres of 5 molar solution of sodium chloride.

Problems:

1. Prepare 500 ml of 1 M solution of sodium hydroxide.
2. Prepare 200 ml of 0.5 M solution of HCl.
3. Prepare 1 lt of 5 M solution of NaOH.
4. Prepare 100 ml of 2 M solution NaCl.
5. Prepare 10 lt of 1 M solution of HCl.

Answers:

(1) 10 gm (2) 9 ml (3) 200 gm (4) 12 gm
(5) 900 ml

Molality

Molality (mol/kg, molal, or m) denotes the number of moles of solute per kilogram of solvent (not solution).

$$\text{Moles of solute} = \frac{\text{Molarity of solution}}{\text{Kilograms of solvent}}$$

For instance: adding 1.0 mole of solute to 2.0 kilograms of solvent constitutes a solution with a molality of 0.50 mol/kg. Such a solution may be described as "0.50 molal". The term molal solution is used as a shorthand for a "one molal solution", i.e. a solution which contains one mole of the solute per 1000 grams of the solvent.

In a dilute aqueous solution near room temperature and standard atmospheric pressure, molarity and molality will be very similar in value. This is because 1 kg of water roughly corresponds to a volume of 1 L at these conditions, and because the solution is dilute, the addition of the solute makes a negligible impact on the volume of the solution. However, in all other conditions, this is usually not the case.

Example 4:

Prepare 1000 ml of one molal solution of sodium carbonate

Molecular weight of sodium bicarbonate = 105 g

Since the density of water is one, hence 1 lt is equivalent to 1000 g of water.

That means if 105 grams of sodium carbonate are dissolved in 1000 g of water that will produce 1 litre of 1 molal solution of sodium carbonate.

Example 5:

Prepare 5 litre of 5 molal solution of sodium carbonate

Molecular weight of sodium bicarbonate = 105

Since the density of water is one, hence 1 lt is equivalent to 1000 g of water.

For 5 molal solutions $105 \times 5 = 525$ g of sodium carbonate is required.

For 5 litre solution $525 \times 5 = 2625$ g of sodium carbonate is required.

That means if 2625 grams of sodium carbonate are dissolved in 5000 g of water that will produce 5 litres of 5 molal solution of sodium carbonate.

Problems

1. What is the molality of a solution that contains 63.0 g HNO_3 in 0.500 kg H_2O?

2. What is the molality of a solution that contains 0.500 mol $HC_2H_3O_2$ in 0.125 kg H_2O?

3. What mass of water is required to dissolve 100 g NaCl to prepare a 1.50 m solution?

4. What mass of water must be used to dissolve 0.500 kg C_2H_5OH to prepare a 3.00 m solution?

5. What mass of H_2SO_4 must be dissolved to 2.40 kg H_2O to produce a 1.20 m solution?

6. What is the number of molecules of C_2H_5OH in a 3 m solution that contains 4.00 kg H_2O?

7. What is the molality of a solution that contains 80.0 g $Al_2(SO_4)$ in 625 g H_2O?

8. What mass of water is required to dissolve 175 g KNO_3 to produce a 2.25 m solution?

9. What mass of $HC_2H_3O_2$ must be dissolved in 800 g H_2O to produce a 6.25 m solution?

10. How many moles of NH_4+ ions are dissolved in 0.750 kg of H_2O when the concentration of $(NH_4) PO_3$ is 0.400 m?

Answers:

(1) 2 mol/kg (2) 2500 mol/kg (3) 110 ml (4) 3.3 lt (5) 283 gm (6) 552 moles (7) 0.5 m (8) 777 ml (9) 300 ml (10) 34

Mole Fraction

The mole fraction X, (also called molar fraction) denotes the number of moles of solute as a proportion of the total number of moles in a solution. For instance, 1 mole of solute dissolved in 9 moles of solvent has a mole fraction of 1/10 or 0.1. Mole fractions are dimensionless quantities. (The mole percentage or molar percentage, denoted "mol %" and equal to 100% times the mole fraction, is sometimes quoted instead of the mole fraction.)

This measure is used very frequently in the construction of phase diagrams. It has a number of advantages: the measure is not temperature dependent (such as molarity) and does not require knowledge of the densities of the phase(s) involved a mixture of known mole fraction can be prepared by weighing off the appropriate masses of the constituents the measure is symmetrical— in the mole fractions X=0.1 and X=0.9, the roles of 'solvent' and 'solute' are reversed.

As both mole fractions and molality are only based on the masses of the components, it is easy to convert between these measures. This is not true for molarity, which requires knowledge of the density.

Example 6:

What is the molality of a solution made by dissolving 50 g of sodium nitrate in 500 g of water?

500 g of water contain 50 g of sodium nitrate

1000 g will contain 50/500 × 1000 = 100 g sodium nitrate

Molecular weight of sodium nitrate = 85

Hence the molality of the above solution is 100/85 = 1.17 molal

Example 7:

How many grams of silver chloride must be dissolved in 200 grams of water to make a 0.5 m (molal) solution?

Molecular weight of silver chloride = 145

For 1 molal solution of silver bromide, 145 g is dissolved in 1 litre of solvent

For 0.5 M solution, 145/2 = 72.5 g of sodium chloride is needed to make 1 litre solution

1 ml of solution contains 72.5/1000 = 0.072 g of silver chloride

For 200 ml, the amount of silver chloride require is 0.072 × 200 = 14.4 g

Hence 14.4 g of silver chloride when it dissolved in 200 ml of water, making 0.5 m solution.

Problems

1. What is the molality of a solution made by dissolving 23.2 g of sodium nitrate in 250.0 g of water?

2. How many grams of silver bromide must be dissolved in 725 grams of water to make a 0.220 m (molal) solution?

3. What mass of solvent must be added to 17.3 g of bromine to make a 0.115 m (molal) solution?

4. What is the mole fraction of ethanol when 23.2 g of ethanol are mixed with 73.1 g of water?

5. How many grams of water must be added to 72.8 grams of sodium chloride to make the mole fraction of sodium chloride 0.200?

6. 285 g of sucrose are added to 1250 g of water. Find both the molality and the mole fraction of sucrose.

7. Calculate the mole fraction of NaOH in a 10.0 m aqueous solution.

Answers:

(1) 1.09 m (2) 29.9 g (3) 0.939 kg (4) 0.110 (5) 89.7 gm (6) 0.0119 (7) 0.153

Normality

The normality of a solution is the number of gram equivalent weight of a solute per litre of its solution, e.g. hydrochloric acid(HCl). One litre of aqueous solution of HCl acid contains 36.5 grams HCl. It is called 1 N (one normal) solution of HCl. It is given by the following formula:

Normality (N) =

$$\frac{\text{Weight of solutes in grams}}{\text{Grams equivalent weight}} \times \text{Volume in litres}$$

Example 8:

How much sodium bicarbonate powder is needed to prepare 60 ml of a 0.07 N solution of $NaHCO_3$?

1 N solution of $NaHCO_3$ contains 84 g/L

Amount of $NaHCO_3$ requires for 0.07N equal to 84 × 0.07 = 5.88 g

Thus 5.88 g of $NaHCO_3$ in 1 lt will produce 0.07 N solution of $NaHCO_3$.

60 ml require 5.88 × 60/1000 = 0.353 g $NaHCO_3$.

Equivalents

The equivalent (symbol: eq or Eq), sometimes termed the molar equivalent is a unit of amount of substance used in chemistry and the biological sciences. Expression of concentration in equivalents per liter (or more commonly, milliequivalents per liter) is based on the same principle as normality. A normal solution is one equivalent per liter of solution (Eq/L). The equivalent is formally defined as the amount of a substance which will either react with or supply one mole of hydrogen ions (H^+) in an acid–base reaction; or react with or supply one mole of electrons in a redox reaction.

Example 9:

1 mol $Ca(OH)_2$ = 2 equivalents $Ca(OH)_2$

There are "TWO" OHO^- released when the hydroxide dissolves.

The calcium hydroxide releases Ca^{2+} and two OH^{1-} ions.

The equivalent weight of calcium hydroxide is 1/2 the mass of a mol of calcium hydroxide.

1 mol $Ca(OH)_2$= 74 grams $Ca(OH)_2$;
1 equivalent $Ca(OH)_2$ = 37 grams $Ca(OH)_2$

Problems

1. How many equivalents are represented by each of the following substances?

   (a) 65.00 ml of 0.75 N H_2CO_3

   (b) 435.00 ml of 6.3 M H_3PO_4

   (c) 0.65 l of a 1.86 N H_2SO_4?

   (d) 40.00 ml of 0.25 M $Ba(OH)_2$?

2. Determine the Normality for each of the following:

   (a) 0.56 eq in 0.45 l of $HC_2H_3O_2$

   (b) 61.2 g in 87.6 ml of $HClO_4$

3. How many ml of 1.60 N NaOH can be prepared from 13.00 g?

4. How many ml of 0.0020 N $Al(OH)_3$ can be made from 100.00 ml of 0.10 M $Al(OH)_3$?

5. 60.0 ml of a 0.16 M solution of H_2SO_4 is diluted to 85.0 ml. Determine the molarity and normality of the diluted solution.

6. 3.42 g of $Mg(OH)_2$ is added to enough water to produce 350.0 ml of solution. This solution is then diluted to 658.0 ml. What is the molarity and normality of the final solution?

Answers

(1) (a) 0.049 eq. (b) 8.22 eq. (c) 1.21 eq. (d) 0.02 eq. (2) (a)1.24 N (b) 6.99 N (3) 203 ml (4) 15000 ml (5) 0.22 M (6) 0.179 N

Milliequivalents

A milliequivalent is 1/1000 of an equivalent. This means an equivalent is 1000 milliequivalents. In terms of grams, the equivalent weight is equal to 1000 milliequivalent weights. This unit is useful because it matches the levels of dissolved ions in small volumes of body fluids.

Example 10:

1 mol H_3PO_4 = 3 equivalents H_3PO_4
The acid releases three H^{1+} and one phosphate PO_4^{2-} ion.
The equivalent weight of phosphoric acid is 1/3 the mass of a mol.
1 mol H_3PO_4 = 98 grams H_3PO_4; 1 equivalent H_3PO_4 = 32 grams H_3PO_4

The relation between equivalents and milliequivalents

1 equivalent H_3PO_4 = 1000 milliequivalent H_3PO_4
1 equivalent mol H_2PO_4 = 32 grams H_3PO_4;
1 milliequivalent mol H_2PO_4 = 32 milligrams H_3PO_4

Example 11:

How many milliequivalents of ferrous are present in 5 gr of ferrous sulfate? (MW = 152 gm/mole)

Eq wt of $FeSO_4$ = gm mol wt/no. of valence = 152 gm/mole/2 = 76

Example 12:

Aluminum (Al^{+3}) has a gram atomic weight of 27. What would be the milliequivalent weight?

Eq weight = weight in gm/no of valence = 27 gm/3 = 9 gm eq weight

mEq = equivalent weight in mg/1000 = 9000/1000 = 9

Example 13:

How many mEq of Na^+ presents in 0.9% 250 cc of normal saline solution? (MW = 58.5 gram/mole)

Equivalent wt of NaCl = gm mol wt/valence = 58.5 gm mol wt/1= 58.5 gm mol wt

Milliequivalent of NaCl = eq wt/1000 = 58.5/1000 = 0.0585

Amount of NaCl in 0.9% 250cc of normal saline solution is = 250 x 0.009 = 2.25 gm, therefore we can say 2.25 units NaCl is dissociate in 2.25 units Na^+ and 2.25 units Cl^- ions.

Total mEq of Na^+ = 2.25 gm/0.0585 g/mEq = 38.46 mEq of Na^+

Example 14:

How many milliequivalents of sodium are present in a 50% of 50cc solution of sodium bicarbonate? (MW = 84 gm/mole)

eq weight = gm mole wt/valence = 84 gm / 1 = 84 g

mEq = eq wt/1000 = 84 / 1000 = 0.084 g

Total mEq of sod = 25 g/0.084 g/eq = 297.61 mEq

REDUCING AND ENLARGING FORMULAS

Determine the total weight or volume of ingredients and convert to the required quantity. The quantities in the original and new formulas will have the same ratio.

To reduce formula in the metric system, divide by a power of 10 by moving the decimal place to the left the required number of places for each ingredient; to enlarge formula. Multiply by a power of 10 by moving the decimal place to the right the required number of places.

Example 1:

Calculate the amounts needed for 50 ml strong sodium salicylate mixture

Sodium salicylate	10 g

Sodium metabisulfate	1 g
D.S. chloroform water	525 ml
Water	1000 ml

1000 ml of mixture contains 10 gm of sodium salicylate

1 ml of mixture contains 10/1000 = 0.01 g of sodium salicylate

50 ml of mixture contain 0.01 x 50 = 0.5 gm

Similarly, calculate the amount of each ingredients require for 50 ml of strong sodium salicylate mixture. The required quantity will be as follows:

Sodium salicylate	0.5 g
Sodium metabisulfate	0.05 g
D.S. chloroform water	26.25 ml
Water	50 ml

Example 2:

Calculate the amounts needed for 100 ml peppermint water

Peppermint	2 ml
Talc	15 gm
Purified water q.s	1000 ml

1000 ml of mixture contain 2 ml of peppermint

1 ml of mixture contain 2/1000 = 0.002 ml of peppermint

50 ml of mixture contain 0.002 × 100 = 0.2 ml of peppermint

Similarly calculate the amount of each ingredients require for 100 ml of peppermint water. The required quantity will be as follows:

Peppermint	0.2 ml
Talc	1.5 gm
Purified water q.s	100 ml

Problems:

1. Reduce this formula to make 100 ml

Liquid coal tar	4 ml
Sulfur	10 gm
Lime water	50 ml
Bentonite magma q.s	120 ml

2. Reduce the formula to make 30 ml

| Ephedrine sulfate | 30 gm |
| Chlorobutanol | 5 gm |

| Sodium chloride | 3.6 gm |
| Purified water q.s | 1000 ml |

3. From the following formula, calculate the quantity of each ingredient required to prepare 1 gallon.

Talc	12 gm
Bentonite	3.5 gm
Zinc oxide	25 gm
Distilled water q.s	100 ml

4. From the following formula, calculate the quantity of each ingredient required to make 1 liter.

Orange oil	12 ml
Lemon oil	3 ml
Coriander oil	1.2 ml
Anise oil	0.3 ml
Alcohol USP q.s	60 ml

5. Reduce the following formula to make 1 pint.

Peppermint oil	2.4 ml
Cinnamon oil	0.16 ml
Diphenhydramine	12 gm
Purified water q.s	500 ml

6. Enlarge the following to make 4 gallons.

Glycerin	15 ml
Propylene glycol	30 ml
Syrup	100 ml
Alcohol q.s	473 ml

7. Reduce the following formula to make 1 pint.

Terpin hydrate	30 gm
Orange tincture	65 ml
Syrup q.s	1000 ml

8. How many mg of zinc oxide are needed to make 4 quarts of the following?

Talc	15 gm
Zinc oxide	75 gm
Purified water q.s	800 ml

Answers:

(1) 3.32 ml, 8.3 gm, 41.5 ml, 100 ml (2) 0.9 gm, 0.15 gm, 0.108 gm, 30 ml (3) 454.2 ml, 132.48 gm, 946.25 gm, 3784 ml (4) 200.04 ml, 50.01 ml, 20 ml, 5 ml, 1000 ml (5) 2.27 ml, 0.15 ml, 11.35 gm, 473 ml (6) 480 ml, 960 ml, 3200 ml, 15140 ml (7) 14.19 gm, 30.75 ml, 473 ml (8) 70.95 gm, 354.75 mg, 3784 ml

"PARTS-PER" NOTATION

The parts-per notation is used in some areas of science and engineering because it does not require conversion from weights or volumes to more chemically relevant units such as normality or molarity. It describes the amount of one substance in another, and is thus related to the mass fraction. It is the ratio of the amount of the substance of interest to the amount of that substance plus the amount of the substance it is in.

- Parts per hundred (denoted by '%' [the percent symbol], and very rarely 'pph') denotes the amount of a given substance in a total amount of 100 regardless of the units of measure as long as they are the same, e.g. 1 gram per 100 gram. 1 part in 100.

- Parts per thousand (ppt) denotes the amount of a given substance in a total amount of 1000 regardless of the units of measure as long as they are the same, e.g. 1 milligram per gram, or 1 gram per kilogram. 1 part in 10^3.

- Parts per million ('ppm') denotes the amount of a given substance in a total amount of 1,000,000 regardless of the units of measure used as long as they are the same, e.g. 1 milligram per kilogram. 1 part in 10^6.

- Parts per billion ('ppb') denotes the amount of a given substance in a total amount of 1,000,000,000 regardless of the units of measure as long as they are the same, e.g. 1 milligram per tonne. 1 part in 10^9.

- Parts per trillion ('ppt') denotes the amount of a given substance in a total amount of 1,000,000,000,000 regardless of the units of measure as long as they are the same, e.g. 1 milligram per kilotonne. 1 part in 10^{12}.

- Parts per quadrillion ('ppq') denotes the amount of a given substance in a total amount of 1,000,000,000,000,000 regardless of the units of measure as long as they are the same, e.g. 1 milligram per megatonne. 1 part in 10^{15}.

Example 1:

How many grams of drug is required to dispense 1 pint of 1 in 25 solution? Strength of solution in mg/ml ?

1 in 25 solution is interpreted as 1 gm of drug in 25 cc solution, therefore we can say 1 pint (480 cc) solution of drug will contain = 480/25 = 19.20 grams of drug.

Example 2:

How much lidocaine is required to prepare 30 cc of 1 in 1000 solution?

1: 1000 is expressed by 1 gm of lidocaine in 1000 cc of solution, therefore 30 cc solution of lidocaine will present in = 30/1000 = 0.03 gram (30 mg) lidocaine.

Example 3:

How much atropine is required to dispense 1 quart of 1 in 100 solutions?

1 in 100 contains 1 gram of drug in 100 cc of solution. We want to prepare 1 quart (960 cc), therefore 960/100 = 9.6 grams of drug.

Problems

1. 25 gm of a chemical is dissolved in 75 grams of water.
   a. What is the concentration of the chemical in parts per hundred (pph)?
   b. What is the concentration of the chemical in parts per thousand (ppt)?
   c. What is the % of solute in this solution?
2. 35 gm of ethanol is dissolved in 115 grams of water. What is the concentration of ethanol in parts per billion (ppb)?
3. The solubility of NaCl is 284 grams/100 grams of water. What is this concentration in ppm?

4. The solubility of AgCl is 0.008 gram/100 grams of water. What is this concentration in ppm?
5. A certain pesticide has a toxic solubility of 5.0 grams/kg of body weight. What is this solubility in ppm?
6. Change 50 ppm to ppb.
7. How many parts per million (ppm) is 1 mg/L?

Answers:

(1) (a) 25 pph (b) 250 ppt (c) 25% (2) 233,333,333.33 ppb (3) 284,000 ppm (4) 80 ppm (5) 5000 ppm (6) 5000 ppb (7) 1 ppm.

SYSTEMS OF MEASUREMENTS

The knowledge and application of various calculations are essential for the practice of pharmacy and related health professions. Many calculations have been simplified by the shift from apothecary to metric system of measurements. However, a significant proportion of calculation errors occurs because of simple mistakes in arithmetic. Further, the dosage forms prepared by pharmaceutical companies undergo several inspections and quality control tests. Such a system of validation is almost impossible to find in a pharmacy or hospital setting. Therefore, it is imperative that the healthcare professionals must be extremely careful in performing pharmacy math.

Imperial System

Before SI units were widely adopted around the world, the British systems of English units and later Imperial units were used in Britain, the Commonwealth and the United States. The system came to be known as US customary units in the United States and is still in use there and in a few Caribbean countries. These various systems of measurement have at times been called foot-pound-second systems after the Imperial units for distance, weight and time even though the tons, hundredweights, gallons, and nautical miles, for example, are different for the US units.

Length

After the 1st July 1959 deadline, agreed upon in 1958, the US and the British yard were defined identically, at 0.9144 meter to match the international yard. Before this date, the most precise measurement of the imperial standard gard was 0.914398416 meter. Table 3.3 gives information about length equivalent units.

Area

Table 3.4 enlists area equivalent units.

Volume (Table 3.5)

In 1824, Britain adopted a close approximation to the gallon known as the imperial gallon. The imperial gallon was based on the volume of 10 lb of distilled water weighed in air with brass weights with the barometer standing at 30 in Hg at a temperature of 62°F. In 1963, this definition was refined as the space occupied by 10 lb of distilled water of density 0.998 859 g/ml weighed in air of density 0.001 217 g/ml against weights of density 8.136 g/ml. This works out to 4.545 964 591 L, or 277.420 cu in. The weights and measures

Table 3.3: Length equivalent units				
Unit	Relative to previous	Feet	Millimeters	Meters
Thou		1/12000	0.0254	thou
Inch	1000 thou	1/12	25.4	
Feet	12 inches	1	304.8	0.3048
Yard	3 feet	3	914.4	0.9144
Furlong	220 yards	660		201.168
Mile	8 furlongs	5,280		1,609.344
League	3 miles	15,840		4,828.032
Maritime units				
Fathom		6.08	1,853.184	1.853184
Cable	~100 fathoms	608		185.3184
Nautical mile	10 cables	6,080		1,853.184
Gunter's survey units (17th century onwards)				
Link		66/100	201.168	0.201168
Pole	25 links	66/4	5,029.2	5.0292
Chain	4 poles	66		20.1168

Table 3.4: Area equivalent units						
Unit	Relation to units of length	Square feet	Square rods	Square miles	Square meters	Hectares
Perch	1 rod × 1 rod	272.25	1	1/10240	25.29285264	0.002529
Rood	1 furlong × 1 rod	10,890	40	1/2560	1,011.7141056	0.1012
Acre	1 furlong × 1 chain	43,560	160	1/640	4,046.8564224	0.4047

Table 3.5: Imperial systems (volume)						
Unit ounce	Imperial	Imperial pint	Milliliters	Cubic inches	US ounces	US pints
Fluid ounce (fl oz)	1	1/20	28.4130625	1.7339	0.96076	0.060047
Gill	5	1/4	142.0653125	8.6694	4.8038	0.30024
Pint (pt)	20	1	568.26125	34.677	19.215	1.2009
Quart (qt)	40	2	1,136.5225	69.355	38.430	2.4019
Gallon (gal)	160	8	4,546.09	277.42	153.72	9.6076

Act of 1985 switched to a gallon of exactly 4.546 09 L (approximately 277.4 cu in).

Mass

In the 19th and 20th centuries, Britain has used three different systems for mass and weight (Table 3.6).

Table 3.6: Imperial systems (weight)		
Unit	Pounds	Grams
Grain	1/7000	0.065
Drachm	1/256	1.78
Ounce (oz)	1/16	28.35
Pound (lb)	1	453.60
Stone (st)	14	6,350.30
Quarter	28	12.70
Hundredweight (cwt)	112	
Ton (t)	2240	1,016.05

Metric system

In the metric system, the three primary or fundamental units are the meter for length, the liter for volume, and the gram for weight. In addition to these basic units, the metric system includes multiples of basic units with a prefix to indicate their relationship with the basic unit, e.g. a milliliter represents 1/1000 or 0.001 part of a liter. A milligram represents 0.001 gram, and a kilogram represents 1000 times the gram. Tables 3.7 to 3.12 of measurements are very important for the pharmacy and healthcare personnel.

The pharmacist should be able to perform interconversions such as going from a microgram to a gram or from a nanogram to a microgram. The following general guidelines may be helpful:

Table 3.7: Metric table					
yotta	(Y)	meaning 10^{24}	deci	(d)	meaning 10^{-1}
zetta	(Z)	meaning 10^{21}	centi	(c)	meaning 10^{-2}
exa	(E)	meaning 10^{18}	milli	(m)	meaning 10^{-3}
peta	(P)	meaning 10^{15}	micro	(μ)	meaning 10^{-6}
tera	(T)	meaning 10^{12}	nano	(n)	meaning 10^{-9}
giga	(G)	meaning 10^{9}	pico	(p)	meaning 10^{-12}
mega	(M)	meaning 10^{6}	femto	(f)	meaning 10^{-15}
kilo	(k)	meaning 10^{3}	atto	(a)	meaning 10^{-18}
hecto	(h)	meaning 10^{2}	zepto	(z)	meaning 10^{-21}
deca	(da)	meaning 10^{1}	yato	(y)	meaning 10^{-24}

To prevent the problem of overlooking a decimal point, precede the decimal point with a zero, if the value is less than one, e.g. writing 0.5 g is better than .5 g. As a practical example, if a prescription is written for oxycodone oral solution .5 mg/.5 ml, one possible mistake could be dispensing 0.5 mg/5.0 ml solution. This under-medication to the patient would most likely be avoided, if zeros are added and the numbers are expressed as 0.5 mg/0.5 ml.

Table 3.8: Units of length

10 millimeters (mm)	1 centimeter (cm)
10 centimeters	1 decimeter (dm) = 100 mm
10 decimeters	1 meter (m) = 1000 millimeters
10 meters	1 decameter (dam)
10 decameters	1 hectometer (hm) = 100 m
10 hectometers	1 kilometer (km) = 1000 m

Table 3.9: Units of area

100 square millimeters (mm)^2	1 square centimeter (cm)^2
100 square centimeters	1 square decimeter (dm)^2
100 square decimeters	1 square meter (m)^2
100 square meters	1 square decameter (dam)^2 = 1 are
100 square decameters	1 square hectometer (hm)^2 = 1 hectare (ha)
100 square hectometers	1 square kilometer (km)^2

Table 3.10: Units of liquid volume

10 milliliters (ml)	1 centiliter (cL)
10 centiliters	1 deciliter (dL) = 100 milliliters
10 deciliters	1 liter = 1000 milliliters
10 liters	1 decaliter (daL)
10 decaliters	1 hectoliter (hL) = 100 liters
10 hectoliters	1 kiloliter (kL) = 1000 liters

Table 3.11: Units of volume

1000 cubic millimeters (mm)^3	1 cubic centimeter (cm)^3
1000 cubic centimeters	1 cubic decimeter (dm)^3
1000 cubic decimeters	1 cubic meter (m)^3

Table 3.12: Units of mass

10 milligrams (mg)	1 centigram (cg)
10 centigrams	1 decigram (dg) = 100 milligrams
10 decigrams	1 gram (g) = 1000 milligrams
10 grams	1 decagram (dag)
10 decagrams	1 hectogram (hg) = 100 grams
10 hectograms	1 kilogram (kg) = 1000 grams
1000 kilograms	1 megagram (Mg) or 1 metric ton(t)

In certain cases, particularly in scientific usage, it becomes convenient to provide for multiples larger than 1000 and for subdivisions smaller than one-thousandth. Accordingly, the following prefixes have been introduced and these are now generally recognized.

Problem:

Convert between the various denominations of each of the basic units of the metric system.

1. 25 cL = _____ L
2. 15 km = _____ m
3. 1,000 mg = _____ gm
4. 500 dL = _____ daL
5. 10 mm = _____ cm
6. 75 mg = _____ μg
7. 250 m = _____ cm
8. 0.00085 dg = _____ μg
9. 450 cc = _____ L

10. 2,500 mg   = _____ gm

11. 5 kL   = _____ dL

12. 8,500 µg   = _____ mg

13. 750 m   = _____ Hm

14. 45 daL   = _____ dL

15. 0.00025 Hg   = _____ µg

16. 0.375 mg   = _____ µg

17. 3 gm   = _____ mg

18. 12 gm   = _____ kg

19. 2,500 mg   = _____ daG

20. 0.025 hL   = _____ dL

21. 2 kL   = _____ cc

22. 70,000 mm   = _____ Hm

23. 5,400,250 µl   = _____ L

24. 0.085 Hg   = _____ gm

25. 375 cm   = _____ Dam

Answers:

(1) 0.25 L (2) 15,000 m (3) 1 gm (4) 5 Dal (5) 1 cm (6) 75,000 mcg (7) 25,000 cm (8) 85 µg (9) 0.45 L (10) 2.5 gm (11) 50,000 dl (12) 8.5 mg (13) 7.5 Hm (14) 4,500 dl (15) 25,000 µg (16) 375 µg (17) 3,000 mg (18) 0.012 kg (19) 0.25 Dag (20) 25 dl (21) 2,000,000 cc (cc = ml) (22) 0.7 Hm (23) 5.40025 L (24) 8.5 gm (25) 0.375 dam

Apothecaries System

Traditional system of weight used for the measuring and dispensing of pharmaceutical items are based on the grain, scruple (20 grains), dram (3 scruples), ounce (8 drams), and pound (12 ounces). The English version of the system is closely related with the English troy system of weights, the pound and grain being exactly the same in both. The apothecaries' system of measures is a similar system of volume units based on the fluid ounce.

In prescription, Roman numbers are used to express weight and measures means two gallon expressed as gal ii. The Roman numbers used are as follows:

Example 1:

If a prescription calls for gr ii thyroid desiccated tablets and the pharmacist has gr ss tablets in stock, how many tablets of gr ss should be provided?

gr ii = 2 grains

gr ss = 1/2 grain

2 /(1/2) = 4 tablets of gr ss

Answer: 4 tablets of gr ss

Example 2:

A doctor ordered morphine sulfate gr 2/5 and the pharmacist has a stock solution of gr 1/8 per milliliter of morphine sulfate. How many milliliters of the stock solution is required to fill the prescription?

gr 2/5 = 0.4 grain needed

gr 1/8 = 0.125 grain per ml

0.125/ml = 0.4/X

X = 0.4/0.125 = 3.2

Answer: 3.2 ml of the stock solution

Example 3:

Convert 1060 grains to ounces, drachms and scruple.

We know that:

480 grains = 1 ounce

So 1060 grains = (1/480)*1060 = 2.20 ounces

60 grains = 1 drachm

So 1060 grains = (1/60)*1060 = 17.66 drachms

20 grains = 1 scruple

So 1060 grains = (1/20)* 1060 = 53 scruples

Answer: 2.20 ounces, 17.66 drachms and 53 scruples.

Example 4:

How many grain doses (single dose= 25 gr) can be obtained from 3 × ii ss of powder?

Solution: 3 × ii ss = 10+1+1+1/2 = 3 12.5

As we know that 1 drachm = 60 grains

So 12.5 drachm = 12.5 * 60 = 750 grains

Single dose = 25 grains (given)

No of doses = total grains available/25 grains

= 750 / 25 = 30 doses

Answer: 30 doses

Avoirdupois System (Table 3.13)

The word avoirdupois is from Old French *aveir de peis*, literally "goods of weight" (Old French *aveir*, "property, goods", also "to have", comes from the Latin *habere*, "to have, to hold, to possess property"; *de* = "from", cf. Latin; *peis* = "weight", from Latin pensum). It is the everyday system of weight used in the United States, and is still widely used to varying degrees by many people in Canada, the United Kingdom, and some other former British colonies despite the official adoption of the metric system (Tables 3.14. and 3.15).

The avoirdupois pound contains 7,000 grains, or 256 drams of 27.344 grains each, or 16 ounces of 437 1/2 grains each. It is used for all products not subject to apothecaries' weight (for pharmaceutical items) or troy weight (for precious metals). It is equal to about 1.22 apothecaries' or troy pounds. Since 1959 the avoirdupois pound has been officially defined in most English-speaking countries as 0.453 kg.

Table 3.13: Avoirdupois system

Unit	Relative	Unit	Relative
dram or drachm	1/256	~1.772 g	1/16 oz
ounce (oz)	1/16	~28.35 g	16 dr
pound (lb)	1	~453.6 g	16 oz
stone (st)	14	~6.35 kg	½ qtr
quarter (qtr)	28	~12.7 kg	2 st
hundred weight (cwt)	112	~50.8 kg	4 qtr
ton (t)	2,240	~1,016 kg	20 cwt

The Household System

Though inaccurate, the use of the household system of measurements is on the rise because of an increased home health care delivery. In this system, the patients use household measuring devices such as the teaspoon, dessertspoon, tablespoon, wine-glass, coffee cup.

Table 3.14: Units of weight

Weight	
20 grains	1 scruple (Ə)
3 scruples	1 dram (Ʒ) = 60 grains
8 drachms	1 ounce (Ʒ) = 480 grains
12 ounces	1 pound (lb) = 5760 grains

Approximate equivalents of milligrams (mg) and grains (gr)

0.2 mg	1/300 gr
0.3 mg	1/200 gr
0.4 mg	1/150 gr
0.5 mg	1/120 gr
1 mg	1/60 gr
3 mg	1/20 gr
6 mg	1/10 gr
10 mg	1/6 gr
15 mg	1/4 gr
25 mg	3/8 gr
30 mg	1/2 gr
60 mg	1 gr
120 mg	2 gr
200 mg	3 gr
300 mg	5 gr
500 mg	7 1/2 gr
600 mg	10 gr
1000 mg	15 gr

Table 3.15: Units of volume

Volume (Liquid)	
1 fluid dram	60 minims (m)
8 fluid dram	1 fluid ounces (fl.oz)
1 fl. oz	480 m = 8 fl. drams
1 pint (pt)	7680 m = 16 fl. oz
1 quart (qt)	2 pt.
1 gallon	4 qt

Table 3.16: Roman numbers in prescription			
1/4	s	5	V
1/2	ss	6	VI
1	I	7	VII
2	II	8	VIII
3	III	9	IX
4	IV	10	X

In the past, a drop has been used as an equivalent of a minim. But such a measure should be discouraged because of many factors affecting the drop size which include the density of the medication, temperature, surface tension, diameter and opening of the dropper, and the angle of the dropper. The official medicinal dropper (USP-NF) has an external diameter of 3 mm, and delivers 20 drops per ml of water at 25°C. Some manufacturers provide specially calibrated droppers with their products. A few examples of medications containing droppers include Tylenol® pediatric drops, Advil® pediatric drops, and Neosynephrine® nasal drops. Several ear, nose and eye medications are now available in calibrated containers which provide drops by gently pressing the containers. Sometimes, the health care professonal has to calibrate the dropper for measuring small quantities such as 0.1 ml or 0.15 ml, when the calibrated dropper is not supplied by the manufacturer. The calibration procedure is outlined in the following section.

Table 3.17 enlists some of the commonly used measurements in house hold system.

Table 3.17: Household system	
1 teaspoonful (tsp)	5 ml
1 dessertspoonful (dssp)	8 ml
1 tablespoonful (tbsp)	15 ml
1 ounce	2 tbsp or 30 ml
1 wine-glass	1 ounce
1 coffee cup	6 fluidounces
1 glass	8 fluidounces
1 quart (qt)	1 liter

Example 5:

A suspension contains 100 mg/5 ml of the drug cefixime. If the patient takes one teaspoonful of the suspension twice daily for ten days, how many grams of the drug does the patient consume?

5 ml × 2 = 10 ml daily

10 × 10 = 100 ml, total dose

0.1 g/5 ml = X g/100

X = 2 g

Answer: 2 g

Example 6:

In calibrating a medicinal dropper, 2 ml of a pediatric solution resulted in 48 drops. If it is desired to administer 0.08 ml of the medication to a baby, approximately how many drops should be given?

By the method of proportion:

48 drops/2 ml = X drops/0.08 ml

X = 1.922 or 2 drops

Answer: 2 drops

Example 7:

If a teaspoonful of paracetamol syrup is to be given three times daily for 5 days, how many fluidounces of the medication should be dispensed?

5 × 3 = 15 ml daily

15 × 5 = 75 ml or 2 1/2 fluidounces

Answer: 2 1/2 fluidounces

Interconversions

In a pharmaceutical or clinical setting, health care professionals encounter more than one system of measurement. Therefore, it becomes necessary to convert all quantities to the same system of measurement. Depending upon the circumstances and the degree of accuracy required, a particular system would be preferred over the others. Some commonly used equivalents in pharmacy practice are shown in Table 3.18.

Example 8:

Tablets are available in strengths of 5 mg and 40 mg of the drug quinapril HCl. Express these strengths in grains.

65 mg/1 grain = 5/X

X = 0.076 or 1/13 grains
65 mg/1 grain = 40/X
X = 0.62 = 1/1.6 = 5/8 grains
Answer: The range of available quinapril tablets in grains is 1/13 to 5/8.

Example 9:

Daypro®, a nonsteroidal anti-inflammatory agent, has a maximum daily dose requirement of 26 mg/kg/day. What is the maximum number of Daypro® 600 mg tablets that can be given to a 127-lb patient?

26 mg/2.2 lb = X mg/127 lb
X = 1501 mg
600 mg/1 tab = 1501 mg/X
X = 2.5 tablets

Table 3.18: Conversion commonly used in practice

Apothecary (fluid)	Metric	Apothecary (mass)	Metric
1 minim (m)	0.062 ml	1 grain (gr)	64.8 mg = 0.064 g
16.23 m	1 ml	1 scruple = 20 gr	1.28 g
1 fluidrachm = 60 m	3.72 ml	1 drachm = 60 gr	3.84 g
1/2 fluidounce = 240 m	14.88 ml	1 ounce = 480 gr	30.72 g
1f = 480 m	29.76 ml	1 pound = 5760 gr	368.64 g
1 pint (O) = 7680 m	476 ml		
1 quart (qt) = 15360 m	952 ml		
1 gallon= 61440 m	3809 ml		

Problems:

1. 1.25 lb   = _____ oz
2. 15,000 gr   = _____ lb
3. 2,188 gr   = _____ oz
4. 116 oz   = _____ lb
5. 5.6 lb   = _____ oz
6. 3.25 lb   = _____ gr
7. 3,500 gr   = _____ oz
8. 4.5 oz   = _____ gr
9. 1.65 lb   = _____ gr
10. 2.8 oz   = _____ gr
11. 800 oz   = _____ lb
12. 218.8 gr   = _____ oz
13. 105,000 gr   = _____ lb

Answers:

(1) 20 (2) 2.143 (3) 5.001 (4) 7.25 (5) 89.6 (6) 22,750 (7) 8 (8) 1,968.75 (9) 11,550 (10) 1,225 (11) 50 (12) 0.5 (13) 15

Problems:

Convert between the AV and metric systems using the ratio and proportion method.

1. 165 lb   = _____ kg
2. 5,000 g   = _____ lb
3. 210 lb   = _____ kg
4. 45 kg   = _____ lb
5. 2.25 lb   = _____ gm
6. 3.5 oz   = _____ gm
7. 2,500 mg   = _____ gr
8. 3.25 kg   = _____ lb
9. 8 oz   = _____ gm
10. 195 lb   = _____ kg
11. 324 mg   = _____ gr
12. 1 g   = _____ gr
13. 400 g   = _____ oz
14. 1 kg   = _____ oz

Answers:

(1) 75 (2) 11.013 (3) 95.455 (4) 99 (5) 1,021.5 (6) 99.225 (7) 38.58 (8) 7.15 (9) 226.8 (10) 88.636 (11) 5 (12) 15.432 (13) 14.109 (14) 35.273

Problems:

Convert the following apothecary problems using the ratio and proportion method.

1. 2,000 gr   = _____ oz (AP)
2. 500 g   = _____ oz (AP)
3. 500 mg   = _____ gr
4. 100 fl oz   = _____ pt
5. 500 fl oz   = _____ gal
6. 4.5 oz (AP) = _____ g
7. 3 gr   = _____ mg
8. 20,000 ml   = _____ gal
9. 3 pt   = _____ ml
10. 119 ml   = _____ fl oz
11. 2.5 gal   = _____ fl oz
12. 5,000 gr   = _____ (AP)
13. 25 pt   = _____ gal
14. 1,500 ml   = _____ pt
15. 6 fl oz   = _____ ml
16. 0.75 gal   = _____ ml
17. 1,000 gr   = _____ oz (AP)
18. 3.25 gal   = _____ pt
19. 350 gr   = _____ mg
20. 2.5 oz (AP) = _____ gr
21. 1.5 tsp   = _____ ml
22. 12.5 ml   = _____ tsp
23. 1.5 fl oz   = _____ ml
24. 500 mg   = _____ gr
25. 500 fl oz   = _____ gal
26. 375 ml   = _____ floz
27. 24 fl oz   = _____ pt
28. 275 gm   = _____ oz (AP)
29. 500 ml   = _____ Tbsp

Answers:

(1) 4.167 (2) 16.077 (3) 7.716 (4) 6.25 (5) 3.906 (6) 139.95 (7) 194.4 (8) 5.284 (9) 1,419 (10) 4.024 (11) 320 (12) 10.417 (13) 3.125 (14) 3.171 (15) 177.42 (16) 2,838.75 (17) 2.083 (18) 26 (19) 22,680 (20) 1,200 (21) 7.5 (22) 2.5 (23) 44.355 (24) 7.716 (25) 3.906 (26) 12.682 (27) 1.5 (28) 8.842 (29) 33.333

ALLIGATION

Alligation is an old and practical method of solving arithmetic problems related to mixtures of ingredients. Alligation is a method used to solve problems that involve mixing two products of different strengths to form a product having a desired intermediate strength. Alligation is used to calculate:

• The amount of diluent that must be added to a given amount of higher strength preparation to make a desired lower strength.

• The amounts of active ingredient which must be added to a given amount of lower strength preparation to make a higher strength.

• The amount of higher and lower strength preparations that must be combined to make a desired amount of an intermediate strength.

There are two types of alligation: **alligation medial**, used to find the quantity of a mixture given the quantities of its ingredients, and a **lligation alternate**, used to find the amount of each ingredient needed to make a mixture of a given quantity.

Alligation Medial

Alligation medial is a technique to determine the resultant concentration when two or more liquids of known concentrations are mixed. As an example, when 5 ml of 2% alcohol is mixed with 10 ml of 4% alcohol, we will know by the alligation medial method that we will obtain 15 ml of 3.33%. Essentially, the resulting strength is the "weighted average" of the percentage strengths of all the individual components used. Thus, the alligation medial is a method where the percentage strength of the mixture may be calculated by dividing the sum of the products of percentage strength of each constituent of the mixture multiplied by its corresponding quantity by the sum of the quantities mixed.

By the method of alligation medial, the percentage strength of a mixture may be calculated using three steps as shown below:

Step 1: Add the quantity of each component used in the mixture.

Step 2: Multiply the quantity of each component used in the mixture by its corresponding percentage strength, and add up the products.

Step 3: Divide the value obtained in Step 2 by the value obtained in Step 1.

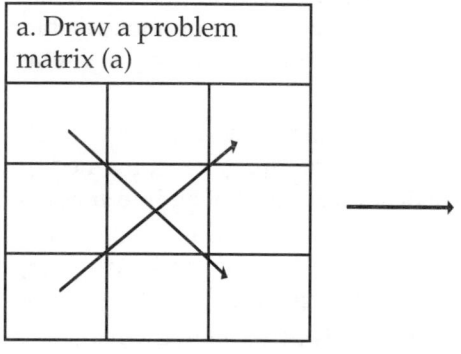

a. Draw a problem matrix (a)

b. Insert quantities as shown

Higher strength		Desired strength – Lower strength
	Desired strength	
Lower strength		Higher strength – Desired strength

The method of alligation medial may be best explained by the following examples.

Example 1:

What is the percentage of alcohol in the following mixture?

Alcohol	2% 5 ml
Alcohol	4% 10 ml

Step 1: 5 ml + 10 ml= 15 ml

Step 2: 5 × 2%	= 10
4 × 10%	= 40
Step 3: 50/15= 3.33%	= 50

Example 2:

What is the percentage of alcohol in the following prescription?

Phenobarbital elixir	60 ml (15% alcohol)
Aromatic elixir	40 ml (22% alcohol)
Terpine hydrate elixir	50 ml (65% alcohol)
Purified water ad	250 ml

Sig. teaspoonful t.i.d.

Step 1: Total quantity 250 ml

Step 2: Quantity of water used in preparation (250 ml - (60 ml + 40 ml + 50 ml) = 100 ml)

$$60 \times 15 = 9.00 \text{ ml}$$
$$40 \times 22 = 8.80 \text{ ml}$$
$$50 \times 65 = 32.50 \text{ ml}$$
$$100 \times 0 = 0 \text{ ml}$$
$$= 50.30 \text{ ml}$$

Step 3: $100 \times 50.30/250 = 20.1\%$

Alligation Alternate

Alligation alternate methods are very commonly employed to obtain a desired concentration of solution by mixing two or more liquids of known concentration. This is a very practical technique to obtain a medicine with prescribed concentration when two or more liquids of other concentrations are already available. By following this technique, we can obtain the prescribed medication without having actually to weigh the raw materials and mix them. Stated in other words, alligation alternate is a mathematical technique to obtain a desired concentration of a mixture when two or more solutions of known concentrations are available. The mixtures can be solutions or ointments. When the alligation alternate technique is used, it is important to remember that the desired solution's concentration has to be somewhere between the available concentrations. It cannot go beyond the boundaries of available concentrations.

The following steps may be used to find the proportional parts of each component to be used in a two-component mixture to obtain the desired strength:

1. Make three columns. In column 1, write the concentrations of the components to be mixed.

c. Subtract along the diagnosis		

2. In column 2, write the desired percentage strength of the mixture to be prepared.

3. In column 3, write the difference in strength by reading diagonally.

4. Find the relative proportions of the components.

d. Read along the horizontals			
Higher strength		Parts of higher	
	Desired strength		
Lower strength		Parts of lower strength	Total of parts of desired strength

Note: The desired strength always goes in the center square of the matrix. The desired strength is the strength of the preparation that you want to make. MAKE is the key word in deciding the desired strength. Usually, the strength on the prescription will be the desired strength.

Example 3:

A pharmacist has a 70% alcoholic elixir and a 20% alcoholic elixir. He needs a 30% alcoholic elixir to use as a vehicle for medications. In what proportion must the 70% elixir and the 20% elixir be combined to make a 30% elixir?

70%		10	10 parts of 70%	
	30%			
20%		40	40 parts of 20%	50 parts of 30%

10 parts of 70% + 40 parts of 20% will produce 50 parts of 30% alcoholic elixer.

Note: This means that if one part of 70% elixir is mixed with four parts of 20% elixir, it will yield five parts of 30% elixir. The arrows in the matrix above have been placed as a reminder that the total number of parts always represent the desired strength.

Example 4:

A hospital pharmacist wants to use three lots of ichthammol ointment containing respectively 50%, 20% and 5 % of ichthammol. In what proportional should they be mixed to prepare a 10% ichthammol ointment?

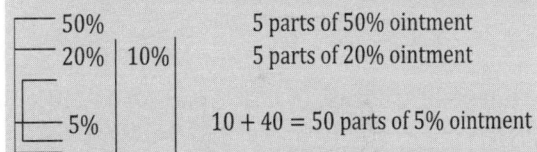

50%		5 parts of 50% ointment
20%	10%	5 parts of 20% ointment
5%		10 + 40 = 50 parts of 5% ointment

1. Write the concentration of the components in desending order on left.

2. Write the desired percentage of the mixture at center.

3. Find the difference of lowest and desired strength and write it against higer strength. Find the difference of higher strength and desired strength and write it against the lowest strength. As demonstrated above.

Check:

$$50 \times 1 = 20$$
$$20 \times 1 = 20$$
$$5 \times 10 = 50$$

Total: $12 = 120$

$$120 + 12 = 10\%$$

Other answers are possible: For the two stronger lots may be mixed in any proportions desired, yielding a mixture that may then be mixed with the weakest lot in a proportion giving the desired strength.

In what proportions may a manufacturing pharmacist mix 20%, 15%, 5% and 3% zinc oxide ointments to produce 10% ointments?

Each of the weaker lots is paired with one of the stronger to give the desired strength and they can be paired in two ways to produce two sets of correct answers.

Answer: Relative amount: 7:5:5:10

20%	7 parts of 20% ointment
15%	5 parts of 15% ointment
10%	
5%	5 parts of 5% ointment
3%	10 parts of 3% ointment

$$20 \times 7 = 140$$
$$15 \times 5 = 75$$
$$5 \times 5 = 25$$
$$3 \times 10 = 30$$

7 parts of 20%, 5 parts of 15%, 5 parts of 5%, 10 parts of 3%, when mixed together will produce 27 parts of 10% ointment.

Problems:

1. How many grams of sulfathiazole should be added to 3400 gm of a 10% sulfathiazole cream to prepare a cream containing 15% sulfathiazole?

2. In what proportions should be 95% alcohol be mixed with 30% alcohol to make 70% alcohol?

3. How many grams of 20% precipitated sulfur ointment and 5% precipitated sulfur ointments should be used to make 908 gm of 8% ointment?

4. How many grams of coal tar solution (LCD) should be added to 2700 gm of an ointment base to prepare a 10% coal tar ointment?

5. How many grams of coal tar should be added to 925 gm of zinc oxide paste to prepare a 6% coal tar ointment?

6. In what proportions should solutions of 12% and 4% be mixed to make a 5% solution?

7. How many grams of petrolatum should be added to 250 gm of 20% sulfathiazole ointment to make a 5% sulfathiazole ointment?

8. How many milliliters of 95% isopropyl alcohol must be mixed with purified water to obtain 7568 ml of 70% isopropyl alcohol?

9. How many milliliters of water should be added to a quart of 75% solution to make 25% solution?

10. How many grams of sulfur should be mixed with some 1:400 sulfur to make 2 ounces (AV) of 1:25 sulfur ointment?

11. How many grams of coal tar should be added to 908 gm of zinc oxide paste to prepare a 9% coal tar ointment?

12. How many milligrams of petrolatum should be added to 340 gm of a 35% sulfur ointment to make 10% sulfur ointment?

13. How many milliliters of water should be added to some 50% isopropyl alcohol to make 2 gallons of 40%?

14. How many milliliters of water should be added to a liter of 1:250 solution to make a 1:4000 solution?

15. How many milliliters of 8% solution can be made, if 1 liter of 30% solution is mixed with water?

16. How many liters of water should be added to a gallon of 80% solution to make 50% solution?

17. How many milliliters of 90% alcohol and 60% alcohol should be added together to make 4 pints of 75% alcohol?

18. How many milliliters of alcohol should be mixed with 1.5 quarts of 30% alcohol to make some 70% alcohol?

19. In what proportions should 90% acetone be mixed with 40% acetone to make 65% acetone?

20. How many milliliters of water should be added to a liter of 75% alcohol to make some 45%?

Answers:

(1) 200 gm (2) 8, 5 (3) 181.6 gm, 726.4gm (4) 300 gm (5) 59.04 gm (6) 1 : 7 (7) 750 gm (8) 5,576.42 ml (9) 1,892 ml (10) 2.13 gm (11) 89.8 gm (12) 850,000 mg (13) 1,513.6 ml (14) 15,000 ml (15) 3,750 ml (16) 2.27 ml (17) 946 ml (18) 1,892 ml (19) 1 : 1 (20) 666.6 ml

SUPPOSITORIES

Suppositories are dosage forms prepared for drug delivery via the rectum. They consist of an active medicament dispersed throughout an inactive base. The bases used in these products can be broadly classified into two groups: Fatty bases, these may be of natural origin, such as theobroma oil (cocoa butter), or synthetic fats such as Witepsol and hydrophilic bases, the most commonly used hydrophilic base is composed of a solid glycerol/gelatin mixture.

Displacement Value (DV)

Suppositories are prepared by dissolving or dispersing an active medicament in a molten base and pouring the mixture into a suppository mould. Suppository moulds are normally available in 1 g, 2 g and 4 g sizes – the approximate weights of theobroma oil suppositories that are produced from them – although the volume of the suppository mould will be constant. However, because the density of the medicament may vary considerably from that of the base, the weight of the base required to make a suppository will vary depending on the medicament used. For example, 2 g of a medicament with twice the density of theobroma oil would occupy approximately the same volume as 1 g of the suppository base. The displacement values (DVs) of medica-

ments are required when calculating the weight of suppository base required to prepare medicated suppositories. The displacement value of a medicament is the number of parts, by weight, of a medicament that will displace one part of suppository base (normally theobroma oil). Displacement values of some important medicaments in reference to cocoa butter are summarized in Table 3.19

Importance of Displacement Value

Suppositories are prepared in the mould by incorporating medicament in suppository base. Suppository moulds are normally available in 1 g, 2 g and 4 g capacity. Here capacity means equal amount of cocoa butter suppositories that can be produced by them with constant volume of the suppository mould. During preparation, we have to add medicament in the suppositories, as the volume of mould is fixed, for addition of medicament into mould we have to displace some amount of base from base required for plain suppositories. However, because the density of medicament may vary considerably from that of base, the weight of base required to make a suppository will vary depending on the medicament used. The displacement value of a medicament is required during the calculation of weight of suppository base required to prepare medicated suppositories.

Calculation of Displacement Value

Displacement value can be calculated by following steps:

i. Calculate the weight of base required for plain suppositories = capacity of mould × total number of suppositories required = A

ii. Calculate the total weight of medicament required = weight of medicament required for one suppository × total no of suppositories = B

iii. Calculate the weight of base used in medicated suppositories = total weight of suppositories–amount of medicament used = C

iv. Calculate weight of base displaced by medicament = total weight of base required for plain suppositories – actual base used = A – C = D

v. Displacement value of medicament = total weight of medicament required/ amount of base displaced = (A – C)/B

The following examples will illustrate the displacement value calculations.

Example 1:

If a prescription requires 400 mg of bismuth subgallate per suppository weighing two grams, what would be the displacement value, if it is known that six suppositories with required bismuth subgallate weigh 13.6 g?

Solution:

Capacity of mould = 2 gm

Theoretical weight of six cocoa butter suppositories without bismuth subgallate = 12 g

Given weight of six cocoa butter suppositories with bismuth subgallate = 13.6 g

Amount of bismuth subgallate in the suppositories = 0.4 × 6 = 2.4 g

Amount of cocoa butter in the bismuth subgallate suppositories = 13.6 – 2.4 = 11.2 g

Cocoa butter displaced by 2.4 g of bismuth subgallate = 12 – 11.2 = 0.8

The displacement value of bismuth subgallate is 2.4/0.8 = 3

Answer: DV = 3

Example 2:

If 12 cocoa butter suppositories containing 40% zinc oxide weigh 17.6 grams, what is the displacement value of zinc oxide? Assume that the suppositories are made in a 1-g mould.

Solution:

Given weight of 12 suppositories with zinc oxide = 17.6 grams

Weight of zinc oxide in the suppositories = (40/100) × 17.6 = 7.04 g

Weight of cocoa butter in the suppositories = (60/100) × 17.6 = 10.56 g

Theoretical weight of 12 suppositories without zinc oxide = 12 g

Cocoa butter displaced by 7.04 g of zinc oxide = 12 – 10.56 = 1.44

Displacement value of zinc oxide = (7.04/1.44) = 4.89 = approx. 5

Answer: DV = Approx. 5

Example 3:

From the information provided below, find the displacement value of phenobarbital sodium. six phenobarbital sodium suppositories, each containing 60 mg of drug, weigh 12 g.

Solution:

The capacity of suppository mould = 2 g.

Given weight of six suppositories with phenobarbital sodium = 12 g

Weight of phenobarbital sodium in six suppositories = 60 mg × 6 = 360 mg or 0.36 g

Weight of cocoa butter in the suppositories = 12 – 0.36 = 11.64 g

Theoretical weight of six suppositories without phenobarbital sodium = 12 g

Cocoa butter displaced by 0.36 g of phenobarbital sodium = 12 – 11.64 = 0.36 g

Displacement value of phenobarbital sodium = (0.36/0.36) = 1

Answer: DV = 1

Calculation of suppository base by using DV

When doctor prescribe any medicament in suppository dosage form, pharmacist have to calculate the amount of base required to dispense the same. Amount of base can be calculated, if the DV of prescribed medicament is known.

i. Calculate the total weight of medicament required = weight of medicament for one suppository × total number of suppositories.

ii. Calculate the weight of base required for plain suppositories = capacity of mould × total number of suppositories required = A

iii. From DV, calculate weight of base displaced by medicament = total weight of medicament required/DV of medicament = B

iv. Calculate the weight of base required for medicated suppositories = weight of base

Table 3.19: Displacement values of certain drugs in suppositories

Drug	Displacement value
Aminophylline	1.5
Aminopyrine	1.3
Aspirin	1.1
Belladonna extract	1.2
Bismuth subgallate	3.0
Bismuth subnitrate	6.0
Boric acid	1.5
Chloral hydrate	1.5
Cocaine hydrochloride	1.5
Codeine phosphate	1.1
Digitalis leaf	1.6
Dimenhydrinate	1.3
Diphenhydramine HCL	1.3
Gallic acid	2.0
Hamamelis dry extract	1.5
Hydrocortisone	1.5
Hydrocortisone acetate	1.5
Ichthammol	1.0
Menthol	0.7
Morphine hydrochloride	1.5
Peru balsam	1.0
Phenobarbital sodium	1.2
Potassium bromide	2.2
Quinidine HCL	3.0
Resorcinol	1.0
Salicylic acid	1.3
Secobarbital sodium	1.2
Tannic acid	1.6
Zinc oxide	5.0
Zinc sulfate	2.8

required for plain suppositories – weight of base displaced by medicament = DV

Example 4:

Calculate the quantity required to make 10 cocoa butter suppositories each containing 400 mg of zinc oxide. (DV = 4.7, capacity of mould = 2 gm)

Solution:

Total weight of medicament required = weight of medicament for one suppository × total number of suppositories = 400 mg × 10 = 4000 mg = 4 g

Weight of base required for plain suppositories = capacity of mould × total number of suppositories required = 2 × 10 = 20 gm

Displacement value of zinc oxide is 4.7 means 4.7 gm of zinc oxide can displace 1 gm of base

Weight of base displaced by 4 gm of medicament = total weight of medicament required / DV of medicament = 4/4.7 = 0.85 gm of base

Weight of base required for medicated suppositories = weight of base required for plain suppositories – weight of base displaced by 4 gm of medicament = 20 gm – 0.85 gm = 19.15 gm

Answer: Base required = 19.15 gm

Medicament required = 4 gm

Example 5:

Calculate the quantities required to make 10 theobroma oil suppositories (2 g mould) each containing 400 mg of zinc oxide (displacement value = 4.7)

Solution:

1. Calculate the total weight of zinc oxide required.

2. Calculate what weight of base would be required to prepare 10 unmedicated suppositories.

3. Determine what weight of base would be displaced by the medicament.

4. Calculate, therefore, the weight of base required to prepare the medicated suppositories.

   Total weight of zinc oxide required = 400 mg × 10 = 4 g

Weight of base required for unmedicated suppositories = 2 g × 10 = 20 g

As the displacement value of zinc oxide = 4.7

This means that 4.7 g of zinc oxide would displace 1 g of theobroma oil.

1 g of zinc oxide would displace 1 ÷ 4.7 g of theobroma oil.

So, 4 g of zinc oxide will displace (4 × 1) ÷ 4.7 g of theobroma oil = 0.85 g

Therefore, the weight of base required to make medicated suppositories = 20 – 0.85 g = 19.15 g

Answer: 19.15 grams

Example 6:

What quantities are required to prepare eight theobroma oil suppositories, in a 4 g mould, containing 1% w/w lignocaine hydrochloride?

Solution:

1. Calculate the total weight of the medicated suppositories.

2. Calculate, therefore, the weight of the drug required (1% of the total weight).

3. Subtract the weight of the drug from the total weight of the suppositories to and the weight of the base required.

Total weight of the suppositories = 32 g

Weight of drug required (–1% w/w) = (32 × 1) ÷ 100 g = 0.32 g

Therefore, weight of base required = 32 g – 0.32 g = 31.68 g

Answer: 31.68 grams

Again, if a glycerogelatin base is used, the appropriate correction factor must be used as a 1 g mould for a theobroma oil suppository will actually hold 1.2 g of glycerogelatin base.

Effect of density of base

Density of base is the main factor for calculation of base for preparation of suppositories. Capacity of mould is considered with reference to theobroma oil, in case of other bases during calculation we have to multiply the density factor with capacity of mould. As in case of glycerogelatin base, it is 1.2 times denser than that of theobroma oil means mould with 1 gm capacity can hold 1.2 gm of glycerogelatin base in comparison to theobroma oil. This factor must be taken into account in displacement value calculation or weight of base calculation.

Example 7:

Calculate the quantity required to make six glycerogelatin suppositories each containing 100 mg aminophylline. (DV = 1.3, capacity of mould = 2 gm)

Solution:

Total weight of aminophylline required = weight of medicament for one suppository × total number of suppositories = 100 mg × 6 = 600 mg

Weight of base required for plain suppositories = capacity of mould × total number of suppositories required × density factor = 2 × 6 × 1.2 = 13.2 gm

Displacement value of aminophylline is 1.3 means 1.3 gm of aminophylline can displace 1 gm of theobroma oil base

Weight of base displaced by 4 gm of medicament = total weight of medicament required / DV of medicament = 4/4.7 = 0.85 gm of base

Weight of base required for medicated suppositories = weight of base required for plain suppositories – weight of base displaced by 4 gm of medicament = 20 gm – 0.85 gm = 19.15 gm

Answer: Base required = 19.15 gm

Medicament required = 4.0 gm

Example 8:

Calculate the quantities required to make six glycerogelatin suppositories (4 g mould), each containing 100 mg aminophylline (displacement value = 1.3)

Solution:

1. Calculate the total weight of aminophylline required.

2. Calculate what weight of glycerogelatin base would be required to prepare 10 unmedicated suppositories.

3. Determine what weight of base would be displaced by the medicament.

4. Calculate, therefore, the weight of base required to prepare the medicated suppositories.

Total weight of aminophylline required = 100 mg × 6 = 600 mg or 0.6 g

Weight of base required for unmedicated suppositories = 4 g × 6 × 1.2 (to take account of the greater density of this base) = 28.8 g

As the displacement value of aminophylline = 1.3

This means that 1.3 g of aminophylline displaces 1 g of theobroma oil

So, 1 g of aminophylline displaces 1 ÷ 1.3 g of theobroma oil

0.6 g of aminophylline displace (1 × 0.6) ÷ 1.3 g of theobroma oil = 0.46 g of theobroma oil

This means that the aminophylline would displace 0.46 g × 1.2 of the glycerogelatin base = 0.55 g

Therefore, the weight of base required to make medicated suppositories = 28.8 g – 0.55 g = 28.25 g

Answer: 28.25 grams

Medicaments included as a percentage w/w. If a medicament is present in a suppository as a percentage w/w, then its displacement value is not required when calculating the respective amounts of medicament and base required to prepare the suppository.

Capsule filling-powder displacement

Example 9:

A pharmacist receives a prescription for forty-eight 15 mg piroxicam capsules. A #1 capsule filled with piroxicam weighs 245 mg tare weight; a capsule filled with lactose weighs 180 mg tare weight. How much piroxicam and lactose are required for the prescription? Prepare sufficient powder for 50 capsules (2 extra).

50 × 15 = 750 mg piroxicam

15 / 245 = x / 180

x = 11 mg

15 mg piroxicam occupies a similar volume as does 11 mg lactose

180 mg – 11 mg = 169 mg lactose/capsule

169 × 50 = 8.45 g lactose required

Problems:

1. How would you prepare 10 theobroma oil suppositories (1 g mould) containing 2.5% w/w bismuth subgallate?

2. How would you prepare six theobroma oil suppositories (2 g mould) containing 10% w/w zinc oxide?

3. Six theobroma oil suppositories (2 g), each containing 125 mg of paracetamol, are to be prepared. The displacement value of paracetamol is 1.5. What quantities of base and medicament are required?

4. You are asked to prepare 11 theobroma oil suppositories (2 g mould) each containing 100 mg of aspirin (DV = 1.1). What weights of base and medicament are required?

5. Prepare 10 theobroma oil suppositories, each containing 50 mg of bismuth subgallate (DV = 2.5). If a 2 g mould is used, what quantities of base and medicament are required?

6. A prescriber requests on glycerogelatin suppositories be made, containing 1% w/w hydrocortisone acetate. If a 4 g mould is used, what quantities of base and medicament are needed?

7. Prepare eight glycerogelatin suppositories (in a 2 g mould) each containing 20 mg of morphine hydrochloride (DV = 1.6).

8. Ten glycerogelatin suppositories, each containing 30 mg phenobarbitone sodium (DV = 1.2), are to be prepared using a 1 g mould. What quantities of base and medicament are required?

9. Prepare 12 glycerogelatin suppositories, in a 2 g mould, each containing 50 mg of diphenhydramine hydrochloride (DV = 1.2).

10. You are required to prepare 10 theobroma oil suppositories (2 g). Each suppository must contain 50 mg of bismuth subgallate (DV = 2.5) and 10 mg of hydrocortisone acetate (DV = 1.5). Calculate the weight of each medicament and of theobroma oil required to prepare the suppositories.

Answers:

(1) 9.75 gm (2) 10.8 gm (3) 11.5 gm (4) 21 gm (5) 19.8 gm (6) 23.72 gm (7) 19.08 gm (8) 11.7 gm (9) 21.6 gm (10) 19.8 gm base and 0.5 gm drug.

PROOF SPIRIT

Alcoholic proof is a measure of how much alcohol (i.e. ethanol) is contained in an alcoholic beverage. The measure is commonly used in the United States, where it is defined as twice the percentage of alcohol by volume. The measurement of alcohol content and the statement of this content on liquor bottle labels is regulated by law. The purposes of such regulations are to tax alcohol and to provide pertinent information to the consumer.

The Customs and Excise Act of 1952 defined spirits of proof strength as follows:

Proof spirit meant that the spirit at a temperature of 51°F weighed exactly twelve-thirteenths of a volume of distilled water equal to the volume of the spirit. It was, in fact, a mixture of spirit and water of a strength of 57.1% of spirit by volume and 42.9% of water.

The strength of alcohol is expressed in terms of proof spirit and proof strength. In India and in Great Britain, 57.15% v/v is considered as 100 proof spirit. In United States, 50% v/v alcohol is considered as 100 proof spirit. For calculation purpose, proof spirit can be expressed as follows:

As per Indian norms

100 proof spirit = 57.1% v/v alcohol

$$1 \text{ proof spirit} = \frac{57.1}{100} \text{ strength of alcohol}$$

$$x \text{ proof spirit} = \frac{57.1}{100} \times x \text{ strength of alcohol}$$

As per United States of America's norms

100 proof spirit = 50.0% v/v alcohol

50.0% v/v alcohol = 100 proof spirit

$$1 \% \text{ v/v alcohol} = \frac{100}{50} = 2 \text{ proof spirit}$$

$x \%$ v/v alcohol = $2 x$ proof spirit

Example 1:

According to USA norms calculate the proof spirit of preparation containing 45% v/v alcohol.

As we know as per USA's norms

100 proof spirit = 50.0% v/v alcohol

Proof spirit = (50.0/100) * % strength of alcohol = 2 * % strength of alcohol

So for 45% v/v alcohol, proof spirit = 2 * 45% strength of alcohol = 90 proof spirit

Answer = 90 proof spirit

Example 2:

According to Indian norms, convert 123 proof spirit into % v/v alcohol.

As per Indian norms

100 proof spirit = 57.1% v/v alcohol

Proof spirit = 1.753* % strength of alcohol

% strength of alcohol = proof spirit /1.753

So for 123 proof spirit

% strength of alcohol = 123 /1.753 = 70.16% v/v alcohol.

Answer: 70.16% v/v alcohol.

Example 3:

Convert 55% v/v alcohol and 65% v/v alcohol into proof spirit.

Proof spirit = 2 * % strength of alcohol

So for 55% v/v alcohol, proof spirit = 2 * 55% strength of alcohol = 110 proof spirit

For 65% v/v alcohol, proof spirit = 2 * 65% strength of alcohol = 130 proof spirit

As per Indian norms for 55% v/v alcohol, proof spirit = 1.753 * 55% strength of alcohol = 96.45 proof spirit

For 65% v/v alcohol, proof spirit = 1.753 * 65% strength of alcohol = 113.94 proof spirit

Answer: According to USA norms, 110 and 130 proof spirit. According to Indian norms, 96.45 and 113.94 proof spirit.

PROOF STRENGTH

100 proof indicates 50% v/v or 57.15% v/v alcohol. Proof strength can be expressed by over proof (o/p) and under proof (u/p). Over proof indicates the % strength of alcohol above 50% v/v or 57.15% v/v alcohol and under proof (u/p) indicates the % strength of alcohol below 50% v/v or 57.15% v/v alcohol. Proof strength is represented in degrees.

Calculation of proof strength:

Proof strength = proof spirit – 100

If the answer is positive then it will be called over proof.

If the answer is negative then it will be called as under spirit.

Example 1:

Calculate proof strength of 135 and 95 proof spirit.

Proof strength = proof spirit – 100
Proof strength = 135 – 100 = 35° o/p
Proof strength = 95 – 100 = -5.0 = 5.0u/p
Answer: 35°o/p and 5.0u/p

Example 2:

Calculate proof strength of 90%v/v alcohol.

As 57.1% v/v alcohol = 100 proof spirit
1% v/v alcohol = 100/57.1 proof spirit
So 90% v/v alcohol = 100/57.1 * 90 = 157.61 proof spirit
Since Proof strength = proof spirit – 100
= 157.61 – 100 = 57.61 over proof spirit
= 57.610 o/p

Example 3:

Calculate the percentage strength corresponding to 470 o/p.

First calculate proof spirit by using formula
Proof spirit = proof strength + 100 (if it is o/p)
Proof spirit = 100 – proof strength (if it is u/p)
Given = 470 o/p.
Proof spirit = proof strength + 100 (if it is o/p)
Proof spirit = 47 + 100 (as it is o/p)
$$= 147$$
We know that:
Proof spirit = % strength * 1.753
% strength = proof spirit/1.753
$$= 147/1.753$$
$$= 83.85\% \text{ strength}$$
Answer: 83.85% strength

Problems:

1. Find out the proof spirit of an elixir containing 30% v/v alcohol?

2. Find out the proof spirit of an alcoholic product containing 60% v/v alcohol sold in France?

3. Find out the proof spirit of a beverage containing 50% v/v alcohol?

4. How many proof gallons are in 10 gallons of alcoholic solution containing 40% v/v alcohol?

5. How much taxable alcohol would be in 2 gallons of 50 proof alcohol?

6. How many proof gallons are there in 1 qt of a preparation that is labeled 75% v/v alcohol?

7. How many proof gallons are there in a pint of an elixir that contains 14% alcohol?

8. How much diluted alcohol USP can be made from 1 gal of 1190 proof alcohol?

Answers:

(1) 52.59 proof spirit (2) 120 proof spirit (3) 100 proof spirit (4) 8 proof gallons (5) 1 proof gallon (6) 0.375 proof gallon (7) 0.035 proof gallon (8) 1.94 gallon

TONICITY

Tonicity is a measure of the osmotic pressure of two solutions separated by a semipermeable membrane. It is commonly used when describing the response of cells immersed in an external solution. Like osmotic pressure, tonicity is influenced only by solutes that cannot cross the membrane, as only these exert an osmotic pressure. Solutes able to freely cross the membrane do not affect tonicity because they will always be in equal concentrations on both sides of the membrane.

There are three classifications of tonicity; these are hypertonic, hypotonic, and isotonic.

Hypertonicity

A hypertonic solution contains a greater concentration of impermeable solutes than the solution on the other side of the membrane. If a cell is placed in a hypertonic solution, there will be a net movement of water out of the cell until the concentration of impermeable solutes in the cell equals that of the hypertonic solution. Finally the cell will shrink.

Hypotonicity

A hypotonic solution contains a smaller concentration of impermeable solutes than the solution on the other side of the membrane. If a cell is placed in a hypotonic solution, there will be a net movement of water into the cell until the concentration of impermeable solutes in the cell equals that of the hypotonic solution. Finally, the cell will swell.

Isotonicity

A condition or property of a solution in which its solute concentration is the same as the solute concentration of another solution with which it is compared. An isotonic solution contains an equal concentration of impermeable solutes as the solution on the other side of the membrane. Ophthalmic, nasal, and parenteral solutions should be isotonic.

There are a number of simple methods developed to adjust tonicity of formulation in pharmacy. The methods of adjusting tonicity could be classified into two types.

In class I methods, some inert substances such as sodium chloride or dextrose are added to the solution to lower its freezing point to match that of blood ($-0.52°C$), i.e. made isotonic by the addition of inert excipient.

In class II methods, a calculated quantity of water is added to the total solute content (drug) of the prescription to make it isotonic, which is then diluted with sufficient isotonic diluting solution to bring it to the final volume These methods are explained below, followed by a simple example illustrating the method.

Freezing-point depression method (cryoscopic method)

Isotonicity adjustments can also be made by the freezing point depression method. The normal freezing (or melting) point of a pure compound is the temperature at which the solid and the liquid phases are in equilibrium at a pressure of 1 atm. The freezing point of a pure compound is described by a unique point in the phase diagram of the compound, and, at that point, the solid and liquid phases are in equilibrium, and the vapor pressure of the liquid phase coincides with the vapor pressure of the pure solid phase.

Pure water has a freezing point of 0°C. When solutes are added to water, its freezing point is lowered. The freezing point depression (or lowering) of a solvent is dependent only on the number of particles in the solution. Therefore, this is a colligative property. Blood plasma has a freezing point of $-0.52°C$. If freezing point depression value of a chemical in certain concentration is known, one can calculate the concentration of that chemical required for isotonicity by setting a proportion as follows:
(Known percentage conc./freezing point depression of the chemical at that concentration) $\times$ (D/0.52°C)

where D = percentage concentration of the chemical required to be isotonic with blood plasma.

Since freezing point depression of a series of compounds at 1% concentration is readily available from standard references, the above expression can be represented as:

$$\frac{1\% \text{ chemical}}{F\Delta T_f \text{ of the chemical}} = \frac{D}{\Delta T_f \text{ of the blood plasma } 0.52°C}$$

where D= percentage concentration of the chemical required to be isotonic with blood plasma or tears.

The following formula is used for the calculation of the quantity of a substance required to make solution isotonic with physiological fluids % w/v of adjusting substance

$$= \frac{0.52 - a}{b}$$

a– Depression in freezing point due to unadjusted solution.

b– Depression in freezing point of 1% adjusting solution.

Example 1:

What concentration of quinine hydrochloride will give isotonic solution with blood plasma? (Freezing point of 1% solution of quinine hydrochloride 0.077°C)

Since weight of substance to be dissolved

= (0.52- depression of freezing point due to ingredient already present)

Depression of freezing point due to ingredient already present = 0.00

Freezing point 1% w/v solution of adjusting substance = 0.077

Because no ingredient is present in the solution. Weight of substance to be dissolved = (0.52-0.00)/0.077 = 6.75% w/v

Answer: 6.75% w/v of Quinine hydrochloride is required.

Sodium chloride equivalents of drug substances

Class I: By definition, the sodium chloride equivalent of a chemical is the amount of sodium chloride (in grams or grains) that has the same osmotic pressure as that of 1 gram of the chemical. The sodium chloride equivalents are symbolized by the letter E. The E value can be found in standard tables that can be found in many pharmaceutics and calculation texts. The E value can also be calculated, if molecular weight and dissociation factor values are known, by the following equation:

$$E = \frac{M.W. \text{ of NaCl}}{i \text{ value of NaCl}} = \frac{i \text{ value of the chemical}}{M.W. \text{ of the chemical}}$$

Where E (sodium chloride equivalents); i value (freezing-point depression of a solution of a particular type of electrolyte at a molar concentration that is isotonic with blood); MW (molecular weight).

Example 2:

Calculate the sodium chloride equivalent of a 1% homatropine hydrobromide. Homatropine hydrobromide has a molecular weight of 358 and having i value of 1.8.

$$E = \frac{M.W. \text{ of NaCl}}{i \text{ value of NaCl}} =$$

$$= \frac{i \text{ value of homatropine hydrobromide}}{M.W. \text{ of homatropine hydrobromide}}$$

$$E = \frac{58.5}{1.8} \times \frac{1.8}{358} = \frac{105.3}{644.4}$$

= 0.16, i.e., 1 gm of homatropin hydrobromide is equivalent to 0.16 gm of NaCl.

Example 3:

Calculate the sodium chloride equivalent of a 1% silver nitrate. Silver nitrate has a molecular weight of 170 and i of 1.8.

$$E = \frac{M.W. \text{ of NaCl}}{i \text{ value of NaCl}}$$

$$= \frac{i \text{ value of silver nitrate}}{M.W. \text{ of silver nitrate}}$$

$$E = (58.5/1.8) \times (1.8/170)$$

= 0.34, i.e., 1 gm of silver nitrate is equivalent to 0.34 gm of NaCl.

Class II: The class II methods involve the calculation of a quantity of water needed to make an isotonic solution for a given amount of drug, followed by dilution with an isotonic solution to make up the volume. These methods were developed to enable pharmacists to prepare parenteral and ophthalmic formulations with simplicity and ease.

The White-Vincent method

In this method, the weight of the drug (w) is first multiplied by its sodium chloride equivalent (E) to obtain the quantity of sodium chloride osmotically equivalent to drug. Because 0.9 g of sodium chloride dissolved in 100 ml results in an isotonic solution, the volume of isotonic solution that can be prepared from weight per gram of drug is given by the following equation:

$$V = wE \times 100/\ 0.9 = 111.1wE$$

Thus, dissolving weight per gram of drug in V ml of water will result in an isotonic solution that can be further diluted with isotonic solutions such as 0.9% sodium chloride or isotonic dextrose solution to make up the volume.

Example 4:

Prepare 100 ml of 2% physostigmine salicylate solution isotonic with blood. Where E of physostigmine salicylate = 0.16.

The volume of water needed to prepare isotonic solution,

$V = 2g \times 0.16 \times 111.1$ ml/g = 35.55 ml.

This solution can be diluted with 64.45 ml of any isotonic diluting solution to obtain 100 ml of 2% isotonic physostigmine salicylate solution. To verify the results, assume that to dilute the above solution with 64.45 ml of isotonic sodium chloride solution, the equivalent amount of sodium chloride added is 0.58 g, which matches with results obtained using the class I methods.

The Sprowls method

In the early days of pharmacy practice, many prescriptions were written to prepare one fluid ounce of a 1% drug solution, thus, the amount of drug (w=0.3 g) and the final volume were fixed (one fluid ounce or 30 ml). Sprowls, recognizing this fact, suggested a modification of the White-Vincent method to further simplify the calculations for the practicing pharmacist. In this method, the amount of drug is fixed at 0.3 g (30 ml of 1% solution), and the volume of water required to prepare the isotonic solution is calculated using equation as described in White-Vincent method. The pharmacist then makes up the volume of the preparation to 30 ml with an isotonic diluting solution to fill the prescription.

Example 5:

Prepare one fluid ounce of 1% physostigmine salicylate solution where 5.3 ml of water is required for 0.3 g of physostigmine salicylate to prepare an isotonic solution.

After the preparation of 5.3 ml solution (using White-Vincent method), it can be diluted with any isotonic diluting solution to make up the volume to one fluid ounce. If one needed to prepare 100 ml of a 1% solution, the volume of water (V) should be multiplied by 3.33 to obtain the amount of water necessary to make it isotonic.

Problems:

1. Find out the proportion of procaine hydrochloride which will yield a solution iso-osmotic with blood plasma. Freezing point of a 1% w/v solution of procaine hydrochloride is –0.122°C.

2. Find out the concentration of sodium chloride required to make a 1% solution of boric acid, iso-osmotic with blood plasma. The freezing point of 1% w/v solution of boric acid is –0.288°C. The freezing point of 1% w/v solution of sodium chloride is –0.576°C.

3. Find out the concentration of sodium chloride required to make a 1.5% solution of cocaine hydrochloride iso-osmotic with blood plasma. The freezing point of 1%

w/v solution of cocaine hydrochloride is –0.09°C. The freezing point of 1% w/v solution of sodium chloride is –0.576°C.

4. Find the concentration of sodium chloride required to make 50 ml of isotonic solution containing 0.5% ephedrine hydrochloride and 0.5% chlorobutol. The freezing point of 1% w/v solution of epinephrine hydrochloride is –0.165°C. The freezing point of 1% w/v solution of chlorobutol is –0.138°C.

5. Find out the proportion of dextrose needed to form a solution iso-osmotic with blood plasma.

Answers:
(1) 4.26% w/v (2) 0.402% w/v (3) 0.668% w/v (4) 0.322 g (5) 5.4 g/100 ml

DOSAGE CALCULATIONS BASED ON AGE

Age of a patient is one of the most important considerations for drug dosage modifications. As explained in the previous section, some of the important pharmacokinetic parameters change with age. In general, the drug elimination (which is comprised of drug metabolism and excretion) is less functional in newborns, and improves with age as they grow into healthy adult individuals. Finally, as they grow further to an age of 65 or above, the elimination declines. A few general equations for the dosage calculations based on age are provided below. However, the use of these equations is rapidly declining. It is important to remember that age is not the only valid criterion for dose modifications. Therefore, after adjusting the dose with one of the formulae given below, it is important to monitor the response in the patient for some more time. The guidelines provided by the manufacturers as usual pediatric dose in the drug inserts and pharmaceutical literature is valuable for drug dosage calculations in children.

Young's equation: (preferably from 1 to 12 years of age) Dose of child = (Age of child in years)/(Age in child years + 12) × Adult dose

Cowling's equation: Dose of child = Age of child in years at next birthday/ 24 × Adult dose

Fried's equation: (preferably from birth to one year of age)

$$\frac{\text{Age in months}}{150} \times \text{Adults dose} = \text{Approx. child dose}$$

Example 1:

An adult dose of drug is 500 mg, what is the dose for a 2-year-old child ? (Young rule)

According to Young's formula
Age in year/ Age + 12 × adult dose
= 2/14 × 500 mg
= 71.42 mg of drug.

Example 2:

If therapeutic dose of drug is 10 mg/kg/ day, how many 250 mg/100 cc ready-infusion bags should be filled? Patient's weight is 156 lb.

Patient weight in kg is 156 lb/2.2 = 70.9 kg. The therapeutic dose of the drug is 10 mg/kg, so patient needs = 70.9 × 10 = 709 mg of the drug.

Therefore the correct answer should be "a" 3-bags.

Example 3:

Calculate the dose of Valium® of a 13-month-old child by the Young's method, if the adult dose is 10 mg. Valium® is available as a 5 mg/5 ml oral solution. How would you administer this medication to the child?

Dose of child = (Age in years)/(Age in years + 12) × Adult dose
Dose of child = [(13/12)]/ [(13/12) + 12] × 10 mg
Dose of child = 0.83 mg
5 mg/5 ml = 0.83 mg in 0.83 ml

Answer: Therefore a medicinal dropper will be calibrated to determine the number of drops which would constitute 0.83 ml and the drug will be administered.

Example 4:

Product information on Lorabid® shows that its usual adult dose is 200– 400 mg q12h. What would be the range of this medication for a patient born on February 9, 1993. How would

you administer the drug from one of the available Lorabid® medications? Assume that the prescription was written on May 1996.

The patient is a child and would be four years old on the following birthday.

Therefore Cowling's equation will be used as follows:

Dose of child = Age in years at next birthday /24 × Adult dose

Dose of child =4 years/24 × 200

Dose of child = 33.33 mg for the lower drug range

Answer: Range of drug for the patient = 33.33 to 66.67 mg

The drug Lorabid® is available as 100 mg/5 ml suspension besides other strengths.

100 mg/5 cc = 33.33 mg/X

Answer: The volume of Lorabid® 100 mg/5 ml required would be 1.67 to 3.34 cc

DOSAGE CALCULATIONS BASED ON BODY WEIGHT

Dose adjustments based on weight are common in children and also in obese patients. From the previous discussion, it is known that the dosing regimen may have to be altered, if the volume of distribution changes. The volume of distribution is a function of the total body water and the extracellular fluids which in turn are related to the body weight. Therefore, the volume of distribution may change with the change in body weight. In the case of an obese patient, the proportion of body fat is greater and the ratio of body water and lean body weight to total body weight is smaller. The percent of body fat and lean body weight can be estimated by the equations,

% Fat = 90 – 2 (Height in inches – Girth in inches at umbilical level at exhalation)

Lean body weight (males) = 50 + 2.3 kg per inch over 5′

Lean body weight (females) = 45.5 + 2.3 kg per inch over 5′

When the percent fat is greater, the extracellular fluid is less. Therefore, there is less distribution of polar drugs. As a result, the plasma concentration of polar drugs will be higher and there may be a need to lower the dose of such drugs. In the case of nonpolar or lipid soluble drugs, their distribution in cellular tissues will be more and there may be a need to increase the dose of such drugs. For this reason, extreme care is needed for changes in the dosing regimen of obese patients. Often, the dosing regimens based simply on milligrams of drug per kilogram of body weight without due consideration of percent fats may lead to erroneous results.

A well-known equation for the dosage calculation based on body weight is the Clarke's equation. The use of this equation is also declining.

Clarke's Equation

Dose of the child = [Weight in pounds × Adult dose]/ [150 lb (average weight of an adult)]

The milligram per kilogram doses of many drugs is greater for children than the adults. For example, the usual dose of digoxin for children in the age group of 2 to 12 is 10 to 15 g per kilogram of body weight per day. For adults, the dose of digoxin is 4 to 5 g per kilogram per day. These doses have shown to provide an average digoxin plasma concentration of 1 to 1.5 ng/ml. The larger mg/kg doses for children are required because of a higher percentage of total body water and extracellular fluid in children as compared to adults. At birth, newborns have approximately 78% body water. In adults, the total body water decreases to about 60%. Because of the higher total body water and the extracellular fluid content, there is more distribution of digoxin, and less appearance of drug in the plasma.

Example 1:

If an adult dose of drug is 750 mg, what is the dose for child weighing 20 lb? According to Clarke's formula

= weight (in lb)/150 × adult dose

= 20/150 × 750 mg = 100 mg dose

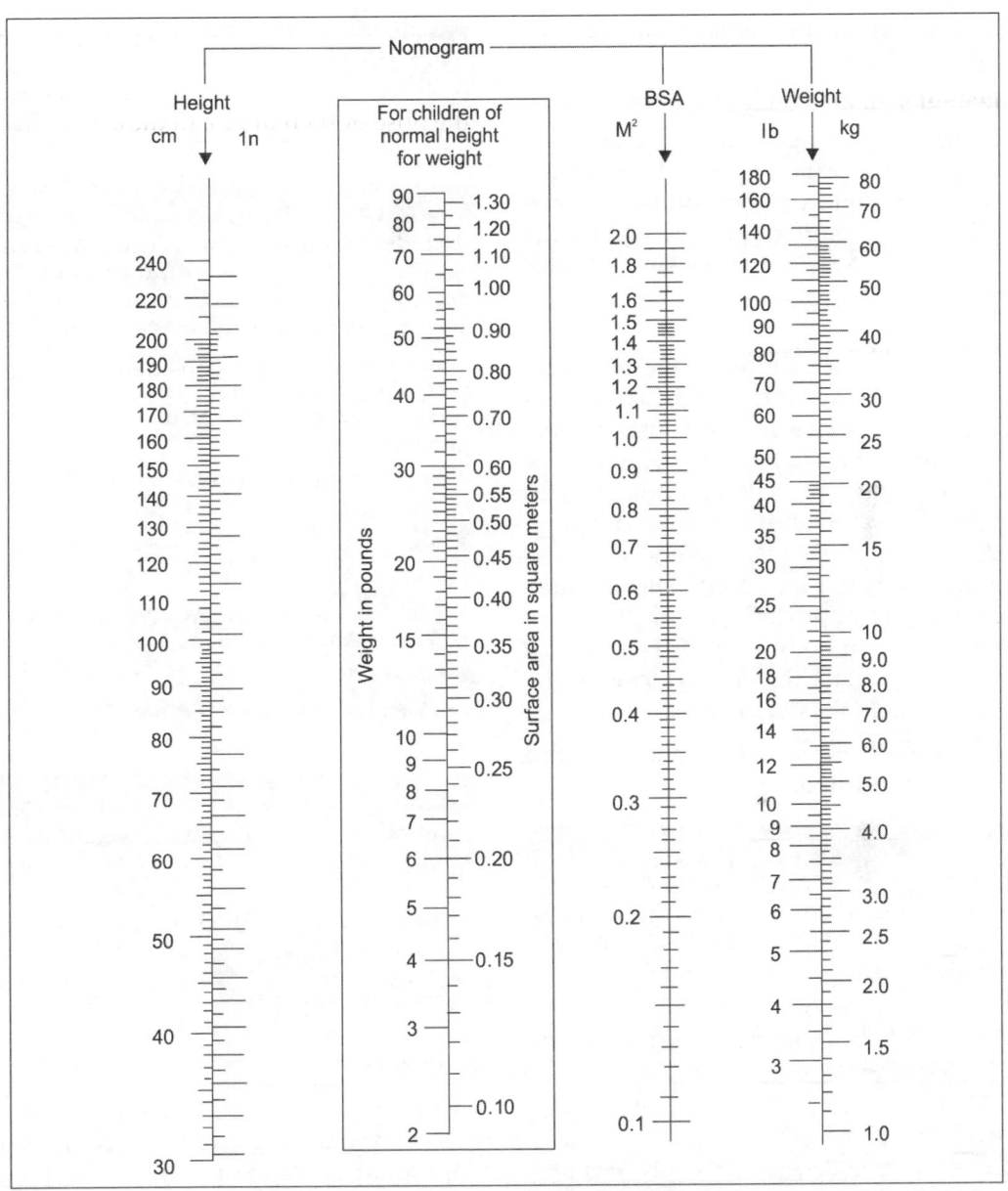

Fig. 3.1: Nomogram (for estimation of body surface area). The BSA is indicated where a straight line connecting the height and weight intersects the BSA column or, if the patient is roughly of normal proportion, from the weight alone (enclosed area).

DOSAGE CALCULATION BASED ON BODY SURFACE AREA

The dose of drugs for children as well as adults may be adjusted based on the body surface area. The normal adult body surface area is 1.73 m². The body surface area may be calculated in many ways. The following equation provides a useful estimate of the surface area when the height (in cm) and weight (in kg) of the patient are known (mosteller formula):

Surface area in m^2 = (height × weight)$^{1/2}$ × 60

Body surface area may also be calculated by using a nomogram. Figure 3.1 shows the nomogram for children and adults. One can find out the body surface area by joining the body weight and height by a straight line, and reading the value at the point where they coincide.

For example, for children if the height in inches is 70 and the body weight in pounds is 42, the body surface area in square meters obtained from Fig. 3.1 is 0.75 m^2. Similary for adult if the height is 90 inches, the body weight of surface area obtained from monogram are 120 lb and 1.8 m^2 respectively. The dose modifications based on body surface area provide a better approximation of dose than the dose based on body weight. The general equation to calculate the child's dose by the surface area method is as follows:

Child's dose = Surface area of child (m^2)/1.73 m^2 × Adult dose

Example 1:

In juvenile arthritis, Advil® is required to be given in a dose of 30 mg/kg/day. How many milliliters of the Advil® suspension (100 mg/5 ml) should be given to a child weighing 74 lb?

74 lb = 74/2.2 = 33.64 kg

In one day, Advil® required is 30 mg per kg or

30/1 kg = X/33.64 kg

X = 1009 mg

100 mg/5 ml = 1009 mg/X

Therefore, X = milliliters of Advil® required = 50.5 ml

Answer: 50.5 ml

Example 2:

Alupent® has a normal adult dose of 20 mg tid for asthma. How much Alupent® should be given to a child weighing 75 lb by the Clarke's equation?

Dose of the child = (Weight in pounds × Adult dose)/150 lb

Dose of the child = (75 lb × 20 mg)/150 lb = 10 mg

Answer: Dose of the child = 10 mg

Example 3:

The height of a child is 120 cm and the weight is 130 lb. The usual adult dose of Elavil® (Amitriptyline HCl) is 75 mg/day. What would be the dose for the child based on body surface area?

When height and weight of a child are known, surface area may be calculated by using the formula:

Surface area in m^2 = (height × weight) 1/2/60

130 lb = 130/2.2 = 59.1 kg

Surface area in m^2 = (120 × 59.1)$^{1/2}$//60 = 1.40 m^2

Child's dose = (Surface area of child (m^2)/1.73 m^2) × Adult dose in mg/day

Child's dose = (1.4 m^2) / (1.73 m^2) × 75 mg/day

Answer: Child's dose = 60.7 mg

Example 4:

If an adult dose of drug is 100 mg, what would be dose for a child that has a body surface area 0.9 m^2?

Body surface area of child/173 m^2 x adult dose

= 0.9/173 x 100

= 0.52 mg of dose.

Problems

Given the following dosage guidelines, determine if the prescriptions below are dosed appropriately. Answer "OK" for appropriate doses, "over" for doses over the recommendation, and "under" for doses under the recommendation.

Acetaminophen: Adults (> 12 yrs) — 325 – 650 mg every 4–6 hours, or 1 gm 3–4 times a day — do not exceed 4 gm/day

Children (< 12 yrs) — 10–15 mg/kg per dose, not to exceed 5 doses in 24 hours

Amikacin: Adults, children and infants — 15 mg/kg/day in 2–3 divided doses

Amoxicillin: Adults (> 12 yrs) — 750–1,000 mg/day in 2 or 3 divided doses

Children (< 12 yrs) — 20–40 mg/kg/day in 3 divided doses

Ampicillin: Children (< 12 yrs) — 50–400 mg/kg per day in 4 divided doses

Adults (> 12 yrs) — 1–12 gm in 4 divided doses

1. Patient — 4 years old having weight of 24 kg

   R_x — Amikacin 140 mg IV q8h

2. Patient — 6 years old having weight of 27 kg

   R_x — Acetaminophen 160 mg/5 ml, 1 tsp po q6h

3. Patient — 17 years old having weight of 150 lb

   R_x — Amoxicillin 250 mg caps, 2 caps po qid

4. Patient — 15 years old having weight of 64 kg

   R_x — Amikacin, 1 gm IV q12h

5. Patient — 10 years old having weight of 38 kg

   R_x — Ampicillin, 350 mg IV q6h

6. Patient — 23 years old having weight of 165 lb

   R_x — Ampicillin 250 mg caps, 1 cap qid

7. Patient — 27 years old having weight of 77 kg

   R_x — Acetaminophen 500 mg tabs, 2 tabs po q4h

8. Patient — 14 years old having weight of 135 lb

   R_x — Ampicillin 250 mg caps, 1 cap qid

9. Patient — 13 years old having weight of 95 lb

   R_x — Amikacin, 70 mg IV q8h

10. Patient — 18 years old having weight of 170 lb

    R_x — Acetaminophen 325 mg, 3 tabs q6h

Answers:

(1) Over 17.5 mg/kg/d (2) Under 5.9 mg/kg/dose (3) Over 2g/d and qid (4) Over 31.25 mg/kg/d (5) Under 36.8 mg/kg/d (6) OK 1gm/d (7) Over 6 gm/d (8) OK 1 gm/d (9) Under 4.8 mg/kg/d (10) OK < 4 gm/d

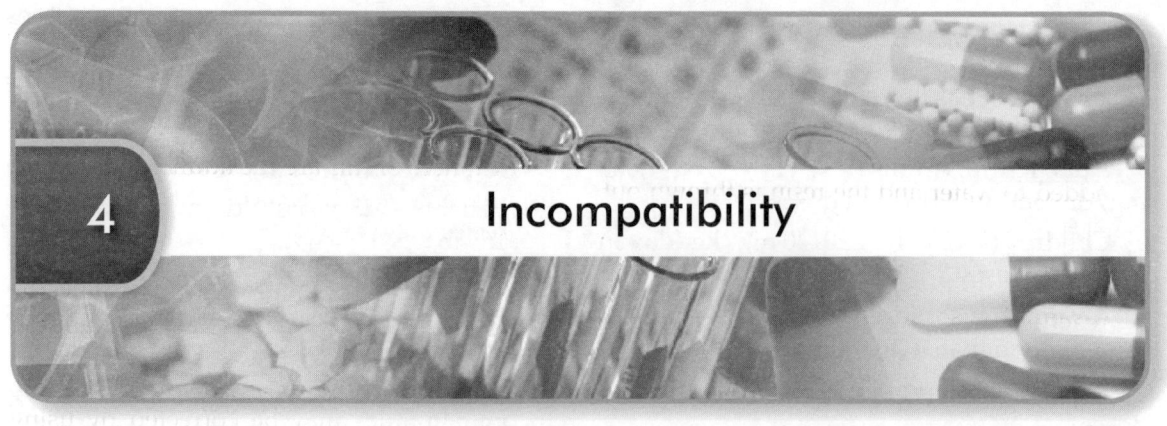

4   Incompatibility

INTRODUCTION

The word "incompatible," means incapable of existing together in agreement or harmony. We call a prescription incompatible when its ingredients are of such a nature that, if brought together, one or more of the following changes would take place: (1) mutual decomposition of the ingredients, with the formation of a new compound; (2) precipitation: chemical or physical; (3) explosion; (4) deflagration; (5) liquefaction, when the ingredients are prescribed in powders; (6) the deterioration of one or more of the ingredients. It may affect the safety, efficacy and appearance of a medicine and the pharmacist must use his pharmaceutical, chemical and pharmacological background and knowledge to anticipate antagonism and decide the most appropriate line of action. Incompatibilities are generally divided into three classes:

1. **Pharmaceutical or physical:** When the change is the result of a physical condition, e.g. when fluid extract of cannabis indica is added to water and the resin is thrown out of solution.
2. **Chemical incompatibility:** Where the change is the result of a true chemical reaction, e.g. when sodium salicylate is prescribed with diluted sulfuric acid, salicylic acid precipitates out, and sodium sulfate is in solution.
3. **Therapeutic:** Where the drugs prescribed have antagonistic medicinal properties, e.g. prescribing drugs like mustard oil (emetic) and domperidone (antiemetic).

The incompatibility, which has been found both useful and practical, is as follows:

1. **Permissible and desirable incompatibility:** When the resulting change is of no significance, or where the new compound is expressly desired by the physician.
2. **Preventable incompatibility:** Where the incompatibility can easily be prevented, either by a change in the order of mixing the ingredients, or by the addition of any ingredients.
3. **Absolute or true incompatibility:** Where the prescription cannot possibly be dispensed in its original form and where one or more ingredients must be left out altogether or other ingredients substituted.

Nowadays, pharmacist hardly notices incompatibilities because proprietary preparations are dispensed or medicines are prepared from official formulae. However, the possibility of incompatibility occurs when proprietary medicines are diluted or mixed together, or stored in unsuitable containers.

PHYSICAL INCOMPATIBILITY

Physical incompatibility differs from chemical incompatibility in the absence of chemical action, and is generally produced when two or more substances are combined together, through differences in solubility, causes a precipitation of solid matter or a separation of part of the liquid.

Instances of this are the addition of an acid to a quinine and liquorice mixture, resulting in precipitation of the glycyrrhizin by the acid or prescribing solutions of chloralhydrate and potassium bromide with an alcoholic preparation, the chloralhydrate separating to the top as an alcoholate, and therefore dangerously in excess for the first few doses. Incompatibilities may be corrected by using any one or more of the following methods:

- **Change the order or mixing of the prescription:** The order of mixing has much to do with the final appearance of the product or mixture. It is always easier to prevent a precipitation than to rectify it, and the order of mixing helps largely in this way, e.g. when concentrated hydroalcoholic solution of volatile oils mixed with water, causes the oil to separate. To prevent this, the hydroalcoholic solution should either be gradually diluted with the vehicle or poured slowly into the vehicle with constant stirring.

- **Emulsification:** When two liquids are immiscible with each other, (like oil and water) and need to blend them into one, they can be made miscible by emulsification or solubilization. An emulsifier is a type of surfactant typically used to keep emulsion (mixtures of immiscible fluids) well dispersed. Emulsifiers typically have a hydrophobic (water-hating) and a hydrophilic (water-liking) end. The emulsifiers will surround oil (or other immiscible molecule) and form a protective layer so that the oil molecules cannot "clump" together. This action helps keep the dispersed phase in small droplets and preserves the emulsion.

- **Addition of an ingredient that does not alter the therapeutic value, such as the addition of suspending agent:** Addition of high concentration of electrolytes to mixtures in which the vehicle is a saturated; aqueous solution of volatile oil causes the oil to separate, to avoid this suspending or an emulsifying agent is used.

- **Change in the form of ingredients by alteration in the solvents or by use of protective agents:** This also requires thorough knowledge of solubility of different drugs. Water dissolves gums, albuminous bodies, mucilages and starch; these solutions are not miscible with alcohol unless diluted.

Alcohol dissolves most organic bodies such as alkaloids, glycosides, organic acids, neutral principles, resins, balsams, camphor and volatile oil. Most of these are thrown out of solution, by diluting with water.

- **Substitution of therapeutically inactive:** Metallic salts soluble in water are not necessarily soluble in alcohol, the converse, however, appears to be true with one important exception, i.e. mercuric iodide is soluble in alcohol, is not appreciably soluble in water, therefore good dispensers always add KI (therapeutically inactive substance) to render same soluble.

Types of Physical Incompatibilities
- Immiscibility
- Insolubility
- Precipitation
- Liquefaction

Immiscibility
Oil and water are immiscible with each other. They can be made miscible with water by emulsification.

Insoluble powders like sulfur and corticosteroids are difficult to wet with water but, this problem is solved by the addition of wetting agents.

Example 1:	
Castor oil	15 ml
Water q.s.	60 ml
Make an emulsion.	

In this prescription, castor oil is immiscible with water. To overcome this incompatibility, an emulsifying agent is used to make a good emulsion.

Insolubility
Insolubility means the inability of material to dissolve in a particular system. The major of incompatibilities are due to insolubility of the inorganic as well as organic compounds in a particular solvent. Liquid preparation contains indiffusible solids like chalk, aromatic chalk powder, calamine, sulphonamides and zinc oxide, a thickening agent is necessary to obtain an elegant product from which uniform dosage can be removed.

Insolubility of Inorganic Compounds
Inorganic compounds usually possess strong binding forces which are ionic or covalent in nature. So these compounds are soluble in polar or semi-polar solvents, like water, alcohol and acetone.

1. Metals and their Salts

Alkali metals
1. The salts of lithium, sodium and potassium are listed in order of their decreasing solubility. The solubility of these cations generally follows heat of hydration and change to ionic radius ratio data.
2. The soluble lithium salts are precipitated from their solutions by soluble carbonate, as lithium carbonate.
3. Soluble phosphates precipitate lithium phosphate.
4. With the exception of the carbonate and phosphate, the common, lithium salts are generally soluble in water and in alcohol.

Example 2:	
Spirit	30 ml
Potassium citrate	3.8 gm
Syrup	30 ml
A teaspoonful after meal	

When the two liquids were mixed, producing a turbidity, and on standing separated into two distinct layers. Potassium citrate is nearly insoluble in alcohol. The alcohol of the spirit has a tendency to precipitate the citrate out of solution. The potassium citrate was dissolved in the syrup and the spirit was then added.

Example 3:	
Potassium bromide	5.6 gm
Sodium bromide	8 gm
Aqueous camphor	160 ml

Camphor is slightly soluble in water. It is almost absolutely insoluble in solutions of salts. In this prescription, it is therefore precipitated out, floating on the top of the liquid or adhering to the bottle as a fine scum. Salts should not be prescribed with camphor water, particularly in concentrated solutions.

Alkali earth metals

Magnesium salts: The soluble magnesium salts, particularly in concentrated solution, are precipitated by the alkaline hydroxides (as magnesium hydroxide); by the alkaline carbonates (as basic magnesium carbonate) and by alkaline phosphates (as magnesium phosphate).

Calcium salts: The soluble calcium salts in concentrated solutions are precipitated by the alkali hydroxides as calcium hydroxide; by alkaline carbonates, phosphates, oxalates, or tartrates as calcium carbonate, phosphate, oxalate, or tartrate. Soluble citrates on heating precipitate the calcium citrate.

Barium salts: Barium salts in aqueous solution are precipitated by sulfuric acid by aqueous solutions of phosphates, tartrates, odates, carbonates, chromates, or tannates, the precipitate being barium sulfate, phosphate, tartrate, oxalate, carbonate, chromate, or tannate.

Example 4:	
Spirit ammon. aromatic	12 ml
Spir. menth. piper	9 ml
Aqueous solution of calcium carbonates	15 ml
Half ounce to be taken after meals.	

A slight precipitate of calcium carbonate will be formed due to the ammonium carbonate in the aromatic spirit. The oils of both spirits will be precipitated by the lime water, making a milky mixture; an inelegant combination but one may be dispensed with a "shake well before use" label.

Example 5:	
Magnesium sulfate	2 gm
Spirit menth. piper	1.5 ml
Water	8 ml
Two teaspoonfuls after every 4 hours.	

There is just about enough water in this prescription to dissolve the magnesium sulfate. It will be a fully saturated solution. But on adding the spirit of peppermint, magnesium sulfate being thrown out of solution. The $MgSO_4$ is insoluble in alcohol. A saturated solution of magnesium sulfate should not be prescribed with alcoholic liquids.

Heavy metals

Zinc salts: Soluble zinc salts are incompatible with soluble hydroxides, carbonates, phosphates, and with borax. With tannic acid, zinc salts give a precipitate only in concentrated solution.

Ferric phosphate (soluble form)

1. The soluble ferric phosphate, is incompatible with mineral acids which precipitate as ferric. phosphate (the insoluble form); the only exception is glacial phosphoric acid, which does not cause a precipitate.

2. Potassium and sodium hydroxide (but not ammonium hydroxide) cause a precipitate of ferric hydroxide.

Arsenic trioxide

1. Incompatible with ferric salts, due to the formation of the insoluble basic ferric arsenite.

2. Incompatible with hypophosphites in acid solution and hypophosphorus acid,

because arsenic trioxide reduced to metallic arsenic.

Arsenic iodide: Arsenic iodide should not be prescribed in solution with alkaloidal salts, as many of them are precipitated.

Silver nitrate: Silver nitrate is dissolved in distilled and freshly boiled water. Its principal incompatibilities are soluble chlorides, which at once precipitate silver chloride, borax (silver borate precipitating) and tannic acid (precipitate of silver tannate).

Alum

1. Alum is incompatible with the alkaline hydrates and their carbonates and lime water, aluminum hydroxide being precipitated.
2. With borax, aluminum borate (and some hydroxide) being precipitated. It is absolute incompatible with soluble sulfates.

Example 6:	
Mercuric chloride	130 mg
Albumin	1.9 gm
Water	300 ml
Teaspoonful three times a day.	

Mercuric chloride combines with albumin form an insoluble compound in water. The presence of an equal weight or more of sodium or ammonium chloride prevents the formation of the precipitate. If this prescription were filled as directed, it would be practically inert. By adding three or four grains of ammonium chloride to the mercuric chloride, dissolving this in about one-half the water and the albumin in the remainder of the water, and mixing these solutions, a nearly clear solution can be obtained.

Example 7:	
Potassium arsenite	4 ml
Mercuric chloride	65 mg
Water	120 ml
Dessert spoonful three times a day.	

In this prescription, there may be a red brown precipitate of the oxychloride of mercury but more generally a white precipitate of calomel forms, as arsenite in an alkaline solution reduces mercuric chloride to mercurous chloride and in excess to metallic mercury. The pharmacist should neutralize the Fowler's solution with hydrochloric acid before adding to the solution of mercuric chloride.

Example 8:	
Zinc chloride	650 mg
Collodion	24 ml
Apply to corn with camel's-hair brush.	

The druggist, anticipating some difficulty in dissolving the zinc chloride directly in the collodion, dissolved the salt in about 0.5 ml water and mixed it with the collodion; thus converting it into a useless mass. The right way is to dissolve the zinc chloride in a few drops alcohol (in which it is very soluble), and then mix the solution with the collodion.

Example 9:	
Aluminum hydroxide	3 parts
Borax	3 parts
Glycerin	1 part
Water	24 parts
Use as a gargle.	

While borax with alum gives a precipitate of aluminum hydroxide, still this prescription may be dispensed. The borax is to be dissolved in the glycerin, the alum in the water, and the solutions mixed.

Example 10:	
Opium poppy	1.6 gm
Silver nitrate	0.78 gm
Mix and make fifty capsules.	
Label: Take as before.	

Powdered opium reduces silver nitrate quickly. The silver nitrate can be mixed with some petrolatum and kaolin and put into no. 5 capsules and then dispensed together with the opium into larger capsules.

2. Non-metals

Iodine: Iodine is insoluble in water, but iodide salts are quite soluble. Iodine is made soluble in water in the presence of potassium iodide due to formation of the iodate ion, which is formed by the union of iodine and iodide ion. Iodine is prescribed practically in two forms—tincture and ointment. The tincture contains potassium iodide and is therefore readily miscible with water.

Example 11:	
Iodine	3.5 gm
Metallic mercury	18 gm
Apply 3 times a day.	

The iodine combines with the metallic mercury and with the oxide of mercury which is usually present in the mercurial ointment to form mercuric iodide. This is much more irritating than either iodine ointment or the mercurial ointment itself. As this prescription is often ordered for epididymitis and orchitis, and as the skin of the scrotum is very tender, it also burns very severely in some cases. If it does, the only thing to do is to wash it off with soap and water and then apply an emollient ointment like cold cream or zinc oxide ointment, or some talcum powder or bismuth subnitrate.

Example 12:	
Iodine	1.8 gm
Turpentine oil	75 ml
Alcohol	375 ml

Great care must be taken not to add the iodine first to the turpentine, as great heat is evolved and the mixture may take fire or explode; the iodine is thereby volatilized as a violet vapor. The right procedure is to dissolve the iodine in the alcohol, and then mix it with the turpentine oil, which is very gradually added. The mixture is not homogeneous, but separates in two layers; there is not enough alcohol to dissolve the turpentine, the latter requiring three volumes of alcohol for solution. The upper layer consists of turpentine oil. Dispense with 'shake' label.

Sulfur

1. Sulfur readily dissolves in hot aqueous solutions of hydrates of potassium, sodium, barium, or calcium, forming polysulfides and thiosulfates.
2. When triturated dry with strong oxidizing agents, as potassium chlorate or permanganate, explosion is liable to occur.
3. It combines with many non-metallic elements.

Example 13:	
Calcium hydroxide	12 mg
Sulfur	21 gm
Water	600 ml
Mix and boil for ten minutes and then filter	
Label: Use as directed	

When lime and sulfur are boiled together, a red solution is formed. The calcium and sulfur unite to form calcium thiosulfate and calcium disulfide or pentasulfide, depending on the proportions. This is the first reaction in making the official precipitated sulfur.

3. Acids

1. Acids combine with metallic oxides, metals, and with some alkaloids to form salts. Basic metallic salts are generally insoluble or sparingly soluble while most acid metallic salts are soluble.
2. Practically all acids decompose carbonates and bicarbonates with effervescence and the liberation of carbon dioxide, and the formation of salts of the corresponding acid.
3. Mineral and common organic acids precipitate potassium tartrate from concentrated solutions of Rochelle salt.
4. Strong mineral acids form esters and ethers with alcohol.
5. Many acids precipitate albuminous substances from aqueous solution. Acic's diminish or prevent the action of pancreatin.

6. Strong acetic acid is a good solvent for resins, gum-resins, camphor, and volatile oils.

7. Citric acid forms citrates with most metallic hydroxides or carbonates, with most acetate, with alkaline sulfides, and with soap.

8. Tannic acid precipitates as tannates nearly all alkaloids from aqueous or dilute alcoholic solutions of their salts; the precipitate is generally soluble in mixtures containing over 15 to 40% alcohol. The presence of some organic acids, acacia, or starch also tends to prevent the precipitation. It precipitates some glucosides (digitalin) and some neutral principles. It precipitates many of the metals, in the form of a tannate, the most important being lead, copper, mercury and silver. With ammonia and potassium hydroxide and carbonate, it gives a slight precipitate. With lime water, it gives a bluish-white precipitate, turning darker. With ferric salts, it gives a bluish-black or green-black solution. With ferrous salts, it is supposed to give a white precipitate.

Example 14:	
Tincture of iodine	4 ml
Salicylic acid	4 ml
Glycerin	15 ml
Water	120 ml
Paint over the affected part several times a day	

The salicylic acid is not readily soluble in the water and glycerin; it requires 460 parts of water for solution. If the acid is dissolved in the glycerin with the aid of heat and the tincture then added gives a clear solution results, but on adding the water, a bulky crystalline precipitate comes down. A better method of filling is to rub the acid with the glycerin and water and then add the tincture. Free iodine reacts with salicylic acid, giving mono-, di-, and tri-iodobenzoic acids and tri-iodophenol.

Example 15:	
Sodium salicylate	8 gm
Lemon syrup	60 ml
Teaspoonful three times a day	

On standing, the citric acid in the syrup combines with the sodium, liberating salicylic acid, which, being only sparingly soluble in water, is precipitated in needle-shaped crystals. This can be dispensed as a shake label.

Example 16:	
Pepsin	1 part
Dilute hydrochloric acid	3 parts
Milk of magnesia q.s.	5 parts
3 times a day after meals.	

This prescription is absolutely incompatible. The hydrochloric acid destroys the magnesium, converting it into magnesium chloride. This is one incompatibility. The other incompatibility is between the milk of magnesia and the pepsin. Pepsin, as we know, is active only in an acid medium. So if we leave out the hydrochloric acid, the activity of the pepsin will be inhibited. The honest way to do is to inform the physician and such combination should never be prescribed.

Example 17:	
Compound rhubarb powder	6 parts
Dilute hydrochloric acid	3 parts
Zingier syrup	1.5 parts
Water	12 parts
3 teaspoonfuls after meals.	

As we know, compound rhubarb powder contains magnesium oxide. This will combine with the hydrochloric acid, forming magnesium chloride, insoluble in water. The physician should be informed of the incompatibility so that he/she may make the proper change in the prescription.

Example 18:	
Lead acetate	2.0 gm
Dilute acetic acid	8 ml
Lemon syrup	2.5 ml
Cinnamon water q. s.	60 ml
Label: Teaspoonful three times a day.	

This gives a white precipitate of lead citrate due to the action of the citric acid in the syrup of lemon acting on lead acetate. If simple syrup flavored with lemon is used no precipitate results.

Example 19:	
Magnesium carbonates	12 gm
Sodium borate	6 gm
Citric acid	5 gm
Distill water	250 ml
Tablespoonful in the morning before breakfast	

The citric acid should be dissolved in the boiling water and then the magnesium carbonate added to this. Carbon dioxide is liberated and magnesium citrate goes into solution. There is not enough of acid to completely dissolve all the carbonate. The addition of borax does not cause any precipitation, although the solution is alkaline. If the borax is added to the solution of citric acid and then the magnesium carbonate a large amount borax is not dissolved as the acid nearly neutralized by the borax.

4. Alkalies

1. Ammonia combines with acids to form salts. It precipitates solution of salts of lead, silver, mercury, bismuth, tin, antimony, copper, cadmium, iron, chromium, cobalt, nickel, manganese, and zinc. The precipitate is a hydroxide, except in case of silver and antimony, when it is an oxide; in case of lead, it is a basic-salt; double compounds are formed in case of mercury. The precipitation many times is prevented or hindered by sugar, glycerin, acacia, citrates, tartrates, and other organic matter.

2. A solution of corrosive sublimate is precipitated by ammonia, giving ammoniated mercury.

Example 20:	
Tincture of ferric chloride	15 ml
Glycerin.	10 ml
Aqueous ammonia solution	8 ml
Water	120 ml
Mix and make a solution.	

The ammonia water combines with the acid in the tincture of iron, forming ammonium chloride and ferric hydroxide. The precipitation of the ferric hydroxide, may be prevented by mixing the glycerin with the tincture before adding the ammonia. If the ammonia is added to the tincture and then the glycerin, the precipitated ferric hydroxide dissolves but slowly in the glycerin. Glycerin, as well as sugar, acacia, honey, and some other organic substances, prevents or hinders the precipitation of many of the metals by alkali hydroxides.

Example 21:	
Lead acetate	1.5 gm
Ammonium carbonate	2 gm
Rose water	220 ml
Make a lotion, apply on lint to allay irritation.	

Reaction between lead acetate and ammonium carbonate resulting in the formation of the soluble ammonium acetate and the insoluble lead carbonate. All lead is precipitated. As it is for external use, it may be dispensed.

Insolubility of Organic Compounds
Organic compounds generally possess both polar and nonpolar parts except hydrocarbons. Hence, their solubility depends on a balance between these parts. Organic molecules which are soluble in water must possess groups which are capable of hydrogen bonding; being polarized or ionized.

1. Hydrocarbons

Fixed oils

1. Fixed oils are readily soluble in or miscible with glycerin. They are not soluble in alcohol, the only exceptions being castor oil and croton oil.
2. With alkaline hydroxides, fixed oils form soaps or emulsion-like mixtures. This is taken advantage of in a number of pharmaceutical preparations.

Volatile or essential oils: Volatile oils are soluble in alcohol and only to a slight extent in water. When water is added to an alcoholic solution of a volatile oil, the volatile oil therefore separate out and a turbidity or milkiness is produced. Clove oil gives a green color with tincture of ferric chloride. Oil of cinnamon gives a brown color.

Petrolatum

1. Petrolatum is not miscible with glycerin, water or alcohol; with the solid petrolatum, small quantities of those liquids can be incorporated.
2. In incorporating alkaloids with petrolatum, it is best to use the free alkaloids instead of the alkaloidal salts, because the free alkaloids are slightly soluble in petrolatum, but not the latter.

Example 22:	
Olive oil	3 ml
Menthol	1.5 ml
Glycerin	12 ml
For external use.	

Menthol is very soluble in olive oil as in all fixed or volatile oils. But the oil is not miscible with glycerin. This prescription does not make a very elegant mixture, but may be dispensed with a shake label.

Example 23:	
Menthol	650 mg
Liquid petrolatum	5 ml
Glycerin	15 ml
Use with atomizer.	

Menthol is very soluble in liquid petrolatum, but liquid petrolatum is not soluble in or miscible with glycerin, but may be dispensed with a shake label.

2. Alcohol

1. Ethyl and isopropyl alcohols show solubility in water. Alcohol with 4 or more carbon atoms shows a sharp decrease in solubility in water. Additional hydroxyl group serve to increase the water solubility of organic compounds of higher molecular weight.
2. Glycerin, polyethylene glycol, gums such as acacia, agar and tragacanth and cellulose derivatives are soluble or dispersible in water.
3. Phenol possesses one hydroxyl group on a benzene ring is slightly soluble in water. Increasing hydroxyl group without the increase in the carbon atoms results in increased solubility.
4. Resorsinol is considered more soluble in water than phenol.

Example 24:	
Iodine	0.72 gm
Lard	3.9 gm
Rub over the affected part	

In making ointments, the medicinal ingredients must be in the form of a powder, soft solid, or solution. Iodine is powdered. It might be dissolved in alcohol and this solution added to the lard. The US Pharmacopoeia directs that iodine should be dissolved in a glycerin solution of potassium iodide, using equal amounts of potassium iodide and iodine and three times as much glycerin as iodide.

Example 25:	
Menthol	1.8 ml
Boric acid	3.8 gm
Tincture of hydrastis	30 ml
Water q.s	120 ml
Use as spray	

In this mixture, the menthol floats on top and the boric acid goes to the bottom. Using alcohol, glycerin, or a fixed oil instead of water will not make a clear solution. The attention of the physician should be called to this prescription.

Compounds Solubilized through Ionization

Many organic compounds are sufficiently acidic or basic to form salts with bases or acids. These salts are considerably soluble in water due to ionization.

1. The organic salts of the alkali metals are capable of ionizing in water, hence shows considerable water solubility.
2. The organic salts of other metals generally do not ionize to any extent, they are not water soluble. Salts formed between organic bases and organic acids are water soluble due to their ionization.
3. Amines form water soluble salts in the presence of mineral and organic acids depending on their basicity. Many of the anesthetics, alkaloids, surface active agents, phenothizine derivatives form water soluble salts in the presence of acids and they tend to precipitate the free base in the presence of alkalies.

Example 26:	
Ephedrine sulfate	0.25 gm
Menthol	0.02 ml
Liquid paraffin (sufficient to make)	30 ml

The ephedrine sulfate is an alkaloidal salt and is not soluble in liquid paraffin, but anhydrous ephedrine is soluble in it. Hence, ephedrine sulfate is substituted with anhydrous ephedrine to make a clear solution

Example 27:	
Phenacetin	3 g
Caffeine	1 g
Orange syrup	12 ml
Water up to	90 ml

In this prescription, phenacetin is an indiffusible substance. Compound powder of tragacanth or mucilage of tragacanth is used as a suspending agent to make a suitable suspension.

Example 28:	
Atropinae sulfate	0.12 p
Olive oil	8.00 p
Apply to neuralgic spots.	

The alkaloidal salts are not soluble in the fixed oils, while the free alkaloids are soluble in fixed oil. Atropine should be used instead of its sulfate.

Example 29:	
Lead subacetate solution	1.2 ml
Mucilage of acacia	15 ml
Distilled water	120 ml
Make a lotion	

When solution of lead subacetate is added to mucilage of acacia, a solid gelatinous mass is formed. In this prescription, if both are diluted with the water and mixed with constant stirring, the acacia is precipitated in small masses. By putting the mucilage into a mortar and adding the solution in small portions with constant stirring, and then adding the water, a good mixture can be made. Neutral lead acetate does not gelatinize mucilage of acacia.

Example 30:	
Tincture guaiac	10 ml
Mucilage of acacia	15 ml
Teaspoonful every three hours	

The alcohol of the tincture throws the acacia out of solution and the mucilage precipitates the resin from the tincture so that a white precipitate forms in the bottom of the bottle. A fresh tincture of guaiac with mucilage of acacia may give a blue color but an old tincture gives a brown red color. With the consent of the physician, the prescription was filled by using glycerin and water instead of mucilage.

Table 4.1: Shows solubility of some substances as specified by pharmacopoeia

Compounds	Water	Alcohol	Ether	Chloroform	Glycerin	Miscellaneous
Acacia	2 parts	Ins.	Ins.	Ins.		
Albumin	Sol.	Ins.	Ins.			
Alcohol	Sol.	Sol.	Sol.	Sol.	Sol.	
Aluminum hydroxide	Ins.	Ins.	Ins.	Ins.		
Caffeine	46	66	530	5.5	9	
Iodide	V.S.	V.S.				
Camphor	Sp.sol.	V.S.	V.S.	V.S.		Sol. in oils
Chloroform	20	Sol.	Sol.	Sol.	Ins.	Sol. in oils
Digitoxin	Sp.sol	Sol.	Sp.sol	Sol.		
Eugenol	Sp.sol	Sol.	Sol.	Sol.		
Gelatin	Swell	Ins.	Ins.	Ins.		
Glycerin	Sol.	Sol.	Ins.	Ins.		
Iodine	2950	125	V.S.	V.S.	80	
Kaolin	Ins.	Ins.	Ins.	Ins.		
Lanolin	Ins.	Sp.sol.	Sol.	Sol.		
Menthol	Sp.sol.	V.S.	V.S.	V.S.		
Phenol	15	V.S.	V.S.	V.S.	V.S.	Sol. in oils

Abbreviations: sol.— soluble; V.S.— very soluble; m.s.— moderately soluble; sp. sol.— sparingly soluble; Ins.— insoluble.

One dram of honey and seven drams of water in place of the mucilage keeps the resinous matter suspended.

Example 31:	
Lead acetate	0.5 gm
Sodium borate	1 gm
Glycerine	20 ml
Water	80 ml
Apply as directed	

If a solution of borax is added to a solution of lead acetate, a white precipitate of lead borate is formed. Or if the glycerin is added to the solution of lead acetate and then the borax solution added, a precipitate is also formed. But, if the glycerin is added to the borax solution, first the borax is decomposed, with the ultimate formation of sodium metaborate and boric acid, making an acid solution which does not cause as much precipitation.

Precipitation

A drug in solution may be precipitated, if the solvent in which it is insoluble is added to the solution. The resins are insoluble in water. When the tincture containing resins is added in water, resin agglomerates forming indiffusible precipitates. This can be prevented by slowly adding the undiluted tincture with vigorous stirring to the diluted suspension or by adding some suitable thickening agent.

Table 4.2 shows the most important instances of solutions which mutually precipi-

	Alkaloidal solutions (generally)	Metallic solutions (generally)	Solutions of lead salts	Solutions of silver salts	Solutions of calcium salts	Solutions of magnesium salts	Solutions of albumin	Solutions of gelatin
Alkalies	P	P	P	P	P	P		
Tannic acid	P	P	P	P			P	P
Carbonic acids and carbonates	P	P	P	P	P			
Sulfuric acid and sulfonates			P	P	P			
Phosphoric acids and phosphates	P	P	P	P	P	P		
Boric acid and borate	P	P	P	P				
Hydrochloric acid and chlorides			P	P				
Hydrobromic acid and bromides			P	P				
Hydriotic acid and iodides	P		P	P				
Sulfides		P	P	P				
Arsenical preparation		P	P	P				
Albumin		P	P	P				

Table 4.2: Precipitant solutions

Abbreviation:(P)Precipitation

tate each other, the letter P meaning "forms a precipitate with."

Liquefaction

When certain low melting point solids are mixed together, a liquid or soft mass known as "eutectic mixture" is produced. This occurs due to the lowering of the melting point of mixture to below room temperature and liberation of water of hydration. Many chemicals form hydrates, compounds with water of hydration.

The medicaments showing this type of behavior are camphor, menthol, thymol, phenol, chloral hydrate and aspirin. This type of substances creates problem when they are dispensed in powder form.

Example 32:	
Menthol	5 g
Camphor	5 g
Ammonium chloride	30 g
Light magnesium carbonate	60 g

In this prescription, menthol, camphor and ammonia chloride get liquified on mixing with each other. To dispense this prescription, menthol, camphor and ammonium chloride are triturated together to form liquid. Add light magnesium carbonate and mix it thoroughly to make free flowing powder.

Example 33:	
Camphor	1 gm
Liquefied phenol	15 ml
For external use.	

When camphor and phenol are rubbed together, a liquid is obtained. In this case, the mixture should be rubbed in a mortar until a perfectly clear solution is obtained. The solid phenol should be taken and not the liquid, as the liquified phenol containing certain amount of water which makes a turbid solution with camphor.

Example 34:		
Chloretone	3	gm
Menthol	0.65	gm
Boric acid	3	ml
For external use.		

When equal parts of chloretone and menthol are rubbed together, a liquid is obtained. In this case, however, the prescription may be dispensed because it contains only 10 grains of menthol. The proper way would be to rub the chloretone with half the boric acid, the menthol with the other half and then mix the two powders. Table 4.3 shows the most important instances of ingrdients which mutually liquefy or forms a soft mass.

Important Physical Incompatibles (Table 4.4)

Aconite: Alkalies, alkaline earths and their carbonates; vegetable astringents, lime water.

Alcohol: With strychnine.

Belladonna: Alkalies, tannin, vegetable astringents, opium, gelsemium.

Bromides: Such agents stimulating the vasomotor nerves, as digitalis, ergot, belladonna, etc., are incompatible with the bromides.

Codeine: With chloral hydrate.

Cocaine: With morphine.

Carbolic acid: With chloral hydrate.

Colchicum: Acid renders the vinous tincture drastic; alkalies render it milder in its operation.

Conium: Strong acids, alkalies, tannin, etc.

Digitalis: Salts of iron and lead, tannin, vegetable astringents.

Gelsemium: Opium, belladonna or its alkaloid atropine.

Hyoscyamus: Acetate of lead, nitrate of silver, sulfate of iron, tannin and vegetable astringents.

Infusions: With metallic salts.

Infusions and bitter tinctures: With metallic salts of iron or lead.

Table 4.3: Ingredients tends to form soft mass or liquified								
	Acetamid	Camphor	Carbolic acid	Chloral hydrate	Menthol	Naphtha	Salol	Resorcinol
Antipyrine	L	P	L	L	P	P	P	L
Carbolic acid	L	L	L	L	L	L	L	L
Chloral hydrate	L	L	L	P	L	P	L	L
Lead acetate	L	P	L	L	P	P	M	P
Menthol	P	L	L	L	P	P	P	L
Pyrocatechin	L	L	L	L	L	L	L	P
Pyrogallol	L	L	L	P	L	P	P	P
Resorcinol	L	L	L	L	L	P	P	P

Abbreviations: L—soft mass or liquid, M—stiff mass which dries, P—slightly damp powder quickly dried

Table 4.4: Examples of some important physical incompatibilities, their causes and method of correction

Type: Immiscibility

Formula	Reason for incompatibility	Correction
Castor oil 15 ml Water 60 ml Make an emulsion.	Oil is immiscible with water	An emulsifying agent, e.g. gum acacia or gum tragacanth may be used to make a good emulsion.

Type: Insolubility	**Subtype: Insolubility of inorganic compounds**	**Sub-subtype: Alkali metals**
Spirit 30 ml Potassium citrate 3.8 gm Syrup 30 ml A teaspoonful after meal	Potassium citrate is nearly insoluble in alcohol. The alcohol of the spirit precipitate the citrate out of solution.	The potassium citrate was dissolved in the syrup and the spirit was then added.

Type: Insolubility	**Subtype: Insolubility of inorganic compounds**	**Sub-subtype: Alkali earth metals**
Spir. ammon. aro. 12 ml Spir. menth. piper 9 ml Aqu. sol.ca. carbo. 15 ml Half ounce to be taken after meals	The oils of both spirits will be precipitated by the lime water.	Precipitants are diluted before mixing and dispensed with a "shake well before use" label.

Type: Insolubility	**Subtype: Insolubility of inorganic compounds**	**Sub-subtype: Heavy-metals**
Mercuric chloride 30 mg Albumin 1.9 gm Water 300 ml Teaspoonful three times a day.	Mercuric chloride combines with albumin to form an insoluble compound in water.	The presence of sodium or ammonium chloride prevents to a considerable extent the formation of the precipitate.

Type: Insolubility	**Subtype: Insolubility of inorganic compounds**	**Sub-subtype: Non-metals**
Iodine 1.8 gm Turpentine oil 75 ml Alcohol 375 ml	Iodine when directly mixed with turpentine oil, the mixture may take fire or explode.	Dissolve the iodine in the alcohol, and then mix it with the turpentine oil, very gradually added.

Type: Insolubility	**Subtype: Insolubility of acids**	
Sodium salicylate 8 gm Lemon syrup 60 ml Teaspoonful three times a day	The citric acid in the syrup combines 'with the sodium, liberating salicylic acid, which, being only sparingly soluble in water	Salicylic acid, being only sparingly soluble in water. This can be dispensed as a shake mixture.

Type: Insolubility	**Subtype: Insolubility of alkalis**	
Tr. ferric chloride 15 ml Glycerin. 10 ml Aq. amm. sol. 8 ml Water 120 ml Mix and make a solution.	The ammonia water combines with the acid in the tincture of iron, forming ammonium chloride and ferric hydroxide precipitate.	The precipitation of the ferric hydroxide, may be prevented by mixing the glycerin with the tincture before adding the ammonia.

contd...

Table 4.4: Examples of some important physical incompatibilities, their causes and method of correction (*contd.*)

Type: Insolubility	Subtype: Insolubility of organic compounds	Sub-subtype: Hydrocarbons
Olive oil 3 ml Menthol 1.5 ml Glycerin 12 ml For external use	The oil is not miscible with glycerin	This prescription may be dispensed with a shake label.
Type: Insolubility	Subtype: Insolubility of organic compounds	Sub-subtype: Alcohol
Menthol 1.8 ml Boric acid 3.8 gm Tr. of hydra. 30 ml Water q.s 120 ml Use as spray	In this mixture, menthol and boric acid are precipitated from their aqueous solution.	Alcohol, glycerin, or a fixed oil instead of water will not make a clear solution.
Type: Insolubility	Subtype: Insolubility of organic compounds	Sub-subtype: compound solubilized through ionization
Ep. sulp. 0.25 gm Menthol 0.02 ml Liq. paraffin 30 ml	The ephedrine sulfate is not soluble in liquid paraffin.	Ephedrine sulfate is substituted with anhydrous ephedrine to make a clear solution.
Type: Precipitation	Subtype: Precipitation by lead salt	
Lead subacet. sol. 1.2 ml Mucilage of acacia 15 ml Distilled water 120 ml Make a lotion	Lead subacetate solution precipitate acacia.	Both lead subacetate and acacia are diluted with the water and mixed with constant stirring.
Type: Liquefaction		
Menthol 5 g Camphor 5 g Amm. chloride 30 g Light mag. carbo. 60 g	Menthol, camphor and ammonia chloride get liquified on mixing with each other.	Add light magnesium carbonate (adsorbent) and mix it thoroughly to make free flowing powder.

Iron: Should not be given with medicine or anything containing tannic acid.

Oils, essential and fixed: With aqueous liquids.

Opium: Alkalies, alkaline earths and carbonates, nitrate of silver, salts of copper, iron, zinc and lead, tannin and gallic acid.

Pepsin: Alkalies, alcohol, tinctures.

Stramonium: Caustic, fixed alkalies or soda and potash.

Strychnine: Alcohol, chloral, hydrocyanic acid, nicotine.

Vegetable preparations: That contain tannic acid are incompatible with salts of iron and lead.

CHEMICAL INCOMPATIBILITY

Chemical incompatibility occurs when two or more substances brought in contact with each other react and form a different compound, entirely different from its components alone, and may be poisonous or non-poisonous. Chemical incompatibilities often occur due to oxidation or reduction, acid base hydrolysis or combination reaction. These reactions may be noticed by precipitation, effervescences, decomposition, color change or by explosion.

Types of Chemical Incompatibility

1. **Tolerated:** In tolerated incompatibilities, the chemical interaction can be minimized by changing the order of mixing or mixing the solutions in dilute forms but no alteration is made in the formulation.

2. **Adjusted:** In adjusted incompaibilities, the chemical interaction can be prevented by addition or substitution of one of the reacting ingredients of a prescription with another of equal therapeutic value.

Chemical incompatibility may be:

- **Intentional:** When the prescriber knowingly prescribes the incompatibility drugs.
- **Unintentional:** When the prescriber prescribes the drugs without knowing that there is incompatibility between the prescribed drugs.

Precipitate Yielding Interactions

The precipitate formed through the chemical incompatibility may be diffusible or indiffusible. The method A and B is followed in dispensing the prescription, yielding diffusible and indiffusible precipitates, respectively.

Method (A)

The method is followed when diffusible precipitates are formed in very small quantity. Divide the vehicle into two equal portions, dissolve one of the reacting substances in one of the portion and the other in the other portion. Mix the two portions by slowly adding one portion to the other by rapid stirring.

Method (B)

The method is followed when indiffusible precipitates are formed in large quantity. Divide the vehicle into two portions. Dissolve one of the reacting substances in one portion. Weigh a suitable quantity of compound tragacanth powder (2 g per 100 ml of finished

product) and transfer in a mortar and use part of second portion of vehicle to produce smooth mucilage. Then add other reacting substances. Mix the two portions by slowly adding one portion to the other with rapid stirring. A secondary label "shake the bottle before use" should be fixed on the container whenever method A or method B is followed in dispensing the prescription.

Alkaloidal Salts with Alkaline Substances

1. The free alkaloids are sparingly soluble in water, except atropine, caffeine, codeine, nicotine, and coniine, but are generally soluble in alcohol, ether, or chloroform.

2. Alkaloids are weak bases. They are almost insoluble in water but, alkaloidal salts are soluble in water. If these salts are dispensed with alkaline preparations, such as strong solution of ammonium acetate, aromatic spirit of ammonia, solution of ammonia and ammonium bicarbonate, the free alkaloid may be precipitated: A few are soluble in excess of solutions of alkali hydrates, e.g. morphine; a few are soluble in excess of ammonia water, e.g. quinine.

Example 1:	
Strychnine hydrochloride solution	6 ml
Aromatic spirit of ammonia	4 ml
Water make up to	1200 ml

Strychnine hydrochloride is an alkaloidal salt whereas aromatic spirit of ammonia is an alkaline substance. When they react together, the strychnine get precipitated because the quantity of strychnine hydrochloride prescribed in the prescription is much more than its solubility in water (1 in 7000). The aromatic spirit of ammonia neither contains negligible amount of alcohol which cannot dissolve the strychnine. Hence, it gets precipitated as diffusible precipitates. Hence, follow method A for precipitate yielding combination.

Example 2:	
Cocaine hydrochloride	0.3 gm
Sodium borate	0.4 gm
Distill water	90 ml

The sodium borate, which has an alkaline reaction, precipitates the cocaine in alkaloidal form. The proper way to do is to substitute an equal quantity of boric acid for the borax, or we may add a little glycerin. The glycerin decomposes the borax, yielding sodium metaborate and boric acid, and the solution being no longer alkaline, no precipitation will take place.

Example 3:	
Morphine sulfate	0.2 gm
Spir. ammon. aromat.	6 ml
Aq. menth. piper	50 ml
3 teaspoonfuls when required.	

This prescription is a dangerous one to dispense. The ammonia will precipitate the morphine. As we know, poisonous principles should never be dispensed in a state of suspension. It is an example of true incompatibility.

Example 4:	
Ammonium carbonate	3 gm
Syr. ipecac	11 ml
Syr. squill	1.5 ml
Water q.s	25 ml
3 teaspoonful in every 3 hours until cough is relieved.	

The acetic acid present in both the syrup of squill and the syrup of ipecac will decompose the ammonium carbonate, producing ammonium acetate and carbon dioxide. The mixture should, therefore, be made in a mortar, and poured into the bottle only after the evolution of CO_2 has ceased.

Example 5:	
Morphine sulfate	0.12 gm
Potassium hydroxide	3.8 gm
Aqueous chloroform	60 ml
Glycerin	3.8 ml

This prescription is incompatible, because the potassium hydroxide, being an alkali, will precipitate the morphine. But, this prescription is not incompatible. True morphine salts are precipitated by potassium and sodium hydroxides, but the precipitates are re-dissolved by an excess of the alkali. In this case, there is more than sufficient quantity of potassium hydroxide which is available which needs to be re-dissolved the precipitated morphine and to keep it in solution.

Alkaloids with Acids

1. Alkaloids combine with mineral acids and acetic and citric acids to form salts which are generally soluble in water or alcohol, but insoluble in ether, chlorofom, benzol, petroleum ether, carbon bisulfide, or oils.

2. In combination with most other organic acids, the alkaloids form salts that are not generally soluble in water.

3. Alkaloids combined with acids and dissolved in water or very dilute alcohol are generally precipitated as free alkaloids by solution of alkali hydroxides or carbonates and by borax.

4. Solutions of lead subacetate, potassium arsenite, sodium phosphate, and sodium arsenate are slightly alkaline and may precipitate the free alkaloid.

Example 6:	
Quinine sulfate	0.3 gm
Ext. glycyrrhizin	15 ml
Syrup	10 ml
Dilute sulfuric acid q.s	

This is an old and well-known prescription incompatibility. The dilute sulfuric acid works double mischief. First, by dissolving the quinine, it renders the mixture intensely bitter; secondly, by precipitating the glycyrrhizin from the fluid extract of glycyrrhiza, the sweetening or disguizing property of the latter is completely destroyed. Omit the sulfuric acid, and dispense the prescription as a "shake" well before use label.

Example 7:	
Picric acid	3 gm
Cocaine	0.38 gm
Water q.s	100 ml
Apply on lint every hour.	

Picric acid has been recommended as an excellent remedy for burns. Picric acid is an excellent precipitant of almost all alkaloids. When picric acid is added to a solution of cocaine hydrochloride, the mixture becomes turbid, and soon the crystals begin to separate out. There can be no option to overcome this incompatibility; the cocaine is to be left out. Of course, the physician is to be informed of the facts in the case.

Example 8:	
Quinine sulfate	0.3 gm
Potassium citrate	3 gm
Citric acid	1.5 gm
Water	150 ml
Label: A dessertspoonful after meals.	

The quinine sulfate dissolves in the water and citric acid, making a clear solution that does not precipitate on standing. On adding the potassium citrate, crystals begin to separate at once. Adding more citric acid will dissolve the precipitate and the addition of another portion of potassium citrate causes a precipitation again. Whatever the precipitate is, it is probably thrown out of solution by making a concentrated solution of potassium citrate, although this does not entirely explain the result since acid clears up the mixture again. The directions are: "shake well".

Alkaloidal Salts with Soluble Salicylates, Benzoates and Iodides

The alkaloidal salts are generally precipitated from aqueous solution, when combined with the soluble salicylates, benzoates, bichromates, iodides, bromides, and by the following general alkaloidal reagents— tartaric acid, picric acid, iodine in solution of potassium iodide, bromine in solution of potassium bromide, potassium mercuric iodide (Mayer reagent).

Example 9:	
Quinine sulfate	0.3 gm
Dilute sulfuric acid	3 ml
Potassium iodide	3 gm
Water q.s	90 ml

This is an example of double incompatibility. The sulfuric acid is incompatible with potassium iodide, forming hydriodic acid, which easily decomposes, the potassium iodide, liberates free iodine, attacks the quinine sulfate, precipitating it as quinine hydriodide (or "iodide"). In this case, it is best to call the physician's attention to the incompatibility. If he/she insists on having the quinine and the iodide in the same mixture, the sulfuric acid must be left out; the quinine is rubbed up with a portion of the water, the potassium iodide dissolved in the remainder, this solution gradually added to the quinine mixture, and the whole dispensed as a "shake" mixture. Only a small quantity of quinine hydriodide will be formed.

Example 10:	
Strychinine sulfate	0.065 gm
Potassium bromide	1.5 gm
Water	150 ml

Potassium bromide is incompatible with strychnine, as it is with most alkaloids, precipitating them in the form of bromides. Chemically pure bromides (and iodides) do not precipitate the alkaloids as readily as do the commercial articles. The latter, in order to be more stable, are crystallized from alkaline solutions, and consequently contain some hydroxide; and alkaline hydroxides are stronger alkaloidal precipitants than the bromides or iodides. To dispense this prescription with the undissolved strychnine bromide would be manifestly unsafe, as too large a dose of strychnine may be poured out in one spoon.

Example 11:	
Mercurial dichloride	0.12 part
Potassium iodide	10.0 parts
Tincture cinchona comp.	10.0 parts
Syrup sarsaparilla. comp	15.0 parts
Water q.s	120.0 parts

The mercurial bichloride and the iodide will precipitate the alkaloids of the cinchona. The bichloride will also be affected by the tannic acid in the cinchona. (Corrosive sublimate is a very delicate agent, and should be prescribed as little in combination as possible.) But, as many physicians insist on prescribing the above mixture, it should be dispensed with a "shake" label.

Example 12:	
Cocaine hydrochloride	0.65 gm
Tincture of iodine	7 ml
Phenol	3.8 ml
Rose water	30 ml
Glycerin	120 ml
Mix and make solution. Label: Spray for throat.	

Iodine makes a compound with cocaine hydrochloride which is insoluble in water or glycerin, although glycerin holds it in suspension. It is doubtful if this compound has much anesthetic effect and the suggestion should be made that separate solutions would be more effective.

Example 13:	
Quinine hydrochloride	0.12 gm
Sodium salicylate	4.0 gm
Water q.s	100 ml

Quinine hydrochloride on reaction with sodium salicylate forms quinine salicylate which gets separated as indiffusible precipitates. Therefore, follow method B for precipitate yielding interactions.

Example 14:	
Caffine citrate	1.0 gm
Sodium salicylate	3.0 gm
Water q.s	90 ml

Caffeine citrate is a mixture of equal weights of caffeine and citric acid. The citric acid present in caffeine citrate reacts with sodium salicylate to liberate salicylic acid which gets precipitated. If caffeine is used instead of caffeine citrate, it forms a soluble complex with sodium salicylate. Hence, substitute caffeine citrate with caffeine to form a clear mixture.

Example 15:	
Potassium iodide	1.5 gm
Tincture of stramonium	8.5 ml
Chloroform water to make	100 ml

Tincture of stramonium contains solanaceous alkaloid, which form indiffusible precipitates of hydroiodides with potassium iodide. So follow method A in dispensing this prescription.

Alkaloidal Salts with Tannic Acid

1. The alkaloidal salts when combine with a drug containg tannins, the alkaloids form tannates which are separated as diffusible precipitates. So follow method A for precipitate yielding interaction.

2. In the presence of acacia, some alkaloids are not precipitated from dilute aqueous solutions by tannic acid, potassium mercuric iodide, or sodium phosphomolybdate.

Example 16:	
Morphine sulfate	0.065 mg
Antimony or potassium tartrate	0.065 mg
Ammonium chloride	3.8 gm
Wild cherry syrup	20 ml

Antimony or potassium tartrates are excellent precipitant of alkaloids and large amount of tannic acid present in wild cherry causes the morphine to precipitate, as morphine tannate. But the precipitates are well suspended in syrup. Nevertheless, the combination is not a good one. If it is dispensed, a "shake" label should invariably accompany it. So follow method B in dispensing this prescription.

Example 17:	
Extract of hyoscyamus	3 gm
Tannic acid	1.5 ml
Lard	12 gm

The extract is to be rubbed up with a little diluted alcohol and incorporated with about half an ounce of the lard; the tannic acid is incorporated with the other half, and mixed the two halves mixed. The tannic acid should not be brought in immediate contact and rubbed with the extract, as the alkaloids of the hyoscyamus hyoscine and hyoscyamine are thus more likely to form insoluble tannate.

Alkaloids with Hydrocarbon

Some alkaloids are soluble in fixed oil whereas their salts are insoluble or sparing soluble in oil and petrolatum.

Example 18:	
Atropine sulfate	0.065 gm
Olive oil	4 ml
Apply with friction	

Atropine sulfate is nearly insoluble in fixed oils. The free alkaloid is soluble in about 38 parts of olive oil, and this is what should be used in filling this prescription. The physician should be notified of the change.

Example 19:	
Cocaine	0.65 gm
Liquid petrolatum	15 ml
Make solution, apply when required	

Cocaine alkaloid is somewhat soluble in liquid petrolatum, requiring about 75 to 100 parts, but not in the proportion given in this prescription. The pharmacist fill it by dissolving the alkaloid in a little oleic acid and adding this to the liquid petrolatum with which it makes a clear mixture. Using forty five minims of acid with a little heat gives a good preparation.

Incompatibility of Purine Base

1. Caffeine does not readily combine with dilute acids, although it unites with concentrated acids. The salts are easily decomposed by water, alcohol, or ether.
2. Caffeine in moderately dilute solutions is not precipitated by the alkali hydroxides or carbonates or the general alkaloidal reagents, but from strong solutions it is precipitated by tannic acid, phosphomolybdic acid, silver nitrate, and mercuric chloride.
3. Warmed with alcoholic potassium hydroxide, it forms carbon dioxide, and a little ammonia.
4. The solubility of caffeine is increased by the presence of sodium salicylate, sodium benzoate, antipyrine, and potassium bromide.

Example 20:	
Caffeine citrate	1 gm
Sodium bromide	3.0 gm
Strontium bromide	1.0 gm
Aquae Foeniculi	15 ml
3 teaspoonfuls every three hours.	

Here, there will be a decomposition between the citrated caffeine and the strontium bromide, with the formation of strontium citrate, which is insoluble in water and precipitates. This prescription was dispensed in a paper box and in a short time it became converted into a wet lumpy mass. Effervescent citrated caffeine is hygroscopic and should be dispensed in well-stoppered bottles only.

Incompatibility of Pyrazolone Derivatives

1. These synthetic derivatives are chiefly non-narcotic analgesics. They produce colors when mixed with oxidizing agents or ethyl nitrite spirit.
2. They are precipitated from aqueous solutions by alkaloidal precipitants.
3. The solid compounds have a tendency to liquefy or form soft mass when triturated with a number of hydrogen bonding substances.
4. Cinchona contains a sufficient amount of tannic acid to make its preparations incompatible with many metallic salts and other compounds.
5. Quinine unites with acids to form salts. Quinine is precipitated from aqueous solution of its salts by all the reagents mentioned for alkaloids.
6. Quinine is precipitated from its concentrated aqueous solutions by benzoates, salicylates, and tartrates.
7. Antipyrine is neutral to litmus, but forms salts with acids by direct addition. An aqueous solution with a strong solution of sodium hydroxide gives a white precipitate. With a solution or tincture of ferric chloride, antipyrine gives a red color.
8. Antipyrine gives a liquid or soft mass when triturated with piperazine and some other solids.
9. Antipyrine increases the solubility of quinine sulfate in water; and at the same time destroys the fluorescence and prevents the green coloration which quinine gives with bromine water followed by ammonia water.
10. The solubility of caffeine is said to be increased by antipyrine.

Example 21:	
Mercuric chloride	0.24 gm
Potassium iodide	3.8 gm
Ferric ammonium citrate	1.5 gm
Tincture nux vomica	3.5 ml
Tincture compound cinchona q.s	100 ml

The sources of incompatibility in this prescription are numerous. First of all it is well to be aware that ammonium ferric citrate, while rapidly and completely soluble in water, is insoluble in alcohol; and as compound tincture of cinchona is made with a menstruum consisting chiefly of alcohol, the salt will not dissolve. Second, the mercuric chloride and potassium iodide precipitate the alkaloids of both the cinchona and the nux vomica. Even if there were no nux vomica in the prescription, the precipitation of the cinchona alkaloids will be in the form of salt. A third cause, black and inky color produced by the action of the tannic acid present in the cinchona, bitter orange-peel, etc., with the ferric salt. The above prescription is a bad combination, and it is advisable to refuse to dispense.

Example 22:	
Cocaine hydrochloride	0.35 gm
Quinine sulfate	0.18 gm
Tannic acid	3.5 ml
Menthol	1.8 ml
Rose water q.s.	50 ml
Use as a gargle.	

The cocaine would be precipitated, as cocaine tannate, which, being insoluble, would have no effect. The quinine would be present partly as quinine sulfate and partly as quinine tannate, both insoluble; the menthol which is here in excessive dose is insoluble in water, and on reaching the pharynx in an undissolved state would prove intensely irritating; even the astringent effect of the tannic acid would be to some extent destroyed, as a part of it would be used up to form insoluble compounds with the alkaloids. In short, the combination is a worthless one and should be avoided.

Example 23:	
Antipyrine	1.9 gm
Syr. Ipecac	1.5 ml
Syr. Wild cherry	12.5 ml
Water q.s	20 ml
Three to four times a day	

A flocculent precipitate is formed, due to the tannic acid of the wild cherry combining with the antipyrine. Antipyrine is precipitated by tannic acid. Though the mixture might be dispensed with a 'shake' label, it is better to call the physician's attention.

Soluble Salicylate Incompatibilities

1. Most acids and acid syrup decompose sodium salicylate precipitating salicylic acid. This type of preparation should not be dispensed.

2. When sodium salicylate administered orally, the acid of stomach contents precipitates salicylic acid which may irritate the gastric mucosa, causing patient discomfort.

3. Sodium salicylate solution, especially if alkaline, absorbs oxygen and become reddish brown. The efficiency of the medicament not seriously impaired by this change, but to avoid causing patient anxiety, a dark coloring matter may be added.

Example 24:	
Quinine sulfate	0.3 gm
Dilute sulfuric acid	3 ml
Sodium salicylate	1.0 gm
Syrup	5 ml
Water q.s	20 ml

Quinine sulfate, water and dilute sulfuric acid in a mortar, form a clear solution, to this clear solution when sodium salicylate is added, a thick mass is resulted. The sulfuric acid here does double mischief; first, it dissolves the quinine sulfate, thus permitting it to fully react with some of the sodium salicylate, forming insoluble quinine salicylate; secondly, it decomposes the rest of the sodium salicylate, forming sodium sulfate and salicylic acid, the latter of which precipitates. In order to dispense this prescription in a more or less presentable form, the sulfuric acid must be left

out. The whole is dispensed with a "shake" label. In this way practically no reaction takes place, the quinine sulfate being kept in suspension instead of being dissolved.

Example 25:	
Antipyrine	3.8 gm
Sodium salicylate	12 gm
Make a powder	

Antipyrine and sodium salicylate should not be prescribed in powder form, as liquefaction often occurs, especially in damp weather.

Example 26:	
Sodium salicylate	12 gm
Lemon syrup	6 ml
Water q.s	20 ml

The citric acid contained in the syrup of lemon will decompose a portion of the sodium salicylate, crystals of salicylic acid floating in the mixture. The prescription should be dispensed with a shake label. Follow method B for precipitate yielding combination.

Incompatibility of soluble salicylates and benzoates with acidic drugs: Salicylic and benzoic acids are poorly soluble in water. In acid medium, soluble salicylates and benzoates precipitate the free insoluble acids.

$$C_6H_5COO\,Na + H \longrightarrow C_6H_5COO\,H + Na^+$$

Free acids or acidic drugs or adjuvants imparting acidic pH values will precipitate the free acid.

Example 27:	
Sodium salicylate	3 gm
Lemon syrup	30 ml
Water to	100 ml

Lemon syrup contains citric acid and, therefore is unsuitable for flavoring sodium salicylate or benzoate containing preparations. If prescribed, it can be replaced by a mixture of lemon tincture and simple syrup. Salicylic acid is separated as indiffusible precipitates. The prescription can be dispensed in two ways. Follow method B for precipitate yielding interaction or replace syrup of lemon with simple syrup and tincture of lemon.

Soluble salicylates with ferric salt: Ferric salts react with sodium salicylate to liberate indiffusible precipitates of ferric salicylate. Therefore, follow method B for precipitate yielding interactions.

Example 28:	
Ferric chloride solution	2 ml
Sodium salicylate	3 g
Water make up to	90 ml

Ferric chloride reacts with sodium salicylate to form ferric salicylate which gets separated as indiffusible precipitates. Therefore, follow method B for precipitate yielding interactions. In the presence of sodium bicarbonate, the precipitates of ferric salicylate remain soluble; hence a clear mixture will be formed. This prescription illustrates the advantage of prescribing sodium bicarbonate along ferric chloride solution and sodium salicylate.

Soluble Iodides Incompatibilities

Iodides undergo oxidation forming iodine which is an undesirable product. Hence, following steps may be taken to avoid this chemical change. Oxidation of iodides with potassium chlorate. When soluble iodides react with potassium chloride, free iodine is liberated.

$$KClO_3 + 3FeI_2 \longrightarrow 3FeOI + 3I + KCl$$

To prevent the incompatibility, the two reacting substances must be dispensed separately.

Oxidation of iodides with ferric salts. When ferric salt reacts with soluble iodide, it gets converted to ferrous salt. There is no satisfactory method to adjust this incompatibility.

$$Fe^{+++} + 2I \longrightarrow Fe^{+++} + I_2$$

To prevent incompatibility, the prescriber may substitute ferric salt with iron and ammonium citrate. Alternatively, the iron is converted into an organic compound which does not yield ferric ions.

Incompatibility of phenolic drugs with ferric Ions: Phenolic drugs as salicylates, resorcinol, adrenaline and oxyphenbutazone, react with ferric ions to give a violet green color. Sources of ferric ions are:

1. As impurities in other chemicals or ingredients used in the formulation.
2. From metallic containers, e.g. tanks, mixers, spautals.
3. Water if not distilled, may contain heavy metal impurities as ferric ion.

Example 29:	
Sodium salicylate	50 gm
Chloroform water (d.s)	500 ml
Water q.s	1000 ml

The discoloration may occur immediately or after storage of the formula. Which can be avoided by avoiding the source of this interaction, or the addition of ions such as tartrate or citrate which complex with ferric ions.

Incompatibility Related to Explosive Compounds

In contact with charcoal, sulfur, organic compounds, or any other readily oxidisable substance, potassium chlorate may explode, especially, if heated or triturated dry. Mixing with any dry substance is inadvisable but, if essential, the ingredients should be powdered separately, using a clean mortar for potassium chlorate and mixed gently with a clean spatula.

The chief members of these two classes are as given in Table 4.5.

Table 4.5: Types of explosive compounds	
Oxidizers	**Oxidizable or combustible**
Nitric acid, chromic acid	Glycerin, sugar, alcohol
Free hydrochloric acid	Oils and ethers
Nitro-hydrochloric acid	Sulfur and Sulfides
Potassium chlorate	Dry organic substances
Potassium permanganate	phosphorus

Example 30:	
Potassium chlorate	0.6 gm
Tannic acid	0.3 gm
Sucrose	0.3 gm
Water	20 ml

The ingredients of this prescription can be compounded with minimum rubbing. Powder all the ingredients and weigh them separately. Mix them on a sheet of paper in ascending order of their weight with a bone spatula without any friction or dispense each ingredient separately with appropriate direction.

Amino Acids Incompatibility

1. Darkening of glycine in water and elixir, due to hydrolysis of sucrose present in elixir with the formation of glucose and levulose.
2. Glycine gives deep wine color with ferric chloride. It disappears with HCl and reappear with NH_3.
3. Glycine gives color with phenol or sodium hypochlorite solution.
4. The water solubility of amines depends on their ability to hydrogen bonding. The aliphatic amines show slightly higher solubility than the aromatic amines.
5. The simple amines are not used to any extent in medicine, but their ionic and organic reactions are very important since the amino grouping occur in many important drug classes like alkaloids, amino acids, aniline derivatives, basic dyes, pyrazolon derivatives and in local anesthetics.
6. Epinephrine is very slightly soluble in water. It is insoluble in oils. An aqueous solution of bases is slightly alkaline. Solution of epinephrine hydrochloride does not form precipitate on the addition of alkaloidal precipitants such as tannic acid and potassium mercuric iodide. Weak alkalis precipitate epinephrine from solution of its salt. Epinephrine is incompatible with iron and its ferrous and ferric salts. Under the influence of light and air, solutions of epinephrine salts are oxidized.

Example 31:	
Pepsin	0.36 gm
Sodium bicarbonate	3.8 gm
Make a powder label: t.i.d. after meals.	

Pepsin is considered absolutely incompatible, therapeutically, with sodium bicarbonate or any other alkali. The digestive power of pepsin is supposed to be destroyed by contact with an alkali.

Example 32:	
Adrenaline	1.5 gm
Aquous hydrogen peroxide	20 ml
For external use.	

This prescription is absolutely incompatible and should not be dispensed. The adrenaline is completely decomposed or oxidized by the hydrogen peroxide.

Example 33:	
Sol. epinephrine	3 ml
Mercuric chloride	0.065 mg
Distill water	20 ml
Use as injection.	

This prescription is absolutely incompatible. The epinephrine is decomposed and the mercuric chloride is reduced to calomel and then to the metallic state.

Incompatibility of Quaternary Ammonium Compound

1. Quaternary ammonium compounds are very soluble in water and readily absorb carbon dioxide from air.
2. Quaternary ammonium salts are usually crystalline salts. These are highly ionized and in water the highly charged cation will react with the anions of weak acids like fatty acids, acidic dyes, antibiotics and barbiturates.
3. Emulsion prepared with alkali metal, ammonia and triethanoamine soaps is incompatible with salts producing polyvalent cations. Due to double decomposition, a polyvalent soap is formed which inverts the emulsion.
4. Germicides action of quaternary ammonium compound may loss by soaps of anionic surfactants.
5. In general, quaternary ammonium compounds are incompatible with anionic surfactants, soaps and synthetic anionic detergents.

Example 34:	
Cetrimide	3.8 gm
Soap	3.8 gm
Cotton seed oil	30 ml
Water	30 ml
Apply with friction	

The interaction occurs upon mixing anionic surfactants with cationic surfactants. This may be manifested, visually, as turbidity or formation of a precipitate. The surface activity of both materials will be drastically reduced. This occurs upon mixing soap with cetrimide. This prescription should not be recommended.

Glycosides Incompatibility

1. Glycosides are decomposed by prolonged contact with mineral acids, alkalies, hot water, or ferments. Some glycosides may be decomposed by one of these agents, others by two or more of them. One of the products formed is glucose or some form of sugar.
2. Tannic acid or lead subacetate generally precipitates the glycosides from their aqueous solutions.
3. The glycosides are not usually precipitated by the alkali hydroxides or carbonates or general alkaloidal reagents.
4. Many of them give color reactions resembling those produced by the alkaloids.
5. Mercuric chloride precipitates from concentrated aqueous solutions nearly alkaloidal salts, some neutral and bitter principles, and some glycosides.
6. Lead acetate gives a precipitate with some coloring matters, gums, resins, neutral principles, glycosides, and alkaloids.

Example 35:	
Tincture of ferric chloride	4 ml
Tincture of digitalis	3 ml
Glycerin	12 ml
Water	12 ml

On mixing, the tincture of iron with the tincture of digitalis, a dark mixture results. This is due to the tannic acid in the digitalis combining with the iron to form iron tannate. Otherwise the prescription is all right. It is best to mix the tincture of iron with the other ingredients, and add the tincture of digitalis in end.

Carbohydrates Incompatibility

1. A solution of sugar when heated with lime, magnesium and other metallic oxides and hydroxides forms saccharates, chemical compounds which are more or less soluble in water.
2. The presence of sugar hinders or prevents the precipitation, or dissolves the precipitate, of many metallic hydroxides or

oxides which are normally formed when alkali hydroxides are added to solutions of metallic salts.

3. Sugar warmed with dilute solution of acids, or heated for some time with water is changed to invert-sugar.

4. When a concentrated solution of sugar and potassium hydroxide is heated, carbon dioxide, acetone, acetic, propionic, and oxalic acids are formed.

5. The presence of honey prevents the precipitation of some of the metallic salts by the alkali hydroxides.

6. Honey decomposes borax, with liberation of boric acid, the reaction being somewhat similar to that between glycerin and borax.

7. Acacia: A solution of this gum forms a thick unsightly precipitate with a solution of lead subacetate (but not with lead acetate), a concentrated solution of borax, ferric salts and alcohol or alcoholic tinctures.

Acacia often acts as a preventative of precipitation. Notably it prevents the precipitation of alkaloids by tannic acid or even potassium mercuric iodide (Mayer's reagent).

8. Starch in aqueous solution is precipitated by strong alcohol, tannic acid, or lead subacetate. Iodine with starch forms the blue black iodide of starch.

Example 36:	
Borax	1.2 gm
Pulverized acacia	1.2 gm
Rose water	150 ml
For external use.	

This is a well-known incompatibility. If the borax is dissolved in a portion of the water and the acacia in another portion and the two solutions are mixed, a thin, gelatinous precipitate will result which will make the mixture altogether unpresentable. There is no

way of obviating the difficulty. It is an instance of true incompatibility.

Incompatibility Anesthetics

1. The alkyl esters of aromatic acids are almost insoluble in water and, hence are unsuitable for injection but, are used in the form of dusting powder, ointments, etc., on wound of the skin or mucous membrane.

2. Procaine in aqueous solution is precipitated by many alkaloidal reagents. The free base is precipitated by an alkalis hydroxide or carbonate. An aqueous solution can be boiled without decomposition.

3. Alypin, this local anesthetic being in the nature of an alkaloid is precipitated by alkaline hydroxides and carbonates and by most of the alkaloidal reagents or precipitants.

Example 37:	
Alypin	0.35 gm
Silver nitrate	0.12 gm
Water	15 ml
Use as injection.	

When alypin is prescribed without any specification, alypin chloride is dispensed, this being the usual combination in which alypin appears on the market. If it is desired to prescribe alypin with silver nitrate, the only way to do is to take alypin nitrate. That avoids the precipitation of silver chloride.

Example 38:	
Anesthesin	2%
Ephedrine sulfate	3%
Normal saline solution q.s	95%
Use as spray in an atomizer.	

The anesthesin will not dissolve completely in the quantity of water present. The use of alcohol or dilute acids to increase the solubility would not be advisable in a solution to be sprayed on the mucous membrane. The use of water soluble anesthesin in place of anesthesin should be recommended to the prescriber.

Incompatibility of Dyes

1. The color of the most of the dyes used in pharmaceutical formulation is influenced by their ionization which depends on pH of the solution. The phenolphthalein dye is colorless in acid solution but red in alkaline mixture.

2. Reducing agents often cause fading, anionic dyes are most stable at acidic pH; for example, in experiments with solutions containg sodium metabisulfied, the pH above which fading began was 5 for amaranth, 3 for orange G, tetrazine feded at pH 4 only.

3. Basic dyes often very sensitive to alkalies, which in some instances (e.g. methylene blue) cause precipitation, and in others like crystal violet convert the dyes to a colorless dye. They are also affectd by acids which may produce mark changes in color.

Example 39:	
Acriflavine (1in 1000 dil)	30 ml
Dakin's solution q.s	120 ml
Apply to sore four times a day	

The chlorine in Dakin's solution reacts with acriflavine, changing the color of the solution. When the prescriber was notified, he/she directed that a 1:1000 solution of acriflavine be dispensed without Dakin's solution.

Example 40:	
Phenolphthalein	0.65 gm
Milk of magnesia	120 ml
Make a solution	

Phenolphthalein almost insoluble in water but soluble in solution of alkalis hydroxide; it is soluble in 15 parts of alcohol. Phenolphthalein gives red color solution in alkaline solution.

Incompatibility of Surface Active Agents

Substances which lower the surface tension of a liquid or the interfacial tension between two liquids are called surface active agents. Some compounds are used as wetting agents, emulsifiers, dispersing agents, emulsifiers, detergents and foaming agents. Surface active agents consist of hydrophilic group which tends to make the compound water soluble and lipophilic group which tends to make it oil soluble. There are three classes of surface active agents, designated as anionic, cationic and non-ionic agents.

- Anionic agents are those in which the negative ion contains the lipophilic group, which is usually long chain hydrocarbon or other oil soluble group. An example of this type is sodium lauryl sulfate.

- In cationic agents, the lipophilic group is part of the positive ion, quaternary nitrogen compounds.

- Non-ionic agents consist of two non-ionisable groups. Usually they are esters of fatty acids with polyatomic alcohols or polymerized glycols. An example is glycol monolaurate.

Aqueous solutions of soap are decomposed by mineral acids, which combine with the base, liberating the free fatty acid. Aqueous solutions of metallic salts give precipitates of metallic oleates with soaps. Soap is frequently alkaline, and so it makes a black mixture with calomel, due to the formation of mercurous oxide. It may precipitate hydroxides or oxides from solutions of metallic salts.

Interaction between Oppositely Charged Surfactants

The interaction occurs upon mixing anionic surfactants with cationic surfactants. This may be manifested, visually, as turbidity or formation of a precipitate. The surface activity of both materials will be drastically reduced. This occurs upon mixing sodium lauryl sulfate with cetrimide.

Interaction between Surfactants and Drugs

Drugs may interact with surfactants carrying opposite charge.

The results of this type of interaction are:

1. Reduction of the therapeutic effectiveness of the drug.
2. Reduction of the surface active property of the surfactant.

Surface active agents and acidic drug or excipient. It occurs with soap surfactants which are salts of weak fatty acids easily displaced by stronger acids. It results in loss of surface activity.

e.g. Na stearate + Salicylic acid $\longrightarrow$ stearic acid (ppt) + sodium salicylate

Surface active agents and heavy metals.

e.g. Na stearate + Ca^{+2} $\longrightarrow$ Ca stearate (insoluble in H_2O)

It can occur by hard water which contains divalent ions.

Example 41:	
Phenol	0.5 gm
Menthol	0.1 gm
Tragacanth	0.5 gm
Olive oil	50 ml
Lime water	100 ml

The free acid in olive oil forms divalent soap with lime water. The divalent soap promote w/o emulsion, whereas with tragacanth o/w emulsion is formed. The prescription should be referred back to the prescriber either to replace lime water with water or to omit tragacanth.

Chemical Incompatibility Causing Evolution of Carbon Dioxide Gas

1. Carbon dioxide is evolved, if a carbonate or bicarbonate is dispensed in a liquid medicine containg an acid or an acidic drug. To prevent leakage or explosion, the reaction must be completed before the preparation is bottled.

2. The ingredients are mixed in a mortar, squat beaker or other wide mouthed open vessel and left until effervescence has ceased. In some instances, the reaction should be hastened by using a hot vehicle.

3. Bismuth subnitrate when combined with sodium bicarbonate in the presence of water, carbon dioxide gas is liberated due to the following reaction.

$$2BiONO_3 + 2NaHCO_3 \longrightarrow (BiO) 2CO_3 + 2NaNO_3 + CO_2 + H_2$$

Example 42:	
Sodium bicarbonate	1.0 gm
Borax	1.0 gm
Phenol	0.5 gm
Glycerin	20 ml
Water	90 ml

When sodium bicarbonate, borax and glycerin mixed together in the presence of water, a reaction takes place with the evolution of carbon dioxide. If the mixture is dispensed as such, there are chances of busting the bottle. Therefore, mix these ingredients in an open vessel until evolution of carbon dioxide ceases. Add phenol and transfer the mixture to a wide mouth bottle.

Important Chemical Incompatibles

- **Acids**: In general with alkalies and weak salts of other acids.
- **Acid chromic**: Mixed with sugar, glycerin or other alcohol producing agents will explode.
- **Acid hydrochloric**: With alkalies and weak salts of other acids.
- **Acid hydrocyanic**: With salts of iron, chlorid, nitrates, sulfates. Mixed with metal-licsalts as well as carbonates, hydrates, nitrate of bismuth or calomel is poisonous.
- **Acid nitric**: Mixed with phosphorus or glycerine will explode and is dangerous.

Nitric acid, muriatic acid and tinct. nux vomica explode after a few hours.

- **Acid nitro-hydrochloric**: Mixed with dry organic substances may explode.
- **Acid salicylic**: Iron and its compounds, lime water, iodide of potassium.
- **Acid tannic**: With glycerin, chlorate of potassium, will explode on addition of water.
- **Acacia gum**: Alcohol, borax, ether and etheral tinctures. Iron, mineral acids and solution of lead.
- **Albumien** and **gelatine** and substances containing them are incompatible with tannic acid, or anything containing it.
- **Arsenic**: Tannic acid, magnesia, lime salts and oxides of iron.
- **Bismuth subnitrate**: Mercury, sulfur, tannin.
- **Camphor**: With water.
- **Chlorates**: With glycerine and tincture of chloride of iron and chloride of lime triturated with sulfur in a mortar have produced explosions.
- **Chloride of iron**: With glycerin and chlorate of potassium if warmed will explode.
- **Chloral hydrate**: Ammonia, alkalies, mercury compounds, alcohol, potassium bromides and cyanides.
- **Chlorides**: Hydrogen peroxide, lead and silver salts.
- **Chloroform**: Amyl nitrite.
- **Hydrogen peroxide**: Alkaline citrates.
- **Iodine tincture**: With ammonia forms the iodide of nitrogen which becomes highly explosive, especially if triturated when mixed with water.
- **Iron salts**: With anything that contains tannic acid.
- **Mucilage**: With iron salts, alcohol and acids.
- **Morphia muriate**: Added to the oxide of silver is explosive, if it be mixed quickly with extract of gentian, but if mixed slowly, it is more safe.
- **Oxidizers**: Such as chromic acid, nitric acid, hydrochloric acid, chloral, potassium nitrate, potassium permanganate, etc. mixed with the readily oxidizable substances, such as oils, phosphorus, ether, turpentine, dry organic substances, tannin, sugar, sulfur, the sulfites, vegetable powders, glycerin, alcoholic or ethereal tinctures result in explosions.
- **Potassium chlorate**: To mix with other salts is dangerous. Mixed with powdered catechu or powdered nut galls it will explode. Mixed with oils and ether it will explode. With alcohol, ammonia, ethereal oils, glycerine and organic substances is dangerous.
- **Potassium permanganate**: Mixed with alcohol, ammonium salts, ethereal oils, glycerin and organic substances is dangerous.
- **Potassium cyanide**: Mixed with metallic salts, such as hydrates, carbonates, subnitrates or subchlorides, as, the carbonates or nitrates of bismuth, or with calomel, is poisonous.
- **Potassium iodide**: Very strong acids and salts of same, alkaloids, iron, potassium chlorate, nitrate of silver, mercurial salts. Mixed with chlorate of potassium it is very poisonous.
- **Silver nitrate**: With acids (with exception of nitric acid) alkalies, bromides, carbonates, iodides, sulfur.
- **Sodium biborate**: Sodium bicarbonate, glycerin and water, if corked, are liable to explode.
- **Sodium bicarbonate**: With acids and their salts, alkaloids, metallic salts, tannic acid.
- **Sodium bromide**: Mineral acids, mercury and its compounds, chlorine water.

- **Sodium hyphophosphite:** With potassium chlorate is explosive, if water is added.

Uva ursi fluid extract: With certain samples of the spirits of nitre or chromic acid with glycerin, permanganate of potassium with glycerine, nitric acid with glycerin, nitrate of silver with creosote, the oxide of silver in pill with extract of gentian, potassium.

Table 4.6: Examples of some important chemical incompatibilities, their causes and method of correction

Type: Alkaloidal salts with alkaline substances

Formula		Reason for incompatibility	Correction
Stryc. hydro. sol.	6 ml	Strychnine hydrochloride when mixed with aromatic spirit of ammonia, strychnine gets precipitated as diffusible precipitates.	Both the reacting substances are diluted with the water and mixed with constant stirring (Method A).
Aro. Sp. of amm.	4 ml		
Water q.s	1200 ml		

Type: Alkaloids with acids

Picric acid	3 gm	When picric acid is added to a solution of cocaine hydrochloride, the mixture becomes at once turbid.	There can be no option to overcome this incompatibility; the cocaine is to be left out as the incompatibility results indiffusible precipitate.
Cocaine	0.38 gm		
Water q.s	100 ml		
Apply on lint every hour.			

Type: Alkaloidal salts with soluble salicylates, benzoates and iodides

Strych. sulp.	0.065 gm	Potassium bromide, precipitating strychnine sulfate in the form of indiffusible bromides.	Substitute strychnine sulfate with half as much as pure strychinine to form a dispensable mixture.
pot. bromide	1.5 gm		
Water	150 ml		

Type: Alkaloidal salts with tannic acid

Ext. of hyoscya.	3 gm	When extracts of hyoscyamus and tannic acid are combined, it forms insoluble precipitates of hyoscymine tannate.	Follow method B for precipitate yielding combination.
Tannic acid	1.5 ml		
Lard	12 gm		

Type: Alkaloids with hydrocarbon

Atropine sulp.	0.065 gm	Atropine sulfate is nearly insoluble in fixed oils.	The free alkaloid is soluble in about 38 parts of olive oil, and this is what should be used in filling this prescription.
Olive oil	4 ml		
Apply with friction			

Type: Incompatibility of purine base

Caffeine citrate	1 gm	Here, there will be a decomposition between the citrated caffeine and the strontium bromide, with the formation of strontium citrate, which is insoluble in water and precipitates.	Follow method B for precipitate yielding combination. Effervescent citrated caffeine is hygroscopic and should be dispensed in well-stoppered bottles only.
Sodium bromide	3.0 gm		
Stro. bro.	1.0 gm		
Aquae foeni.	15 ml		
3 teaspoonfuls every three hours.			

contd...

4.6: Examples of some important chemical incompatibilities, their causes and method of correction (*contd.*)

Type: Incompatibility of pyrazolone derivatives

Mer. chloride	0.24 gm	The mercuric chloride and potassium iodide precipitate the alkaloids of both the cinchona and the nux vomica.	The above prescription is a bad combination, and it is advisable to refuse to dispense.
Pot. iodide	3.8 gm		
Fer. amm. cit.	1.5 gm		
Tr. nux vomica	3.5 ml		
Tincture compound cinchona q.s	100 ml		

Type: Soluble salicylate incompatibilities

Antipyrine	3.8 gm	Antipyrine and sodium salicylate should not be prescribed in powder form, as liquefaction often occurs.	Mixed with an adsorbent like magnesium carbonate or kaolin to produce free flowing powder and filled in suitable container.
Sodium salicylate	12 gm		
Make a powder			

Type: Incompatibility of soluble salicylates and benzoates with acidic drugs

Sodium salicylate	12 gm	The citric acid contained in the syrup of lemon will decompose a portion of the sodium salicylate, crystals of salicylic acid floating in the mixture.	The prescription should be dispensed with a shake label.
Lemon syrup	6 ml		
Water q.s	20 ml		

Type: Soluble salicylates with ferric salt

Ferric chl. sol.	2 ml	Ferric chloride reacts with sodium salicylate to form ferric salicylate which gets separated as indiffusible precipitates.	Therefore follow method B for precipitate yielding interactions.
Sodium salicylate	3 g		
Water make up to	90 ml		

Type: Soluble iodides incompatibilities

Ferr. chl. sol.	1.5 ml	Ferric chloride solution reacts with potassium iodide to liberate free iodine.	To prevent the liberation of iodine, ferric chloride is converted into organic compound before addition of KI.
Pot. iodide	3 gm		
Pot. citrate	6 gm		
Water q.s	90 ml		

Type: Incompatibility causing evolution of carbon dioxide gas

Sodium bicar.	1.0 gm	When sodium bicarbonate, borax and glycerin mixed together in the presence of water, a reaction takes place with the evolution of carbon dioxide.	Therefore, mix these ingredients in an open vessel until evolution of carbon dioxide ceases.
Borax	1.0 gm		
Phenol	0.5 gm		
Glycerin	20 ml		
Water	90 ml		

Type: Incompatibility of phenolic drugs with ferric ions

Sodium salicylate	50 gm	Phenolic drugs as salicylates, react with ferric ions (present in water or other chemicals) to give a violet green color.	It is prevented by the addition of ions such as tartrate or citrate which complex with ferric ions.
Chloroform water (double strength)	500 ml		
Water to	1000 ml		

contd...

4.6: Examples of some important chemical incompatibilities, their causes and method of correction (*contd.*)

Type: Incompatibility related to explosive compounds

Pota.chlorate	0.6 gm	When prescribed compounds mixed together, there are chances of explosion.	Mix them on a sheet of paper in ascending order with a bone spatula without any friction or dispense each ingredient separately with appropriate direction.
Tannic acid	0.3 gm		
Sucrose	0.3 gm		
Water	20 ml		

Type: Amino acids incompatibility

Pepsin	0.36 gm	Pepsin gets deactivated in presence of alkalies.	The prescription may be referred back to the physician for necessary changes.
Sodium bicar.	3.8 gm		
Make a powder			
One t.i.d. after meals.			

Type: Incompatibility of quaternary ammonium compound

Cetrimide	3.8 gm	The interaction occurs upon mixing anionic surfactants with cationic surfactants. This may be manifested, visually, as turbidity or formation of a precipitate. The surface activity of both materials will be drastically reduced. This occurs upon mixing soap with cetrimide.	The prescription may be referred back to the physician for necessary changes.
Soap	3.8 gm		
Cotton seed oil	30 ml		
Water	30 ml		
Apply with friction			

Type: Glycosides incompatibility

Tr. of ferric chloride	4 ml	Tannic acid in the digitalis combining with the iron to form black precipitate of iron tannate.	It is best to mix the tincture of iron with the other ingredients, and add the tincture of digitalis last.
Tincture of digitalis	3 ml		
Glycerin	12 ml		
Water	12 ml		

Type: Carbohydrates incompatibility

Borax	1.2 gm	Borax reacts with aqueous solution of acacia results indiffusible gelatinous precipitate of acacia which will make the mixture altogether unpresentable.	There is no way to overcome the difficulty. It is an instance of true incompatibility.
Pulverized acacia	1.2 gm		
Rose water	150 ml		
For external use.			

Type: Incompatibility anesthetics

Alypin	0.35 gm	Silver nitrate is reduced to silver oxide. Which comes out of the mixture as indiffusible precipitate.	If alypin is replaced by alypin chloride, with silver nitrate form alypin nitrate and silver chloride. That avoids the reduction and precipitation of the silver nitrate to silver oxide.
Silver nitrate	0.12 gm		
Water	15 ml		
Use as injection			

Type: Incompatibility of dyes

Acriflavine	30 ml	The chlorine in Dakin's solution reacts with acriflavine, changing the color of the solution.	Acriflavine should be dispensed in 1:1000 solution without Dakin's solution.
Dakin's sol. q.s	120 ml		

contd...

4.6: Examples of some important chemical incompatibilities, their causes and method of correction (*contd.*)			
Type: Incompatibility of surface active agents			
Phenol	0.5 gm	The free acid in olive oil form	The prescription should be
Menthol	0.1 gm	divalent soap with lime water.	referred back to the prescriber
Tragacanth	0.5 gm	The divalent soap promote w/o	either to replace lime water with
Olive oil	50 ml	emulsion, whereas with tragacanth	water or omit tragacanth.
Lime water	100 ml	o/w emulsion is formed.	

THERAPEUTIC INCOMPATIBILITIES

Substances are said to be therapeutically incompatible when their action on the human system is mutually antagonistic; the pharmacist does not spend much time over this class. With the exception of rectifying a lethal dose, therapeutic incompatibilities are often intentional. Therapeutic incompatibility results due to the following reasons:

- Error in dosage
- Wrong dose or dosage form
- Contraindicated drugs
- Synergistic and antagonistic drugs
- Drug interactions.

Error in Dosage

Prescription error most commonly arises when a drug or dosage error is made either in prescribing or compounding. They sometimes occur if the physician makes an error in writing the prescription which the pharmacist fails to recognize or correct. Occasionally, pharmacist may interpret the prescription or label it incorrectly. One of the most common errors is the result of mistaking or misspelling the name of manufactured product or in writing it so illegibly that the wrong product is dispensed.

Example 1:	
Strychnine sulfate	0.02 gm
Iron or ammonium citrate	0.5 gm
Make capsule	

This prescription calls for a 10 times over dose of strychnine and probably represents a decimal point error. The physician intended to prescribe 0.002 gm but misplaced the decimal. He should call for permission to change the dose.

Wrong Dose or Dosage form

There are certain drugs which have similar names and there is always a danger of dispensing the wrong dose, e.g. prednisone and prednisolone, digoxin and digitoxin. Sometimes the prescription dosage exceeds the permitted daily dose given on label or in official references.

Example 2:	
Codeine phosphate	15 mg
Ammonium chloride	500 mg
Two caps q, h for cough	

This represensts an improper frequency of dosage of codeine. The USP recommends the prescribed dose every four hours. The prescriber intended to write q.4hr for cough and should be consulted.

Contraindicated Drugs

There are certain drugs which may be contra-indicated in a particular disease or a particular patient who is allergic to it. For example, corticosteroids are contraindicated in patients with active peptic ulcer. The penicillin and sulfa drugs are contraindicated for allergic patients.

Example 3:	
Sulfadiazine	250 mg
Sulfamerazine	250 mg
Ammonium chloride	500 mg
Take two capsules after every 6 hours	

Ammonium chloride is a urinary acidifier. It would cause deposition of sulfonamide in crystal in the kidney. Hence, the prescription should be referred back to the physician.

Synergistic and Antagonistic Drugs

Drugs with same pharmacological actions are prescribed together, near their full or maximum individual dose. Drugs of such combinations usually should be prescribed in reduced amounts since the sum of their therapeutic activity may be too great. This is especially true if the combination is additive or synergetic. The combined action greater than normal would be expected.

Prescriptions with more than one ingredient may sometimes produce both rapid and prolong action, if a rapid acting drug is prescribed with a drug having prolong action, e.g. combination of procaine penicillin and penicillin.

If the full doses of two antagonistic drugs are prescribed together, it is possible that the resulting prescription will have no therapeutic action. The prescribing of stimulants with sedative, demulcents with irritants, purgatives with antidiarrheal or emetics with antiemetics.

Example 4:	
Acetyl salicylic acid	0.6 gm
Probencid	0.5 gm

Acetyl salicylic acid and probenecid are used in the treatment of gout. However, the combination of these leads to neutralization. So refer back to the physician for necessary correction.

Drug Interactions

The effect of one drug is altered by the prior or administration of another drug. The drug interactions can usually be corrected by the proper adjustment of dosage, if the suspected interaction is detected.

Example 5:	
Tetracycline hydrochloride	250 mg
Take one capsule every six hours with milk.	

Tetracycline is inactivated by calcium present in the milk. So tetracycline should not be taken with milk. In this prescription, the therapeutic incompatibility is unintentional. So the prescription may be referred back to the physician to change the direction.

Contraindication for Drugs in their Secondary Action

- **Apocynum cannabinum:** Contraindicated in anemia when the pulse is full and strong.
- **Bromide of potassium:** Contraindicated in pale, anemic people.
- **Cactus grandiflor us:** Contraindicated in increased arterial tension, exaltation of nerve force and excess of strength in heart action.
- **California laurel (Umbellularia Californica):** Contraindicated in active inflammation of the intestinal tract and stomach.
- **Capsicum:** Contraindicated in fevers, inflammation, recent cases of hemorrhoids and where there is marked burning, sensation in the rectum.
- **Chloral hydrate:** Contraindicated where there is marked depression, cerebral anemia, in weak heart, especially in alcoholism.
- **Cinnamomum:** Contraindicated in all gastro-intestinal tract inflammation.
- **Colchicum:** Contraindicated in great debility, profuse diarrhea, asthenic form of gout.
- **Colocynthis:** Contraindicated in fever and inflammation.
- **Conium:** Contraindicated in debility.
- **Convallaria majalis:** Will not agree when tongue is clean and red or there are red edges on tongue showing irritation. Useful

where there is a heavy coated tongue, pale and flabby. Do not use when tongue shows irritation of the digestive organs. Also in fatty degeneration of the heart.

- **Copaiba:** Contraindicated in inflammatory stage of gonorrhea with great irritation and profuse discharge. In some cases, not to be used at all.

- **Elaterium:** Contraindicated in cases of debility and in acute intestinal inflammation.

- **Emetics:** Contraindicated, as a rule, where there is marked determination of blood to the brain. In apoplexy, cerebral congestion, pregnancy, hernia, aneurism or some other defect of the circulatory apparatus. In marked gastro-intestinal irritation or inflammation advanced stage of inflammatory fever and in cases of marked debility.

- **Ergot:** Contraindicated as a parturient when os is hard and rigid; when there is an obstruction of the soft parts or excessive debility.

- **Epsom salts:** Contraindicated in great debility brought on by old age or wasting disease. Do not use in cholera. Dangerous to use when suffering from chills.

- **Ferric acetate:** Contraindicated in gastric catarrh.

- **Fowler's solution:** Contraindicated when there is irritability of the sympathetic and nerve centers.

- **Galium:** Contraindicated in disease of a passive nature on account of its refrigerant and sedative effects on the system.

- **Gelsemium:** Contraindicated when eyes are dull, pupils dilated and circulation feeble. Under these circumstances, it is poison even in small doses.

- **Guaiac:** Contraindicated in fever or vascular excitement.

- **Ipecac:** Contraindicated in nausea from organic disease of the stomach.

- **Jaborandi:** Contraindicated when pulse is weak; weak heart. Never give in large doses unless specially indicated; it may cause diarrhea and other disagreeable symptoms. Always be careful in giving it when the heart is feeble.

- **Juniperus:** Contraindicated in inflammatory conditions of the urinary tract.

- **Lobelia:** Contraindicated in general relaxation, in dyspnea from fatty or enlarged heart or enfeebled heart with valvular incompetence.

- **Myrrh:** Contraindicated in fever and inflammation.

- **Opium:** Contraindicated where there is congestion or a tendency to congestion. When there are kidney affections or when face is flushed, contracted pupils, pulse full and bounding, tongue red and turgid, eyes blood-shot, pain in head with wild delirium, in such cases it may kill and will always do harm. In dry skin, dry and dirty tongue and where there is a lack of secretion.

- **Origanum:** Contraindicated in active inflam-mation.

- **Passiflora:** Contraindicated when tongue is dirty and heavily coated. In insomnia with flushed face and determination of blood to the brain. In such cases, gelsemium is useful.

- **Peppermint:** Contraindicated where there is pain or pressure on the stomach, inflammation of the gastrointestinal tract indicated by dry, possibly contracted tongue, with red edges and tip.

- **Pichi:** Contraindicated in structural degeneration of the kidneys. In Bright's disease.

- **Podophyllum:** Contraindicated when pulse is small and wiry; also where there is irritation of the intestinal tract.

- **Potassium acetate:** Will not act well when tongue is red and pointed.

- **Potassium iodide:** Contraindicated when tongue is red and pointed.
- **Pulsatilla:** Contraindicated in fevers, inflammation and determination of blood to the head.
- **Quinia:** Contraindicated when pulse is hard, vibratile, wiry. If skin and tongue are dry, it will not give good results. If stomach is alkaline, it will not be absorbed. Here, it should not be given or else preceded by acid or lemonade.
- **Rochelle salts:** Contraindicated when there are deposits of phosphates in the urine.
- **Rhus aromatica:** Contraindicated in active inflammation. Use in glycerin and not in water.
- **Salicylic acid:** Contraindicated when tongue is red and pointed.
- **Santal oil:** Contraindicated in gonorrhea, if there is swelling of the testes.
- **Savine:** Contraindicated in active inflammation.
- **Scammonium:** Contraindicated in debility and inflammation.
- **Senega:** Contraindicated in fevers.
- **Serpentaria:** Contraindicated in asthenic conditions.
- **Spotted spurge:** Contraindicated in acute diarrhea or dysentery.
- **Squill:** Contraindicated in inflammation of the urinary organs and fevers.
- **Strophanthus:** Contraindicated in any circulatory and respiratory troubles of vasomotor origin. In active hyperemia, also in tendency to visceral hemorrhage. In ascites of tumors, hepatic, splenic and pelvic.
- **Sulfur:** Contraindicated in fevers and inflammation.
- **Thuja:** Contraindicated in inflammation of the urinary tract.
- **Turpentine:** Contraindicated in all active inflammatory conditions of the urinary organs.
- **Veratrum viride:** Contraindicated where inflammation has resulted in marked structural changes. In asthenic cases and where there is irritation of the stomach.
- **Zingiber:** Contraindicated in any inflammation, especially of the gastrointestinal tract.
- **Zinc sulfate:** Contraindicated, if irritant poisons have been taken.

Doses Variation at Different Ages

From 20 to 45 years adult doses are given; 50 years 5/6; 60 years 4/5; 80 years 2/3 of adult doses.

Doses for children under 12 years: The dose of most medicines must be diminished in proportion of the age, to the age increased by 12. Thus at 4 years the dose will be 1/4 of that of adults, viz.: 4/4+12=4/16 or 1/4; at 6 years it will be 6/6+12=6/18 or 1/3. Narcotics use even less than above, especially in infants.

Hypodermic injections: As a rule, hypodermic injections should be about 1/2 of that by mouth. By rectum about 4/5 of that by mouth.

Comparison of doses: Approximately, a drop corresponds with a minim; a teaspoonful with a fluid drachm; a dessert spoonful with 3 fluid drachms; a tablespoonful with 1/2 ounce; a wineglassful to 2 ounces; a tea cupful with a gill or 4 fluid ounces.

Solutions: Rules in regard to making solutions. Taking 1 grain as a base of 1% solution; we mean 1 grain of drug or 1 drop of a drug to 100 drops of water. Therefore, 1:1000 would mean 1/10 of a grain or minim to 100 drops of water, etc.

Table 4.7: Examples of some therapeutic incompatibilities, their causes and method of corrections

Formula	Reason for incompatibility	Correction
Type: Error in dosage		
Strychnine sulfate 0.02 gm Iron or amm. cit. 0.5 gm Make capsule.	This prescription calls for a 10 times over dose of strychinine and probably represents a decimal point error.	The physician intended to prescribe 0.002 gm but misplaced the decimal. He should call for permission to change the dose.
Type: Wrong dose or dosage form		
Codeine phosphate 15 mg Amm. chloride 500 mg Two capsuls q.h for cough.	This represents an improper frequency of dosage of codeine. The USP recommends the prescribed dose every four hours.	The prescriber intended to write q.4hr for cough and should be consulted.
Type: Contraindicated drug		
Sulfadiazine 250 mg Sulfamerazine 250 mg Amm. chloride 500 mg Take two capsules after every 6 hours.	Ammonium chloride is a urinary acidifier. It would cause deposition of sulfonamide in crystal in the kidney.	Hence the prescription should be referred back to the physician.
Type: Synergistic and antagonistic drugs		
Acetyl sal. acid 0.6 gm Probencid 0.5 gm	Acetyl salicylic acid and probenecid in the combination leads to neutralization.	This prescription should refer back to the physician for necessary correction.
Type: Drug interactions		
Tetracy. hy.chlo. 250 mg Take one capsule every six hours with milk.	Tetracycline is inactivated by calcium present in the milk.	Tetracycline should not be taken with milk.

Table 4.8: Summary of common incompatibilities and recommended corrections

Types	Therapeutic	Physical				Chemical			
Recommended procedure	Over or under dose, wrong dose	Insolubility	Precipitation	Immiscibility	Liquefaction	Precipitation	Effervescence	Color change	Production of toxic agents
Consult physician	♠	♣	♣	♣	♣	♥	♥	♠	♠
Use special pharmaceutical techniques.									
Modify order of mixing ♦	♣	♠	♠	♠	♣	♥	♣	♠	♣
Dispense with "shake well" label ♦	♣	♥	♥	♥	♣	♥	♣	♣	♣

contd...

Table 4.8: Summary of common incompatibilities and recommended corrections (*contd.*)

Types	Therapeutic	Physical				Chemical			
Recommended procedure	Over or under dose, wrong dose	Insolubility	Precipitation	Immiscibility	Liquefaction	Precipitation	Effervescence	Color change	Production of toxic agents
Dispense with "store in refrigerator" label ♦	♣	♣	♣	♣	♣	♣	♣	♠	♣
Allow to react than package ♦	♣	♣	♥	♣	♥	♣	♥	♥	♣
Protect from air, light and moisture ♦	♣	♣	♣	♣	♥	♣	♥	♥	♣
Addition of an ingredient (C)									
Add suspending agent ♦	♣	♥	♠	♣	♣	♥	♣	♣	♣
Add emulsifying agent ♦	♣	♥	♣	♠	♣	♥	♣	♣	♣
Add solubuliser or miscibility agent	♣	♠	♥	♥	♣	♥	♣	♣	♣
Add stabilizer ♦	♣	♣	♣	♣	♥	♥	♣	♥	♣
Omission of an ingredient (C)									
Leave out troublesome ingredient	♣	♥	♥	♥	♥	♥	♥	♥	♥
Filter of inactive sediment	♣	♥	♥	♣	♣	♥	♣	♥	♣
Divide into two prescriptions	♣	♥	♥	♥	♥	♥	♥	♥	♣
Change of vehicle (C)									
Increase volume, increase dose	♣	♠	♠	♠	♠	♥	♣	♣	♣
Decrease volume, decrease dose	♣	♠	♠	♠	♣	♥	♣	♣	♣
Change solvent same dose	♣	♠	♠	♠	♣	♥	♣	♣	♣
Change of ingredient (C)									
Use form most compatible with other ingredients ♦	♣	♥	♥	♥	♣	♠	♠	♠	♠

contd..

Types	Therapeutic	Physical				Chemical			
Recommended procedure	Over or under dose, wrong dose	Insolubility	Precipitation	Immiscibility	Liquefaction	Precipitation	Effervescence	Color change	Production of toxic agents
Use form stable in vehicle ♦	♣	♥	♥	♥	♣	♥	♥	♥	♥
Change in dosage form (C)									
Use more suitable dosage form	♣	♥	♥	♥	♥	♥	♥	♥	♥
Use different brand	♣	♥	♥	♥	♥	♥	♥	♥	♥

Table 4.8: Summary of common incompatibilities and recommended corrections (*contd.*)

(C) = consult physicians if therapeutically significant drug or dosage change is required. ♠ = Preferred procedure. ♥ = Acceptable procedure. ♣ = Procedure not applicable. ♦ = Procedure usually not requiring physician approval.

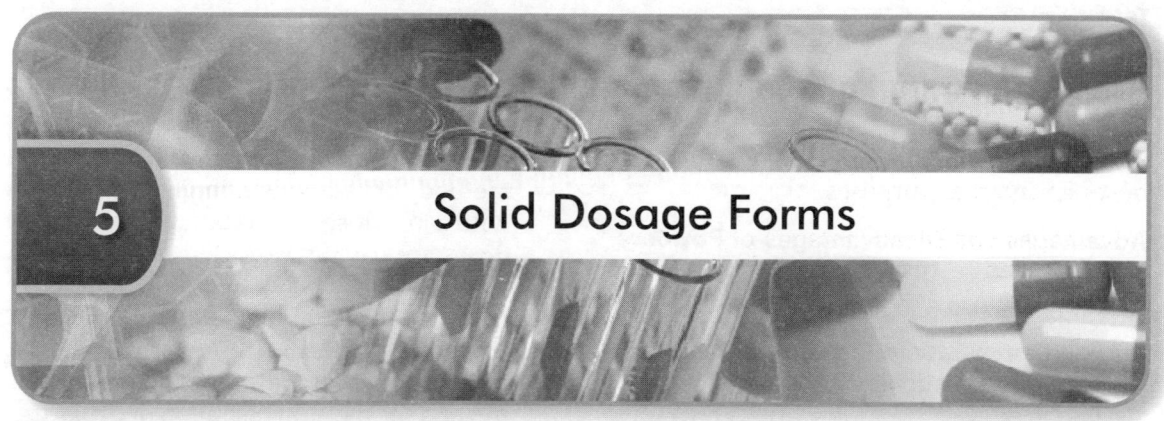

5 Solid Dosage Forms

INTRODUCTION

The solid dosage forms are available mostly in unit dosage forms like tablets, capsules, pills, lozenges or powders. They are stable, effective and patients have no problem in their handling and administration. This chapter focuses on conventional solid dosage forms and is divided into the following three sections:

1. Powders and granules
2. Tablets
3. Capsules

POWDERS AND GRANULES

Powders are solid dosage forms. They are supplied either in the bulk or as unit doses in the fine state of subdivision of active drug or

137

may be a mixture of the active drug and other ingredients. Usually, bulk powders are intended for external applications and unit doses for internal purposes.

Advantages and Disadvantages of Powders and Granules

Advantages

1. Solid preparations are more stable than liquid preparations.
2. Powders and granules are convenient forms to dispense large dose of drugs.
3. Orally administered powders and granules of soluble medicaments have a faster dissolution rate than tablets or capsules, as they must first disintegrate before the drug dissolves.
4. Powders offer a lot of flexibility in compounding solids.
5. Pleasant to use.
6. Absorb skin moisture.
7. Decreasing skin friction.
8. Discouraging bacterial growth.
9. Administered with relative ease.

Disadvantages

1. Bulk powders or granules are far less convenient for patients to carry than a small container of tablets or capsules.
2. The masking of unpleasant tastes may be a problem with this type of preparation.
3. Bulk powders or granules are not a good method of administering potent drugs with a low dose. This is because individual doses are usually extracted from the bulk using a 5 ml spoon, which is subject to variation in spoon fill (e.g. level or heaped spoonfuls).
4. Powders and granules are not a suitable method for the administration of drugs that are inactivated in the stomach; these should be presented as enteric-coated tablets.
5. Powders and granules are not well suited for dispensing hygroscopic or deliquescent drugs.
6. May block pores causing irritation.
7. Possibility of contamination.
8. Light fluffy powders may be inhaled by infants leading to breathing difficulties.
9. Not suitable for application to broken skin.
10. Variable dose accuracy.

Classification of Powders

Powders are broadly classified in three classes (Table 5.1):

1. Bulk powders for internal use.
2. Bulk powders for external use.
3. Divided or unit doses powder.

Table 5.1: Classification of powders		
Type	**Product illustration**	**Description**
1. **Bulk powders for internal use:** They are mixture of finely divided drugs and/or chemicals in a dry form that may be intended for internal use (oral powders).		
Oral powder	 Oral powder for reconstitution	Oral powders are preparations consisting of solid, loose, dry particles of varying degrees of fineness. They contain one or more active substances, with or without excipients and, if necessary, coloring matter authorized by the competent authority and flavoring substances. They are generally administered in or with water or another suitable liquid. They may also be swallowed directly. They are presented as single-dose or multidose preparations. Multidose oral powders require the provision of a measuring device capable of delivering the quantity prescribed. Each dose of a single-dose powder is enclosed in an individual container, e.g. a sachet or a vial.

contd...

Type	Product illustration	Description
Table 5.1: Classification of powders (*contd.*)		
Powder spray	Powder spray	In contrast to dusting powders, powders dispensed under pressure will deliver targeted and uniform application at the desired site. Also, in an aerosol container medicated powders may be maintained in a sterile condition. The powder particles must be in a definite size range to prevent clogging of the valve orifice and to provide uniformity of application. In general, powders that are to be packaged as powder sprays must not contain particles greater than 50 microns, if they are to be sprayed successfully.
Dry-powder inhalers	Dry-powder inhalers	The use of dry-powder systems for pulmonary drug delivery is now extensive. This dosage form has developed into one of the most effective methods of delivering active ingredients to the lung for the treatment of asthma and chronic obstructive pulmonary disease.
Effervescent powders	Effervescent powder in bulk packaging	Effervescent powders are presented as single-dose or multidose preparations and generally contain acid substances and carbonates or hydrogen carbonates which react rapidly in the presence of water to release carbon dioxide. They are intended to be dissolved or dispersed in water before administration.

2. **Bulk powders for external use:** They are mixture of finely divided drugs and/or chemicals in a dry form that may be intended for external use available in multiple doses (dusting powders).

Type	Product illustration	Description
Dusting powders	Dusting powder	Dusting powders contain ingredients used for therapeutic, prophylactic or lubricant purposes and are intended for external use. Only sterile dusting powders should be applied to open wounds. Such preparations should be prepared using materials and methods designed to ensure sterility and to avoid the introduction of contaminants and the growth of microorganisms.
Insufflations	Powder insufflator	Insufflations are extremely fine powders to be introduced into body cavities. To administer an insufflation, the powder is placed in the insufflator, and when the bulb is squeezed, the air current carries the fine particles through the nozzle to the region for which the medication is intended. All extemporaneously compounded insufflations must be passed through a 100 mesh sieve. Pressurized packages provide an elegant approach to the administration of insufflations.

contd...

Type	Product illustration	Description
Dentifrices	Dentifrices powder	Dentifrices may be prepared in the form of a bulk powder, generally are pharmaceutical compound used for cleaning and polishing the teeth. It typically contains a mild abrasive, detergent, flavoring agent, fluoride, and binder. Other common ingredients are deodorants, humectants, desensitizers, and various medications to prevent dental caries.

Table 5.1: Classification of powders (*contd.*)

3. **Divided powder:** Divided powders are similar formulations to bulk powders but individual doses are separately wrapped. Traditionally in papers (unsatisfactory for most products, especially if the ingredients are hygroscopic, volatile or deliquescent). Modern packaging materials of foil and plastic laminates have replaced paper wrapping because they offer superior protective qualities and are amenable to use on high speed packaging machines.

Type	Product illustration	Description
Douche powders	Vaginal douche powder in unit dose	Douche powders are completely soluble and are dissolved in water prior to use as antiseptics or cleansing agents for a body cavity. They most commonly are intended for vaginal use, although they may be formulated for nasal, otic, or ophthalmic use.
Powders for injection	Injectables in unit dose	They may be classified as bulk or divided powders. Injections of drugs that are unstable in solution must be made immediately prior to use and are presented as sterile powders in ampoules. Sterile water for injection is added from a second ampoule and the injection is used immediately. The powder may contain suitable excipients in addition to the drug, e.g. sufficient additive to produce an isotonic solution when the injection is reconstituted.
Effervescent powders	Effervescent powder in unit dose	Effervescent powders are presented as single-dose or multidose preparations and generally contain acid substances and carbonates or hydrogen carbonates which react rapidly in the presence of water to release carbon dioxide. They are intended to be dissolved or dispersed in water before administration.

Size Classification of Powders

Pharmaceutical powders are formulated to be exist as fine particles. The powders are then smooth to the touch and nonirritating to the skin. Powders generally range from 0.1 to 10 micron in size. The size of the particles are often expressed as a number which corresponds to the mesh screen size of a sieve. The screen size indicates the number of openings in the mesh screen per inch. For example, a # 40 sieve has 40 openings per inch in the screen mesh. Particles that can sift through that mesh are said to be "40 mesh" size. Below is a list of mesh sizes and the size of the mesh opening in millimeters (1/1000 of a meter) or microns (1/1,000,000) of a meter. Of course there is a correlation between the size of the mesh opening and the particle size of the sifted powder. As the opening

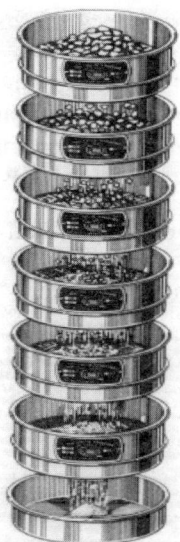

Fig. 5.1: Arrangement of sieves in ascending order from top to bottom

Table 5.2: Mesh opening size of different sieves		
Mesh size number	**Mesh opening size**	
	Millimeters	Micrometers
2	9.52	9520
4	4.76	4760
8	2.38	2380
10	2.00	2000
20	0.84	840
30	0.59	590
40	0.42	420
50	0.297	297
60	0.250	250
70	0.210	210
80	0.177	177
100	0.149	149
120	0.125	125
200	0.074	74

Table 5.3: Classification of powder depending on their size		
Description term	**Mesh opening size (microns)**	**Mesh size number**
Very Coarse	> 1000	2 – 10
Coarse	355 – 1000	20 – 40
Moderately Coarse	180 – 355	40 – 80
Fine	125 – 180	80 – 120
Very Fine	90 – 125	120 – 200

becomes smaller, so will be resulting particle size. Most of the particles of a sifted powder will have approximately the size as the mesh opening. Table 5.2 contains mesh opening size of different sieves. Table 5.3 showing a size classification of powders. According USP, powders are classified into following categories.

1. **Very coarse (no. 8) powder:** All particles pass through a no. 8 sieve (2.38 mm) and not more than 20% pass through a no. 60 sieve.

2. **Coarse (no. 20) powder:** All particles pass through a no. 20 sieve (0.84 mm) and not more than 40% pass through a no. 60 sieve.

3. **Moderately coarse (no. 40) powder:** All particles pass through a no. 40 sieve (0.42 mm) and not more than 40% pass through a no. 80 sieve.

4. **Fine (no. 60) powder:** All particles pass through a no. 60 sieve (0.25 mm) and not more than 40% pass through a no. 100 sieve.

5. **Very fine (no. 80) powder:** All particles pass through a no. 80 sieve (0.18 mm). There is no limit to greater fineness.

The USP 24/NF19 uses descriptive terms to define powder fineness. The Table 5.3 shows the correlation between different grade powders.

A good powder formulation has a uniform particle size distribution. If the particle size distribution is not uniform, the powder can segregate according to the different particle sizes which may result in inaccurate dosing or inconsistent performance. A uniform particle size distribution insures a uniform dissolution rate, if the powder is to dissolve a uniform sedimentation rate, if the powder is used in a suspension, and minimizes stratification when powders are stored or transported. Reducing the particle size of a powder will result in a uniform distribution of particle sizes. The process of reducing the particle size is called comminution.

In extemporaneous compounding, there are three methods of comminution:

1. **Trituration** is the continuous rubbing or grinding of the powder in a mortar with a pestle. This method is used when working with hard, fracturable powders.

2. **Pulverization** by intervention is used with hard crystalline powders that do not crush or triturate easily, or gummy-type substances. The first step is to use an "intervening" solvent (such as alcohol or acetone) that will dissolve the compound. The dissolved powder is then mixed in a mortar or spread on an ointment slab to enhance the evaporation of the solvent. As the solvent evaporates, the powder will recrystallize out of solution as fine particles.

3. **Levigation** reduces the particle size by triturating it in a mortar or spatulating it on an ointment slab or pad with a small amount of a liquid in which the solid is not soluble. The solvent should be somewhat viscous such as mineral oil or glycerin. This method is also used to reduce the particle size of insoluble materials when compounding ointments and suspensions.

Powder Mixing

Powder mixing is an important step in the manufacturing process of pharmaceuticals. Mixing can be described as a combination of three phenomena, namely:

1. **Diffusion** (viz. the motion of a particle with respect to its neighbors);

2. **Convection** (viz. the motion of a group of particles in relation to their neighbors); and

3. **Shearing** (viz. a change of distribution layers of ingredients in space).

Blending is intended to ensure a uniform distribution of all components in the end product. In this way, each sample will contain an appropriate amount of the active components. There are many factors that influence mixing quality such as mixing time, speed of mixing rotation, the type of the mixer, dry or wet mixing process, and so on. Reduction of particle size is often accomplished with the use of a mortar and pestle. Figure 5.2 depicts the three types of mortars and pestles commonly used in pharmaceutical compounding— glass, wedgewood, and ceramic. Large scale powder mixing can be performed with high performances stainless steel mixers and blenders like double cone, V blenders, planetary mixers, IBC tumblers, and high shear: latest mixer can offer a variety of batch mixers ranging from 2 to 2000 liter capacity.

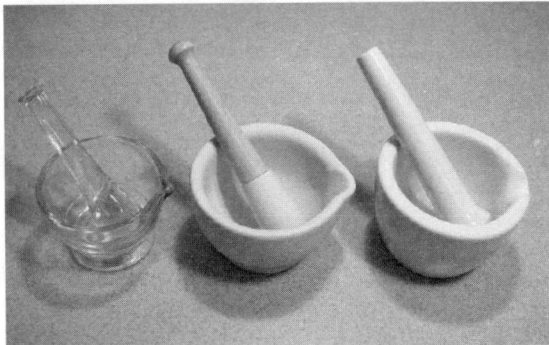

Fig. 5.2: Different types of mortar and pestle used in powder mixing and size reduction

Preparation of Powders
Preparation of dusting powder

Dusting powders are fine medicinal (bulk) powders intended to be dusted on the skin by means of sifter-top containers. A single medicinal agent may be used as a dusting powder; however, a base is frequently used to apply a medicinal agent and to protect the skin from irritation and friction. Bentonite, kaolin, kieselguhr, magnesium carbonate, starch, and talc are used as inert bases for dusting powders. Powder bases absorb secretions and exert a drying effect, which relieves congestion and imparts a cooling sensation. All extemporaneous dusting powders should be passed through a 100–200 mesh sieve to ensure that they are grit free and will not further mechanically irritate traumatized areas.

General Method for Preparing Bulk or Dusting Powders

1. Weigh the powder present in the smallest volume (powder A) and place in the mortar.
2. Weigh the powder present in the next largest volume (powder B) and place on labeled weighing paper.
3. Add approximately the same amount of powder B as powder A in the mortar.
4. Mix well with pestle.
5. Continue adding an amount of powder B that is approximately the same as that in the mortar and mix with the pestle, i.e. doubling the amount of powder in the mortar at each addition.
6. If further powders are to be added, add these in increasing order of volume as in parts 3, 4 and 5 above.

Preparation of divided powder

Divided powders or charts are single doses of powdered medicines individually wrapped in cellophane, metallic foil, or paper. The divided powder is a more accurate dosage form than bulk powder because the patient is not involved in measurement of the dose. Cellophane and foil-enclosed powders are better protected from the external environment until the time of administration than paper-enclosed powders. Divided powders are commercially available in foil, cellophane or paper packs. All drugs are reduced to a fine state of subdivision before weighing, the weighed powders are blended by geometric dilution or mixing in ascending order of amount.

General method for producing unit dose powders

1. Remember, for ease of handling the minimum weight of powder in a unit dose paper is 200 mg.
2. Calculate to make an excess of the number of powders requested.
3. Determine whether a single or double dilution of the active ingredient is required.
4. Mix the active ingredient and the diluents in a mortar using the 'doubling-up' technique.
5. Work on a clean dry glass tile. Select a suitable size of paper (e.g. 10 × 10 cm), turn in one edge and fold down.
6. Place the paper on the glass tile, with the folded edge away from the compounder, and each edge slightly overlapping, next to the balance pan to be used for weighing.
7. Weigh out the individual powder from the bulk powder, and transfer to the center of the paper (if placed too near the fold, the powder will fall out during opening).
8. Fold the bottom of the powder paper up to, and underneath, the flap folded originally.
9. Fold down the top of the paper until it covers about two-thirds of the width of the paper. This top edge of this fold should help to hold the contents of the paper in the center of the paper.
10. Fold the two ends under, so that the loose ends slightly overlap, and then tuck one flap inside the other.
11. Wrap each powder in turn, making sure they are all of the same size.
12. Stack the powders in pairs, flap to flap.
13. Tie together with a rubber band (not too tightly).
14. Place in a rigid cardboard box.
15. The label should be placed on the outer pack such that when the patient opens the box, the label is not destroyed.

General Labeling Considerations for Powder and Granules

- Title
- Quantitative particulars (quantitative particulars are not required as the product is official)
- Product-specific cautions (or additional labeling requirements)

- 'For external use only' will need to be added to the label as the product is a dusting powder for external use or as directed.
- 'Store in a dry place' will need to be added to the label as the product is a powder.
- 'Not to be applied to open wounds or raw weeping surfaces' will need to be added to the label as the product is a dusting powder.
- Discard date.
- The name and address of the pharmacy and the words 'Keep out of the reach of children' are pre-printed on the label.
- The directions for use of the oral powder.
- The conditions under which the oral powder should be stored.

Example 1: Dusting powder

Ingredients	Quantity
Camphor	0.1 gm
Starch	0.6 gm
Zinc	0.3 gm

Method
1. Weigh the camphor and try to pulverize in the mortar with pestle.
2. Add few drops of alcohol and pulverize.
3. Mix starch and zinc oxide and gradually add to camphor while trituration until uniformity.
4. Pass through 90-mesh sieve.

Storage: Store in an airtight container and in a dry and cool place.

Use: Counter irritant

Example 2: Gregory powder, compound BP

Ingredients	Quantity
Heavy magnesium carbonate	325 gm
Light magnesium carbonate	325 gm
Rhubarb, in powder	250 gm
Ginger, in powder	100 gm

Method
1. Remember to incorporate the powder in order of bulk, adding at each addition, a quantity that approximately doubles the bulk already in the mortar.
2. Use a mortar that comfortably holds all of the mixture and do not grind too vigorously because heavily rubbed powders become compacted and less easily miscible with water.
3. Although, normally each ingredient should not be weighed until it is required, it may be necessary, until familiarity with the bulks of common medicaments has been acquired, to weigh the entire ingredient first, so that, the relative and total bulks can be estimated and the order of mixing and size of mortar determined.
4. Occasionally, loosen the powder from the bottom of the mortar and scrape it from the sides. To scrape quickly, use a large flexible spatula. Shape it to the side of the mortar and move it in a clockwise direction repeat after moving the mortar anti-clockwise.
5. Light magnesium carbonate was added to the mixture after passing through 250 sieves.

Storage: Store in an airtight container and in a dry and cool place.

Use: Rhubarb increases the flow of saliva when chewed and acts as a stomachic in atonic dyspepsia. Large doses are purgative; they increase peristalsis without producing inflammation of the intestines.

Example 3: Six seidlitz powder, compound BP

Ingredients	Quantity
Sodium potassium tartrate	7.5 gm
Sodium bicarbonate	2.5 gm

Method
1. As sodium tartrate and sodium bicarbonate are both hygroscopic in nature, it is advisable to double-wrap both powders, using an inner wrapper of waxed paper.

2. Normal powder folders are too small for the no. 1 powder. After stage 2 of the wrapping procedure, invert the packet and turn each end back over the edge of a large spatula.

3. Although no. 2 powder is much smaller, it is neater to make both packets of the same size.

4. When staking, the pair's should consist of a no. 1 and a no. 2 powder. The normal type of powder box is not big enough for these powders.

Storage: Stored in an airtight container and in a dry and cool place.

Use: Laxative

Example 4: Chlorhexidine dusting powder (BP, 1988)	
Ingredients	Quantity
Chlorhexidine dusting powder	5 g
Sterilizable maize starch Sufficient to produce	1000 g

Method

Triturate the chlorhexidine hydrochloride with the sterilizable maize starch, pass the powder through a sieve of suitable mesh size (250 µm may be available), distribute the sieved powder in quantities not greater than 30 g in suitable containers and heat the containers so that the whole of contents is maintained at 150°C to 155°C for one hour.

Storage: Dusting powder should be kept in a wide-mouthed airtight container.

Use: Antimicrobial

Example 5: Talc dusting powder (BP, 1988)	
Ingredients	Quantity
Starch, in powder	100 g
Purified talc, sterilized	900 g

Method

Triturate the starch with the purified talc, and pass the powder through a sieve of suitable mesh size (250 µm may be suitable). The purified talc may be sterilized by heating at a temperature not less than 160°C for not less than 1 hr; alternatively, the final product may be subjected to a suitable sterilization procedure.

Storage: Powder should be kept in a wide-mouthed airtight container.

Use: Use as directed.

Example 6: Dover's powder (Ipecacuanha and opium powder) (IP 1966)	
Ingredients	Quantity
Prepared ipecacuanha	100 g
Powder opium	100 g
Lactose finely powder	800 g

Method

1. Prepared ipecacuanha is ipecacuanha reduced to fine powder and adjust either by admixture in suitable proportion of powdered exhausted ipecacuanha or by the addition of powdered lactose to contain 2.0% of the total alkaloids of ipecacuanha.

2. Finally mix all the ingredients.

Storage: Preserve ipecacuanha and opium powder in a well-closed container.

Use: Antipyretic

Example 7: Gregory's powder (IP 1966)	
Ingredients	Quantity
Rhubarb finely powdered	250 g
Light magnesium carbonate	325 g
Heavy magnesium carbonate	325 g
Ginger finely powdered	100 g

Method: Mix the above stated ingredients.

Storage: Preserve rhubarb compound powder in well-closed container, protect from light.

Use: Purgative.

Example 8: Divided powder	
Ingredients	**Quantity**
Magnesium trisilicate	0.2 gm
Tribasic calcium phosphate	100 gm
Activated charcoal	0.2 gm

Method

1. Mix the ingredients to full homogeneity.
2. Divided as mentioned above (by weighing).
3. Fill in packets as follows:
   a. Fold down 1 cm margin from the weighing paper.
   b. Distribute the divided dose over the paper.
   c. From left fold the lower end of the paper until it lies exactly in the crease of the original top fold.
   d. Make additional fold.
   e. Bring the two ends to each other dividing the paper to three equal part.

Storage: Store in an airtight container and in a dry and cool place.

Use: Antacid, antiflatulent.

GRANULES

Granules are particles ranging in size from about 4 to 10 mesh. Granules generally are made by first blending the powders together and then moistening the mixture to form a pasty mass. The mass is passed through a sieve and then dried in air or in an oven. They are prepared as a convenience for packaging, as a more stable product due to less surface exposure and as a popular dosage form. Granulations are also used as intermediates in the preparation of capsules and tablets, since they flow more smoothly and predictably than do small powder particles. The most popular compounded granulation is the effervescent powder (sometimes called effervescent salts). These granulations are popular due to their taste and psychological impression. When added to water, the granules produce effervesces of carbon dioxide.

Advantages and Disadvantages of Granules

Advantages

1. Granules are more flowable compared to powders.
2. Segregation of the constituents of the powder mixture could be avoided by granulation. Segregation occurs due to difference in particle size or densities.
3. Granules are more stable against humidity and atmosphere and less likely to make cake or harden upon standing. (Due to less exposed surface area compared to powders.)
4. Granules are more easily wetted by liquids than light and fluffy powders (which tend to float on the surface).
5. Granules are more preferable for dry products intended to be constituted into solution or suspension (mostly antibiotics for stability reasons).

Disadvantages

1. The masking of unpleasant tastes may be a problem with this type of preparation.
2. Granules are not a good method of administering potent drugs with a low dose.
3. Granules are not a suitable method for the administration of drugs that are inactivated in the stomach.
4. Instability in presence of moisture.
5. Problems in packaging and storage.

Classification of Granules

Several categories of granules may be distinguished (Table 5.4):
1. Effervescent granules
2. Coated granules
3. Gastro-resistant granules
4. Modified-release granules.

General Method for Producing Granules

1. Mix the ingredients taking great care to distribute the dye evenly, if any.
2. Add purified water, in small amounts, until the powder becomes coherent. If the

Table 5.4: Classification of granules

Type	Product illustration	Description
Effervescent granules		Effervescent granules are uncoated granules generally containing acid substances and carbonates or hydrogen carbonates which react rapidly in the presence of water to release carbon dioxide. They are intended to be dissolved or dispersed in water before administration.
Coated granules		Coated granules are usually multidose preparations and consist of granules coated with one or more layers of mixtures of various excipients. The substances used as coatings are usually applied as a solution or suspension in conditions in which evaporation of the vehicle occurs.
Gastro-resistant granules		Gastro-resistant granules are delayed-release granules that are intended to resist the gastric fluid and to release the active substance(s) in the intestinal fluid. These properties are achieved by covering the granules with a gastro-resistant material (enteric-coated granules) or by other suitable means.
Modified-release granules		Modified-release granules are coated or uncoated granules which contain special excipients or which are prepared by special procedures, or both, designed to modify the rate, the place or the time at which the active substance or substances are released. Modified-release granules include prolonged-release granules and delayed-release granules.

mass is too wet the granules will be too large; if it is too dry there will be too much loose powder.

3. Place a sieve having 280 μm mesh size over a sieve having 710 μm mesh size and press the mixture through the top sieve with a flat scoop or a spatula. Fine granules and powder fall through the lower sieve leaving practically uniform granules on its surface.

4. Spread the powder thinly on a large tray or grease proof paper and dry at not more than 60°C in a drying oven.

Example 1: Methylcellulose granules BP

Ingredients	Quantity
Methylcellulose 2500, in powder, or methylcellulose 4500, in powder	64 g
Amaranth, food grade of commerce	20 mg
Saccharin sodium	100 mg
Vanillin	200 mg
Acacia, in powder	4 g
Lactose	Sufficient to produce 1000 g

Method

1. Mix the ingredients taking great care to distribute the dye evenly.
2. Add purified water, in small amounts, until the powder becomes coherent.
3. Pass the damp mass through sieve no. 10 to obtained granales of uniform size. The size distribution of the granules largely depends on the physical property of the paste it should be neither too soft nor too dry.
4. Spread the powder thinly on a large tray of white demy or grease proof paper and dry at not more than 60°C in a drying oven.

Storage: Methylcellulose granules should be kept in a wide-mouthed airtight container.

Usual dose range and use: As a laxative, 1 to 4 g daily.

Effervescent Granules

They are granules of drug in a dry mixture usually composed of sodium bicarbonate, citric acid and tartaric acid, when added to water, the acids and the base react to liberate CO_2, resulting in effervescence. A combination of tartaric acid and citric acid is used as an effervescent base rather than either acid alone, because when tartaric acid is used alone, chalky friable granules are produced, and citric acid alone results in sticky mixture too difficult to granulate.

Advantages and Disadvantages of Effervescent Granules

Advantages

1. Attractive dosage form for the public.
2. The carbonated solution masks undesirable taste of the drug.
3. The liberated CO_2 gas is used as a therapeutic agent; it increases gastric secretions and hence facilitates digestion, and it acts as antinauseant.
4. Using granules rather than powders decreases the rate of solution and prevents uncontrollable effervescence.

Disadvantages

1. Instability in presence of moisture.
2. Problems in packaging and storage.
3. It is important to protect effervescent granules from moisture during manufacture and storage to prevent premature reaction between acid and base.

Methods of Preparation of Effervescent Granules

There are two methods of preparation of effervescent granules:

1. Dry fusion method
2. Wet method

1. Dry Fusion Method

- In the fusion, one molecule of water present in each molecule of citric acid acts as the binding agent for the powder mixture.
- After weighing the required amount of powders, they are mixed together to ensure the uniformity of the mixture.
- Then the powder is placed on a porcelain dish on boiling water bath and stirred with the help of a glass rod. The heat causes the release of the water of crystallization from the citric acid which in turn dissolves a portion of the powder mixture, setting of the chemical reaction and the consequent release of some carbon dioxide. This causes the softened mass of powder to become somewhat spongy.
- When of the proper consistency as bread dough, it is removed from the oven and rubbed through an acid resistant sieve to produce granules, are dried at temperature not more than 54–60°C and transferred to containers which are then promptly and tightly sealed.

❖ The fused method is used in the preparation of most commercial effervescent powder.

2. Wet Method

1. All powders are dried to constant weight at temperature 100–105°C.

2. Pulverize each powder through sieve no.90 and weigh the calculated amount separately.

3. Pass the pulverized powder through sieve no. 90 and weigh the calculated amount from each powder separately.

4. Mix the powder together and by the aid of alcohol 96% (drop adding) make the mass coherent between your fingers and the mixing is continued until the mass will retain its shape when moulded into a ball.

5. The mass is forced through sieve no. 10 then dry in ovens at temperature not exceeding 50°C.

6. After drying the granules sieved through sieve no. 20 to leave the fine particles, and packed in well closed wide mouth bottles.

Example 2: Sodium citrate and tartrate BPC	
Ingredients	Quantity
Sodium bicarbonate	510 gm
Tartaric acid	270 gm
Citric acid	180 gm
Sucrose	150 gm

Method

1. Calculate for slight excess due to the mechanical loss (loss arised from handling the materials and during the preparation) and the chemical loss (arised from liberation of CO_2 and H_2O, the chemical loss nearly equals to 1/7 formula).

2. It has been found that citric acid monohydrate and tartaric acid used in the ratio of 1:2, respectively, produces a powder with good effervescent properties. Citric acid monohydrate is not used alone because it results in a sticky mixture that will not easily granulate. Tartaric acid is not used alone because the granules are too friable and crumble. The amount of sodium bicarbonate to be used may be calculated from the reaction which occurs when the granules come in contact with water.

Storage: Effervescent granules should be kept in an airtight container.

Usual dose range and use: As an antacid.

Packaging of Powders and Granules

Oral powders may be dispensed in doses premeasured by the pharmacist, that is, divided powders or in bulk.

- Traditionally, divided powders have been wrapped in materials such as bond paper and parchment. However, the pharmacist may provide greater protection from the environment by scaling individual doses in small cellophane or polyethylene envelopes.

- Divided powders are dispensed in the form of individual doses and generally are dispensed in papers, properly folded.

- They also may be dispensed in metal foil, small heat-sealed plastic bags, or other containers.

- Hygroscopic and volatile drugs can be protected best by using a waxed paper, double-wrapped with a bond paper to improve the appearance of the completed powder. Parchment and glassine papers offer limited protection for these drugs.

TABLETS

A tablet is a pharmaceutical dosage form. It comprises a mixture of active substances and excipients, usually in powder form, pressed or compacted from a powder into a solid dose. The excipients can include diluents, binders or granulating agents, glidants (flow aids) and lubricants to ensure efficient tabletting; disintegrants to promote tablet break-up in the digestive tract; sweeteners or flavors to enhance taste and pigments to make the tablets visually attractive. A polymer coating is often applied to make the tablet smoother and easier to swallow, to control the release rate of the active ingredient, to make it more resistant to the environment (extending its shelf life), or to enhance the tablet's appearance.

Ideal Properties of Tablets

1. **Therapeutic compliance:** Optimal drug dissolution and hence, availability from the dosage form for absorption.

   Consistent with intended use (i.e. immediate or extended release).
2. **Accuracy and uniformity of drug content**: Stability, including the stability of the drug substance, the overall tablet formulation, disintegration and the rate and extent of drug dissolution from the tablet for an extended period.
3. **Patient acceptability**: As much as possible, the finished product should have an attractive appearance, including color, size, taste, etc. as applicable, in order to maximize patent acceptability and encourage compliance with the prescribed dosing regimen.
4. **Manufacturability**: The formulation design should allow for the efficient, cost-effective, practical production of the required batches.

Advantages and Disadvantages of Compressed Tablets

Advantages

1. A wide range of tablet types are available, offering a range of drug release rates and durations of clinical effect. Tablets may be formulated to offer rapid drug release or controlled drug release.
2. Tablets may be formulated to release the therapeutic agent at a particular site within the gastrointestinal tract to reduce side effects, promote absorption at that site

and provide a local effect (e.g. ulcerative colitis). This may not be easily achieved by other dosage forms that are administered orally.
3. Tablets may be formulated to contain more than one therapeutic agent (even if there is a physical or chemical incompatibility between each active agent). Moreover, the release of each therapeutic agent may be effectively controlled by the tablet formulation and design.
4. With the exception of proteins, all classes of therapeutic agents may be administered orally in the form of tablets.
5. It is easier to mask the taste of bitter drugs using tablets than for other dosage forms, e.g. liquids.
6. Tablets are generally an inexpensive dosage form.
7. Tablets may be easily manufactured to show product identification, e.g. exhibiting the required markings on the surface.
8. The chemical, physical and microbiological stability of tablet dosage forms is superior to other dosage forms.

Disadvantages

1. The manufacture of tablets requires a series of unit operations and therefore there is an increased level of product loss at each stage in the manufacturing process.
2. The absorption of therapeutic agents from tablets is dependent on physiological factors, e.g. gastric emptying rate, and shows inter-patient variation.
3. The compression properties of certain therapeutic agents are poor and may present problems in their subsequent formulation and manufacture as tablets.
4. The administration of tablets is difficult for certain groups, e.g. children.

Types of Tablets

Tablets may be classified according to the method of manufacture, as compressed, coated or uncoated tablets (Table 5.5). Tablets can be produced in a wide variety of sizes, shapes, and surface markings, depending upon the design of the punches and dies. Capsule-shaped tablets are commonly referred to as caplets. Boluses are large tablets intended for veterinary use, usually for large animals.

Type	Product illustration	Description
Compressed tablets		These tablets are formed by compression and contain no special coating. They are made from powdered, crystalline or granular materials, in combination with binders, diluents, etc.
Multiple compressed tablets	 Cross Section — Top view Tablet showing the multiple coating.	These tablets are prepared by subjecting the tablet powder to more than one compression cycle. The result may be a multilayered tablet or a tablet-within-a-tablet. Multilayer tablets are mainly used for incompatible substances.
Sugarcoated tablets	 Different layers in sugar coating	Compressed tablets may be coated with a sugar layer that is colored or uncolored. Sugar coats are water soluble. The coat protects the drug from the environment and provides a barrier for bad tasting or smelling drugs.
Film coated tablets	 Different film coated tablets	Film coated tablets are compressed tablets coated with a thin layer of a polymer to protect their contents from moisture or to mask the taste of the ingredients. These coats rupture in the gastrointestinal tract, exposing the drug.
Gelatin coated tablets	 Gelcaps	The innovator product gelcaps, is a capsule-shaped compressed tablet coated with a gelatin layer. This allows the product to be smaller than an equivalent capsule filled with an equivalent amount of powder.

Table 5.5: Classification of tablets

contd...

Table 5.5: Classification of tablets (*contd.*)

Type	Product illustration	Description
Enteric coated tablets	**Fig. A Fig. B** Figure A showing the GIT as enteric tablets dissolved in intestine, Fig. B showing enteric coated tablet.	These tablets are intended to pass unchanged through the stomach to the intestines, where the tablets disintegrate and drug dissolution occurs. This helps to protect drug molecules that are susceptible to degradation in gastric acid and drugs that can irritate the gastric mucosa. It can also be used to control the delivery of certain drugs to the intestines to enhance absorption.
Buccal or sublingual tablets	Tablet with sublingual route	Buccal tablets are inserted in the buccal pouch, and sublingual tablets are inserted beneath the tongue. Where rapid drug availability is required such as in the case of nitroglycerin tablets, these tablets are administered sublingually. They are sometimes also referred to as instant disintegrating or dissolving tablets. Examples are isoprenaline sulfate (bronchodilator) and glyceryl trinitrate tablets (vasodilator). These tablets are usually small and flat. Sometimes sweeteners are added.
Chewable tablets	Chewable tablets contain sweetening agents	Chewable tablets, when chewed, produce a pleasant tasting residue in the mouth, when swallowed does not leave a bitter or unpleasant aftertaste. These tablets have been used in tablet formulations for children, especially multivitamin formulations, and for the administration of antacids and selected antibiotics. Chewable tablets prepared by compression usually contain mannitol, sorbitol, or sucrose as binders and fillers, colors and flavors to enhance their appearance and taste.
Effervescent tablets	Tablet liberates carbon dioxide	These tablets are compressed effervescent powders. They are usually dissolved in a glass of water before administration. The resultant solution is usually a flavored, drink. This type of tablet offers quick dissolution of the active ingredient in water, if the tablet is broken by the internal liberation of carbon dioxide. This also increases palatability.

contd...

Table 5.5: Classification of tablets (*contd.*)

Type	Product illustration	Description
Lozenges	Lozenges	Lozenges are compressed tablets that do not contain a disintegrant. Some lozenges contain antiseptics (e.g. benzalkonium) or antibiotics for local effects in the mouth. The second type of lozenge produces a systemic effect, e.g. a lozenge containing vitamin supplements (multivitamin tablets). Lozenges must be palatable and slowly soluble. Flavors are normally included to make the lozenge more acceptable. Compressed lozenges are called troches in the USP.
Molded tablets	Damp mass is molded into tablets	Molded tablets can be prepared from mixtures of medicinal substances and a diluent, usually consisting of lactose and powdered sucrose in varying proportions. The powders are dampened with solutions containing high percentages of alcohol. The dampened powders are pressed into molds, removed, and allowed to dry. Solidification depends upon crystal bridges built up during the subsequent drying process and not upon the compaction force.
Immediate release tablets	Fast dispersible tablets contain superdisintegrant, absorb water and swells, and finally disintegrate.	These tablets are designed to disintegrate and release the drug immediately.
Extended release tablets	Drugs dissolved or dispersed in matrix causes delayed release.	Extended release tablets, sometimes also called sustained release tablets, are designed to release a drug in a predetermined manner over an extended time.

Excipients Used in the Manufacture of Tablets

The design of the formulation and selection of excipients is especially critical in tablet dosage forms. Products can vary from a relatively simple aspirin tablet containing aspirin and starch to more complex systems that might contain fillers, binders, disintegrating agents, glidants, lubricants, and coating agents. Modified release introduces even more complexity. The appropriate selection of excipients and their concentration are critical to both the ability to manufacture tablets and to their performance as a drug delivery system. Typically the following excipients are used in the manufacture of conventional tablets:

1. Diluents/fillers;
2. Lubricants;
3. Disintegrants;
4. Binder;
5. Glidants; and
6. Miscellaneous.

Diluents/fillers

Diluents are employed in the formulation of tablets (by all methods) to increase the mass of the tablets that contain a low concentration of therapeutic agent and thereby render the manufacturing process more reliable and reproducible. The ideal diluent would be chemically and physiologically inert, and would not interfere with the bioavailability of the active ingredient. Diluents must exhibit good compression properties and should be economical. Examples of diluents for tablets are enlisted in Table 5.6.

Lubricants

Lubricants reduce friction during the compression and ejection cycle. In addition, they aid in preventing adherence of tablet material to the dies and punches. Therefore most lubricants are hydrophobic and as such tend to reduce the rates of tablet disintegration and dissolution. Consequently, excessive concentrations of lubricant should be avoided. Table 5.6 enlists some of the commenly used lubricant tablets.

Glidants

Glidants act to enhance the flow properties of the powders within the hopper and into the tablet die in the tablet press. The reduced friction between the powders/granules and the surfaces of the hopper and dies has been suggested, due to the ability of the glidants to locate within the spaces between the particles/granules. To achieve this, it is therefore necessary for the glidant particles to be firstly small and, secondly, to be arranged at the surface of the particles/granules. Glidants are typically hydrophobic and therefore care should be taken to ensure that the concentration of glidants used in the formulation does not (in a similar fashion to lubricants) adversely affect tablet disintegration and drug dissolution.

Disintegrants

Disintegrants are employed in tablet formulations to facilitate the breakdown of the tablet into granules upon entry into the stomach. If the formulated tablet is hydrophobic and/or it has been manufactured using a high compression force, disintegration of the tablet will be unacceptably low. In these situations, disintegrants are an essential formulation component, enabling tablet disintegration within the specifications defined in the various pharmacopoeias (typically disintegration of conventional tablets must occur within 15 minutes). There are several mechanisms by which disintegrants elicit their effect:

- Disintegrants may increase the porosity and wettability of the compressed tablet matrix. In doing so, gastrointestinal fluids may readily penetrate the tablet matrix and thereby enable tablet breakdown to occur, e.g. starch, MCC and sodium starch glycolate.
- Disintegrants may operate by swelling in the presence of aqueous fluids, thereby enhances tablet disintegration due to the increase in the internal pressure within the tablet matrix, e.g. sodium starch glycolate croscarmellose sodium (a cross-linked

sodium carboxymethyl cellulose) and crospovidone.

- Tablet disintegration may also be mediated by the production of gas whenever the tablet contacts aqueous fluids. This is the mechanism of disintegration of effervescent tablets.

Binders

Binders give adhesiveness to the powder during the preliminary granulation and at the time of compression of granules into tablets. While binders may be added dry but they are more effective when added in solution. The most effective dry binder is microcrystalline cellulose, which is commonly used for preparing tablets by direct compression. Binding agents can be added in two ways depending on the method of granulation:

1. As a powder as in slugging or in dry granulation methods.
2. As a solution to the mixed powders as in wet granulation.

Methods Used for the Manufacture of Tablets

There are three methods by which tablets are manufactured:

1. Wet granulation
2. Dry granulation
3. Direct compression.

The choice of manufacturing process employed is dependent on several factors, including the compression properties of the therapeutic agent, the particle size of the therapeutic agent and excipients and the chemical stability of the therapeutic agent during the manufacturing process. Table 5.8 enlists the unit operation process involved in different granulation techniques. Generally, the manufacture of tablets consists of a series of steps:

1. Mixing of the therapeutic agents with the excipients.

2. Granulation of the mixed powders (note: this is not performed in direct compression).
3. Mixing of the powders or granules with other excipients (most notably lubricants).
4. Compression into tablets.
5. The details of each of these steps will vary depending on the manufacturing method used.

1. Wet Granulation

Wet granulation is the most commonly used method for the manufacture of tablets. As water is frequently used as the granulation fluid (and heat is employed to dry the formed granules), it is important to ensure that the therapeutic agent is chemically stable during the granulation process. Tablets manufactured by wet granulation exhibit sufficient mechanical properties to be subsequently exposed to other unit operations, e.g. film coating. Granule (and hence tablet) quality is directly affected by the choice and concentration of binder and by the type and volume of granulation fluid employed. Due to the number of unit operations required, the manufacture of tablets by wet granulation is not as efficient as other methods, e.g. direct compression.

Advantages and disadvantages of wet granulation

Wet granulation is a popular technique within the pharmaceutical industry for the manufacture of tablets. There are several advantages and disadvantages associated with this technique.

Advantages

- Reduced segregation of formulation components during storage and/or processing, leading to reduced intra- and inter-batch variability.
- Useful technique for the manufacture of tablets containing low concentrations of therapeutic agent.
- Employs conventional excipients and therefore is not dependent on the inclusion

of special grades of excipient (e.g. the requirement for spray-dried excipients in the direct compression method of tablet manufacture).

- Tablets produced by wet granulation are amenable to post processing unit operations, e.g. tablet-coating techniques.

Disadvantages

- Require several processing steps
- Presence of solvents in the process, leads to a number of concerns, e.g. drug degradation may occur in the presence of the solvent. This is particularly relevant if water is used as the granulation medium due to the susceptibility of some drugs to hydrolysis. To overcome this concern, a hydroalcoholic (water/alcohol) or an alcohol (ethanol or isopropanol) granulation medium should be used.
- The drug may be soluble in the granulation fluid. During the drying process, the drug will then precipitate/crystallise, resulting in possible changes in the polymorphic form. If the drug and some excipients are soluble in the granulation medium, subsequent drying will result in deposition of these components on the surface of the insoluble particles and, in doing so, this may enhance the hardness of the granule

(and hence both the physical and the biological properties of tablet).

- Heat is required to remove the solvent. This may result in the degradation of thermolabile therapeutic agents. In addition, drying is a costly operation and, furthermore, if alcohols are used as the granulation medium, there are issues regarding solvent recovery and flammability.

2. Dry Granulation

Granulation by compression or slugging is one of the dry methods that have been used for many years for moisture- or heat-sensitive ingredients. The blend of powders is forced into dies of a large heavy-duty tableting pressed and compacted. The compacted masses are called slugs. An alternative technique is to squeeze the powder blend into a solid cake between rollers. This is known as roller compaction. The slugs or roller compacts are then milled and screened in order to produce a granular form of tableting material that flows more uniformly than the original powder mix. Table 5.6 enlists the excipients used in dry granulation.

Advantages and disadvantages of dry granulation

The popularity of dry granulation for the manufacture of tablets has decreased in recent

Table 5.6: Excipients used in dry granulation				
Diluents/filler	Disintegrants	Lubricants	Glidants	Miscellaneous excipients
Anhydrous lactose or lactose monohydrate	Starch	Stearates (magnesium stearate, stearic acid)	Talc	Colors, sweetening agents, etc.
	MCC		Colloidal silicon dioxide	
Starch	Sodium starch glycolate	Glyceryl fatty acid esters (glyceryl behenate, glyceryl)		
		Palmitostearate		
Dibasic calcium phosphate, and	Croscarmellose sodium	PEG		
MCC.	Crospovidone	Polyoxyethylene stearates,and		
		sodium lauryl sulfate.		

years, having been superseded by direct compression. However, both slugging and roller compaction are still employed in tablet manufacture. As with wet granulation, there are several advantages and disadvantages associated with these techniques.

Advantages

- Both roller compaction and slugging require conventional (i.e. non-specialist) grades of excipients.
- These methods are not generally associated with alterations in drug morphology during processing.
- No heat or solvents are required.

Disadvantages

- Specialist equipment is required for granulation by roller compaction.
- Segregation of components may occur post-mixing.
- There may be issues regarding powder flow.
- The final tablets produced by dry granulation tend to be softer than those produced by wet granulation, rendering them more difficult to process using post-tabletting techniques, e.g. film coating.
- Slugging and roller compaction lead to the generation of considerable dust. Therefore, there may be a reduction in the yield of tablets.

3. Direct Compression

The manufacture of tablets using wet granulation or dry granulation methods requires series of unit operations, both time-consuming and potentially costly. A potentially more attractive option for the manufacture of tablets involves powder mixing and subsequent compression of the powder mix, thereby obviating the need for granulation (and related unit operations). This process is termed direct compression. The mechanisms of particle–particle interactions in tablets produced by direct compression are similar to those operative in tablets produced by dry granulation and roller compaction. Table 5.7 enlists the exceipients used in direct granulation.

Advantages and Disadvantages of Tablet Manufacture by Direct Compression

The advantages of the direct compression method may at this stage be obvious; however, it is important to note that this method does suffer from several disadvantages.

Advantages

- There are fewer processing steps (unit operations) and therefore the method is potentially more cost-effective than other methods.
- Direct compression does not require the use of water or other solvents. This therefore negates potential problems regarding the stability of therapeutic agents in the presence of the solvents. In addition, heating (a costly unit operation) is not required in direct compression.
- Lubrication is performed in the same vessel as powder mixing, thereby reducing

Table 5.7: Excipients used in the manufacture of tablets by direct compression			
Diluents/filler	Disintegrants	Lubricants	Glidants
Spray-dried lactose (e.g. Lactopress spray-dried, MCC, dicalcium phosphate (e.g. encompress grades), mannitol, sorbitol, lactopress Spray-dried 250	MCC (e.g. avicel pH-102), pregelatinised starch (e.g., starch 1500), sodium starch glycolate, croscarmellose sodium crospovidone	Magnesium stearate, stearic acid, sodium Stearyl fumarate	Talc, colloidal silicon dioxide

both transfer losses and contamination of equipment.

Disadvantages

- Special grade excipients are required.
- The quality of the final dosage form is dependent on the powders being easily mixed and remaining homogeneously mixed.
- There may be issues regarding powder flow into the tableting machine.
- The final tablets produced by direct compression tend to be softer than those produced by wet granulation, rendering them more difficult to process using post-tableting techniques, e.g. film coating.
- If the loading of the therapeutic agent in the final formulation is high (10% w/w), the compression properties of the powder are significantly affected by the compression properties of the therapeutic agent.
- Direct compression is not used, if a colourant is required in the formulation due to the mottled appearance of the resulting dosage form.

Tablet Compression

All tablets are made by a process of compression. Solid, in the form of relatively small particles, is contained in a die and a compressing force of several tonnes is applied to it by means of punches. The shape of the die governs the cross-sectional shape of the tablet, and the distance between the punch tips at the point of maximum compression governs its thickness. The conformation of the tablet faces, usually flat or convex, is a reflection of those of the punches. The tip of the lower punch moves up and down within the die, but never actually leaves it. The upper punch descends to penetrate the die and apply the compressive force. It is then withdrawn to permit ejection of the tablet, brought about by an upward movement of the lower punch. There are two types of tablet press, viz. excentric press and rotary press. The excentric press has one die and one pair of punches. The rotary press has a larger number of dies which are fitted, with their corresponding punches, into a rotating turret. Irrespective of the type of press that is used, the process of tablet compression can be divided into three stages as follows.

Stage 1. Filling

The lower punch falls within the die, leaving a cavity into which particulate matter flows under the influence of gravity from a hopper. Though tablets are usually described in terms

Table 5.8: Typical unit operations involved in wet granulation, dry granulation, and direct compression

Wet granulation	Dry granulation	Direct compression
• Milling and mixing of drugs and excipients.	• Milling and mixing of drugs and excipients.	• Milling and mixing of drugs and excipients.
• Preparation of binder solution.	• Compression into slugs or roll compaction.	• Compression of tablets.
• Wet massing by addition of binder. solution or granulating solvent.	• Milling and screening of slugs and compacted powder.	
• Screening of wet mass.	• Mixing with lubricant and disintegrant.	
• Drying of the wet granules.	• Compression of tablets.	
• Screening of the dry granules.		
• Blending with lubricants and disintegrant to produce 'running powder'.		
• Compression of tablets.		

of weight, the die is filled by a volumetric process. The volume is determined by the depth to which the lower punch descends in the die. Unless this volume is filled properly on each occasion, then the mass of the tablet will vary, and with it the drug content of each tablet. Therefore, uniform filling is essential.

Stage 2. Compression

The upper punch descends, and its tip enters the die, confining the particles. This process is facilitated by the particles fragmenting and/or deforming. Once the particles are close enough together, interparticulate forces then cause the individual particles to aggregate, forming a tablet.

Stage 3. Ejection

The upper punch is withdrawn from the die, and so the force being applied to the tablet is removed. The effect of this might cause the deformed particles to return to their former shape, which would result in a decrease interparticulate contact and hence tablet strength. It is essential that this does not occur. As the upper punch leaves the die, the lower punch moves upwards, pushing the tablet before it. Figure 5.3 illustrates the principle of compression in a single-punch machine. Successful ejection demands lack of adhesion between the tablet and the die wall. Therefore for a particulate solid to be successfully transformed into tablets, three key properties need to be present:

1. Good particle flow.
2. The ability of the particles to cohere under the influence of a compressing force. This coherence must be retained after the compressing force has been removed.
3. The ability of the tablet to be ejected from the die after the compressing force has been removed.

Tablet Coating

The objective for tablet coatings is provided:

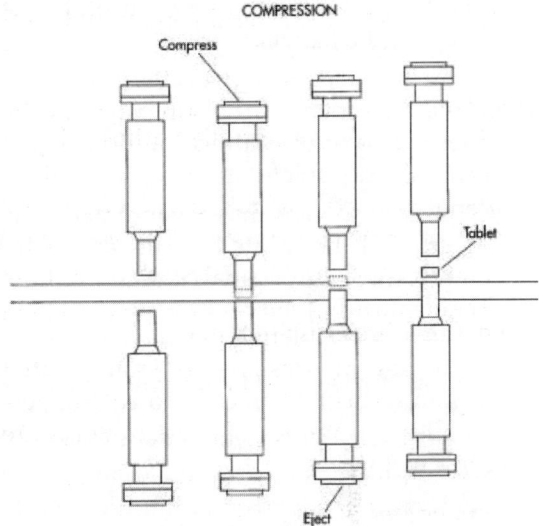

Fig. 5.3: Illustrates the principle of compression in a single-punch machine. First, the mixture is fed into a dye cavity. Then, a punch descends into the cavity and compresses the mixture into a tablet. As the punch retracts, another punch below the cavity rises to eject the tablet

- To protect the drug from degradation in the stomach (an enteric coating).
- To prevent drug-induced irritation at a specific site within the gastrointestinal tract, e.g. the stomach for non-steroidal anti-inflammatory drugs.
- To provide controlled release of the drug throughout the gastrointestinal tract.
- To target drug release to a specific site in the gastrointestinal tract, e.g. the delivery of drug to the colon for the treatment of inflammatory conditions.
- To mask the taste of drugs.
- To improve the appearance of the tablet.

General Description of Tablet Coating

The main steps involved in the coating of tablets are as follows:

- The tablets (or granules) are placed within the coating apparatus and agitated.

- The coating solution is sprayed on to the surface of the tablets.
- Warm air is passed over the tablets to facilitate removal of the solvent from the adsorbed layer of coating solution on the surface of the tablets.
- When the solvent has evaporated, the tablets will be coated with the solid component of the original coating solution.

Tablet Coating in Practice

There are several designs of systems that are used in industrial practice to coat tablets (or granules). Examples of these systems are described below.

1. Pan coater

The pan coating system is generally composed of a metal pan (drum) into which the tablets are placed and that may be rotated at a range of speeds (Fig. 5.4). The coating solution is sprayed on to the surface of the tablets within the pan whilst the drum is rotated. Simultaneously warm air is passed over the surface of the tablets to facilitate the evaporation of the solvent in which the coating material has been dissolved. Control of the coating process is obtained by modifying the following parameters:

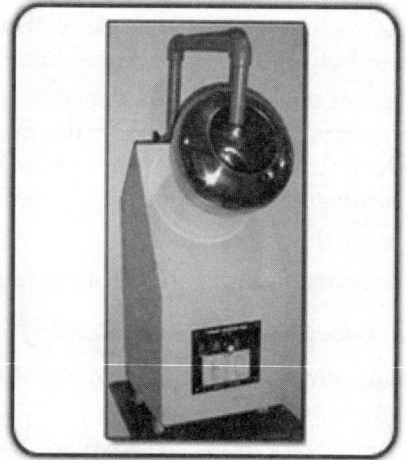

Fig. 5.4: Pan coater

- Rotation rate of the drum/pan
- Airflow rate
- Temperature of the air
- Concentration of sugar/polymer within the coating solution/emulsion.

2. Air suspension coaters

Air suspension coaters are highly efficient coating systems in which the coating solution is sprayed on to tablets (or granules) that have been suspended in a positive (warmed) airflow. This ability simultaneously suspend and coat tablets leads to high coating efficiency. There are several process factors that control both the efficiency of the coating process and the quality of the formed coat. These are: (1) evaporation rate of the solvent; (2) fluidised air volume; (3) specific humidity; and (4) coating spray rate and duration.

a. Sugar Coating

The sugar coating protects the enclosed drugs from the enviorment and mask the objectionable taste and odor of the drugs, sugar coating also enhances the tablet appearance and permit imprinting of manufacturing information. Sugar coating process involves building up layers of coating material on the tablet cores as they are tumbled in a revolving pan by repetitively applying a coating solution or suspention and drying off the solvent. Sugar coating process involves following operation.

1. **Sealing/waterproofing**: Sealing coat provides an adequate moisture barrier. Commenly used materials for sealing coat are shellac, PVP (polyvinylpyrrolidone) or other polymaric materials, such as cellulose acetate phthalate and polyvinly acetate phthalate.

2. **Subcoating**: The next satge is to built up a subcoat that provides a good bridge between the main coating and the sealed core, as well as round off any sharp corners.

3. **Smoothing or grossing**: Subcoating is followed by smoothing or grossing. This stage is accomplished by again applying one or two layers of clear syrup.
4. **Coloring**: This gives tablet its color, identity and also mask the color of polymaric material used in previous coating. The tablets are then left for several hours before being transferred to the next step that is polishing.
5. **Polishing:** The polish consisting of dilute wax solution (e.g. carnauba or beswax in patroleum spirit) applied sparingly until a high luster is produced.

b. Film Coating

Film coating has increased in popularity for various reasons. The film process is simpler and, therefore, easier to automate. It is also faster than sugar coating, since weight gains of only 2 to 6% are involved, as opposed to more than 50% with sugar coating. In addition, moisture involvement can be avoided (if absolutely necessary) by using non-aqueous solvents. Moreover, distinctive identification tablet markings are not obscured by film coats. Two major groups of film coating materials may be distinguished: (a) those that are non-enteric, cellulose derivatives, and (b) those that can provide an enteric effect and are commonly esters of phthalic acid. Within both groups, it is general practice to use a mixture of materials to give a film with the optimum range of properties. Films may contain a plasticizer that prevents the film from becoming brittle with consequent risk of chipping. The choice of plasticizer depends on the particular film polymer.

The nature of the solvent system may markedly influence the quality of the film and, to optimize the various factors, mixed solvents are usually necessary. More specifically, the rate of evaporation and, hence, the time for the film to dry, has to be controlled within fine limits, if a uniform smooth coat is to be produced. The solvent mixture must be capable of dissolving the required amount of coating material yet give rise to a solution within a workable range of viscosity. Until recently, alcohols, esters, chlorinated hydrocarbons, and ketones have been among the most frequently used solvents. Because of the need to develop a uniform color, the colorants used in film coating are more likely to be lakes than dyes. In lakes, the colorant has been absorbed on to the surface of an insoluble substrate. Table 5.9 indicates the differences between sugar coating and film coating.

Table 5.9: Differences between sugar and film coating		
Features	**Sugar coating**	**Film coating**
Tablets		
Appearance	Rounded with high degree of polish	Retains contour of original core. Usually not as shiny as sugar coat types.
Weight increase due to coating materials	30–50%	2–3%
Logo or 'break' lines	Not possible	Possible
Other solid dosage forms	Coating possible but little industrial importance	Coating of multiparticulates very important in modified release forms.
Process		
Stages	Multistage process	Usually single stage
Typical batch coating time	Eight hours, but easily longer	1.5–2 hours
Functional coatings	Not usually possible apart from enteric coating	Easily adaptable for controlled release

c. Modified-release Coatings

A coating may be applied to a tablet to modify the release pattern of the active ingredient.

Two general categories, enteric coating and controlled-release coating, are distinguished. The former are insoluble in the low pH environment of the stomach but dissolve readily in the small intestine with its elevated pH. They are used to minimize irritation of the gastric mucosa by certain drugs and to protect others that are degraded by gastric juices.

Problems Associated with Tablet Coatings

There are several problems associated with tablet coatings, including: (1) poor adhesion of the coating to the tablet; (2) tablet abrasion; (3) filling tablet markings; (4) rough surface; (5) formation of cracks in the coating; (6) variations in the color of the coating. Poor adhesion of the coating to the tablet, this phenomenon may be due to:

- High relative humidity within the coating chamber when organic solvent is used for tablet coating.

- High coating spray rate.

- Concentration of polymer in the coating solution/emulsion is too low.

- Temperature of air is too low, resulting in a slow rate of solvent evaporation (particularly valid for coating systems that employ solvents of low vapor pressure, e.g. water).

- Air fluidization rate or pan rotation rate is too slow.

- The tablet substrate has minimal curvature. Typically curved surfaces are easier to coat than flat surfaces.

Compendial Standards and Quality Assurance

Compressed tablets may be characterized or described by a number of specifications. These include the diameter, shape, thickness, weight, hardness, disintegration time, and dissolution characteristics. The diameter and shape depend on the die and the punches selected for the compression of the tablet. The tablets may be scored in halves or quarters to facilitate breaking, if smaller doses are desired. The top or lower surface may be embossed or engraved with a symbol or letters that serve as an additional means of identifying the source of the tablets. These characteristics along with the color of the tablets tend to make them distinctive and identifiable with the active ingredient they contain. Table 5.10 includes USP-recommended tests and specifications for quality control and quality assurance of tablets.

Property	Test	Equipment used	Specification
Uniformity of dosage units	Weight		Take 20 tablets and weight individually. Calculate average weight and compare the individual tablet weight to the average. The tablets pass the USP test if not more than 2 tablets are outside the percentage limit and if no tablets differ by more than 2 times of the percentage limit. Limits according to USP: Weight of tablet 130 mg or less — % error = ±10%
		Electronic balance	Weight of tablet 130–324 mg — % error = ±7.5% Weight of tablet 324 mg or more — % error = ±5%

Table 5.10: USP-recommended tests and specifications for quality control and quality assurance of tablets

contd...

Table 5.10: USP-recommended tests and specifications for quality control and quality assurance of tablets (*contd.*)

Property	Test	Equipment used	Specification
	Drug content	UV spectrophotometer	Randomly select 30 tablets, 10 of these asseyed individually. Tablets pass the test if 9 of 10 tablets must contain not less than 85% and not more than 115% of the labeled quantity. The content uniformity test has been extended to monographs on all coated and uncoated tablets and all capsules intended for oral administration where the range of sizes of the dosage form available includes a 50 mg or smaller size. A UV spectrophotometer is commonly used for the estimation of drugs.
Drug release	Disintegration	Disintegration apparatus	It is the time required for the tablet to break into particles, the disintegration test is a measure only of the time required under a given set of conditions for a group of tablets to disintegrate into particles. At present disintegration test, the particles that will pass through a 10-mesh screen. The basket rack immersed in a bath held at 37°C and the volume of fluid is such that on the upward stroke the wire mesh remains at least 2.5 cm below the surface of the fluid. Complete disintegration occurs when no residue of the tablet still present on the screen except the insoluble ingredients as the shell or the coat of the tablet. 1. Start the disintegration test on 6 tablets. 2. If one or two tablets from the 6 tablets fail disintegrate completely within specified time repeat the same test on another 12 tablet (i.e. the whole test will consume 18 tablets). 3. Not less than 16 tablets disintegrate completely within the time, if more than two tablets (from the 18) fail to disintegrate, the patch must be rejected.

contd...

			Table 5.10: USP-recommended tests and specifications for quality control and quality assurance of tablets (*contd.*)
Property	**Test**	**Equipment used**	**Specification**
	Dissolution	Dissolution apparatus	Since drug absorption and bioavailability depend on quality of drug in the dissolved state, therefore, suitable dissolution characteristics are important properties of a satisfactory tablet. According to USP, there are two types of dissolution apparatus recomended for dissolution study.
			Basket type: The basket is immersed in a dissolution medium contained in a 1000 ml flask. The falsk is maintained at 37°C by a contant temperature bath. The motor is adjusted to turn at specified RPM. Samples of the fluid are withdrawn at diffrent time intervals to determine the drug content.
			Paddle type: This is same as above instruments except the basket is replaced by a paddle.
			Dissolution specifications state that a certain percentage of drugs must dissolve in a specified time. Dissolution study needs to be performed at 37°C and at simulated gastric or intestinal fluid or as specified in official pharmacopeia.
Other tests	Moisture content	IR moisture balance	Minimum quantity of moisture is necessary for a successful tablet but too much moisture will result sticking, picking, microbial contamination and other stability problems.
			Moisture content of granules can be determined by IR moisture balance. There are no official limits for moisture content of granules: it depends on types of products and method used for tablet manufature.
			However, it must comply with minimum standard specified in BMR.
	Particulate impurities	Tablet sorting equipment.	The genreral appearance of a tablet is essential for customer acceptance. The control of general appearance includes the determination of sizes, shapes, color, presence of impurity.
			Each tablet should be inspected for the presence of black/foreign particles.
			No impurities should be permitted.

contd...

Table 5.10: USP-recommended tests and specifications for quality control and quality assurance of tablets (*contd.*)

Property	Test	Equipment used	Specification
	Packaging and storage (Leakage test)	 Leak test apparatus	The test may be performed by subjecting the strips to a vacuum in a vacuum desicator, the strips being immersed in water or another procedure frequently employed is to simply autoclave the strips, if leakage is present that causes water to enter inside the strip which can be easily observed. The limits for leaker test must meet standard monographs.
	Tablet hardness	 Monsanto hardness tester	The instrument measures the force required to break the tablet when the force generated by a coil spring is applied diametrically to the tablet. Tablet requires certain amount of strength to withstand the mechanical shock during manufacturing, dispensing and transporting. • 5 kilograms minimum and 8 kilograms maximum. • Make hardness test on 5 tablets and then take the average hardness.
	Thickness	 Vernier caliper	Tablet thickness is determined with a caliper or thickness gauge that measures the thickness in millimeters. Plus or minus 5% may be allowed, depending on the size of the tablet.
	Friability requirements	 Friability apparatus	Subjects a number of tablets to abrasion and shock by utilizing a plastic chamber that revolves at 25 rpm, dropping the tablets a distance of 6 inches with each revolution. After a given number of rotations, the tablets are weighed and the loss in weight indicates the ability of the tablets to withstand this type of wear. It must be ≤ 1% but if more we do not reject the tablets as this test is non-official. • Perform this test using 20 tablets that were used first in the weight variation test.

Example 1: Calcium gluconate tablets (ip 1966)	
Ingrdients	**Quantity**
Calcium gluconate	0.5 g
Sucrose	1.0 g
Menthol oil	0.0015 ml

Method

1. Mix the calcium gluconate and sucrose.
2. Mixture of drugs in powder form is mixed, if necessary with suitable inert substance to act as diluents, absorbent, adhesive or disintegrating agent and the material in the requisite degree of fineness in intimately mixed and damped with a suitable moistening agent selected with regard to its effect on the chemical and physical nature of the material.
3. The granules are dried in a current of air, at a suitable temperature generally not exceeding 60°C, and again passed through a sieve.
4. The addition of small proportion of lubricant to the dried granules may be required to prevent them from sicking to the punches and dies during compression.
5. Finally add the menthol oil, previously dissolved in small quantity of alcohol into the prepared dried granules.
6. Mix and compress the mixture.

Storage: Store in airtight and cool place.

Use: Calcium gluconate is used to prevent and to treat calcium deficiencies.

Example 2: Direct compression tablet containing a low dose, highly soluble active ingredient		
Formula	**Quantity %**	**Use**
Diphenhydramine HCl powder	10.0	Active
Microcrystalline cellulose (Avicel; pH 102)	25.0	Filler (direct compression)
Lactose	62.2	Filler
Croscarmellose sodium (Ac-di-Sol)	2.00	Disintegrant
Colloidal silicon dioxide	0.20	Glidant
Magnesium stearate	0.30	Lubricant
Stearic acid	0.30	Lubricant

Method

1. Screen all the ingredients through a 20-mesh sieve.
2. Blend everything except the lactose, stearic acid, and magnesium stearate in a V-shaped blender for 3 min.
3. Add lactose to the batch and blend for 10 min.
4. Add stearic acid to the batch and blend for 3 min.
5. Add magnesium stearate to the batch and blend for 5 min.
6. Tablet using flat-faced bevel-edge tooling with appropriate size.

Storage: Store in airtight box and preserve in a controlled temperature.

Use: Common cold and analgesic.

Example 3: Wet granulated tablet containing a high dose, partially soluble active		
Formula	**Quantity %**	**Use**
Theophylline anhydrous	30.0	Active
Anhydrous lactose	65.5	Filler (direct compression)
Croscarmellose sodium (Ac-di-Sol)	3.00	Disintegrant
Stearic acid	1.00	Lubricant
Granulating fluid (10% PVP solution)	Qs	Binder

Method

1. Screen all the ingredients through a 20-mesh sieve.
2. Blend everything except stearic acid in a V-shaped blender for 20 min.

3. Granulate powder with PVP solution.

4. Screen granules to appropriate size and dry.

5. Add stearic acid to dried granules and blend for 3 min.

6. Tablet using flat-faced bevel-edge tooling with appropriate size.

Storage: Store in airtight and preserve in a controlled temperature.

Use: For relief and/or prevention of symptoms of asthma and reversible bronchospasm associated with chronic bronchitis and emphysema.

Packaging and Storing Tablets

- Tablets are stored in airtight containers and protected from extremes direct sunlight and temperature. Products that are prone to decomposition by moisture generally are co-packaged with a desiccant packet.

- Drugs that are adversely affected by light are packaged in light-resistant containers. With a few exceptions, tablets that are properly stored will remain stable for several years or more.

- In dispensing tablets, the pharmacist should use a similar type of container as provided by the manufacturer. The patient should maintain the drug in the dispensed container.

- Storage conditions, as recommended for the particular product, should be maintained by the pharmacist and patient.

- The pharmacist should also be aware that the hardness of certain tablets might change upon aging, usually resulting in a decrease in the disintegration and dissolution rate of the product. The increase in tablet hardness can frequently be attributed to the increased adhesion of the binding agent and other formulation components in the tablet.

- Certain tablets containing volatile drugs, such as nitroglycerin, may experience the migration of the drug between tablets in the container, resulting in a lack of uniformity among the tablets. Further, when packing materials such as cotton come in contact with nitroglycerin tablets it may absorb varying amounts of nitroglycerin, rendering the tablets sub-potent.

- The USP directs that nitroglycerin tablets should be preserved in airtight containers, preferably of glass, at controlled room temperature. The USP further directs that nitroglycerin tablets must be dispensed in the original, unopened container, labeled appropriately.

LOZENGES

Lozenges are solid preparations, each containing one or more medicaments, usually in a flavored bases, which are intended to dissolve slowly in the mouth. They do not contain flavoring agent other than those indicated in the individual monograph. They may be prepared by molding or by compression.

General Method of Preparation

1. Mix the ingredients of lozenges in a mortar to produce a mass of the desired consistency.

2. Roll out the mass on lozenges board previously dusted with powdered talc to uniform thickness.

3. Cut out the cake for as many as lozenges as possible.

4. Place the lozenges on a slab dusted with starch and dry in a hot air oven at 40°C for 1 day in order to obtain desired hardness.

5. Dispense the lozenges in flat boxes which are made of metal.

Compressed Lozenges

They are prepared by the method used in the preparation of tablets by compression. These are generally contain a sweetening agent ar.d flavoring agent. Compressed lozenges shoula comply with the requirements for standard for content of active ingredient and uniformity of weight.

Labeling: Comply with the general requirements for labeling.

Storage: Lozenges should be kept in a cool and dry place and should be packed in airtight container.

Example 1: Compound bismuth lozenges (BP, 1988)	
Ingredients	Quantity
Bismuth subcarbonate	150 mg
Heavy magnesium carbonate	150 mg
Calcium carbonate	300 mg
Rose oil, of commerce	0.00006 ml

Method: The lozenges may be prepared by incorporating the ingredients in a base consisting of 7 parts of acacia, in fine powder, and 100 parts of sucrose, in fine powder, by weight, and by molding the resulting mixture with water followed by drying in hot air or by dry compression after admixture with a suitable excipient, such as sucrose. Each lozenge weighs about 1.6 gm.

Storage: Compound bismuth lozenges should be protected from light.

Use: Used to treat diarrhea and gastric ulcers.

CAPSULES

Capsules are solid-dosage forms that are most commonly composed of gelatin and are designed to contain a drug-containing formulation. Two types of capsule are available: hard and soft gelatin capsules. Hard gelatin capsules are less flexible and are composed of two pieces, termed as the cap and the body, whereas soft gelatin capsules are more flexible and are composed of one piece capsule shell. A wide range of formulation types may be included within the interior of the capsule. For example, powders, tablets, semisolids and non-aqueous liquids/gels may be filled into hard capsules, with powders being the most common formulation option. Soft gelatin capsules are usually filled with non-aqueous liquids containing the therapeutic agent either dispersed or dissolved within this carrier. Capsules offer the pharmaceutical scientist with an alternative method for the formulation of solid-dosage forms. Several categories of capsules may be distinguished (Table 5.11).

Advantages and Disadvantages of Capsules
Advantages

The formulation of capsules may be preferred for several reasons:

- The use of capsules avoids many unit operations that are associated with the manufacture of tablets, e.g. compression, granulation, drying.
- Capsules (generally soft gelatin capsules) may be formulated to increase the oral bioavailability of poorly soluble therapeutic agents. This is particularly the case when formulated as a liquid-filled hard gelatin or soft gelatin capsule.
- Capsules are a convenient method by which liquids may be orally administered to patients as a unit dosage form.
- Capsules are difficult to counterfeit.
- The stability of therapeutic agents may be improved in a capsule formulation.
- Capsules are a convenient means of formulating substances of abuse, e.g. temazepam.
- Capsule may be formulated to offer rapid drug release or controlled drug release.

Disadvantages

- Filling equipment is slower than tableting, although that gap has narrowed in recent years with the advent of high-speed automatic-filling machines.
- Generally, hard gelatin capsule products are more costly to produce than tablets.
- Highly soluble salts (e.g. iodides, bromides, and chlorides) are not suitable

Table 5.11: Different categories of capsules

Type	Product illustration	Description
Hard gelatin capsules	Hard gelatin capsules showing cap (dark grey) and body (light grey)	Hard gelatin capsules are solid dosage forms in which one or more medicinal and inert substances are enclosed within small shells of gelatin. Capsule shells are produced in varying size, shape, thickness, softness, and color. Hard shell capsules, which have two telescoping parts — the body and the cap — are commonly used in extemporaneous hand filling operations as well as in small and large-scale manufacture of commercial capsules. They usually are filled with powder mixtures and granules. After filling, the two capsule parts are joined for tight closure. They may also be sealed and bonded through a variety of special processes for added quality assurance and capsule.
Soft capsules	Soft gelatin capsules	Soft capsules have thicker shells than those of hard capsules. The shells consist of a single part and are of various shapes. Soft capsules are usually formed, filled and sealed in one operation, but for extemporaneous use the shell may be prefabricated. The shell material may contain an active substance. Liquids may be enclosed directly; solids are usually dissolved or dispersed in a suitable vehicle to give a solution or dispersion of a paste-like consistency. There may be partial migration of the constituents from the capsule contents into the shell and vice versa because of the nature of the materials and the surfaces in contact.
Modified-release capsules	Modified release filled with multiple coated granules.	Modified-release capsules are hard or soft capsules in which the contents or the shell or both contain special excipients or are prepared by a special process designed to modify the rate, the place or the time at which the active substance(s) are released. Modified-release capsules include prolonged-release capsules and delayed-release capsules.
Gastro-resistant capsules	Enteric or gastro-resistant capsule	Gastro-resistant capsules are delayed-release capsules that are intended to resist the gastric fluid and to release their active substance in the intestinal fluid. Usually, they are prepared by filling capsules with granules or with particles coated with a gastro-resistant coating, or in certain cases, by providing hard or soft capsules with a gastro-resistant shell (enteric capsules). For capsules filled with granules or filled with particles covered with a gastro-resistant coating, a suitable test is carried out to demonstrate the appropriate release of the active substance(s).
Cachets	Cachets	Cachets are solid preparations consisting of a hard shell containing a single dose of one or more active substances.

to dispense in hard gelatin capsules. Their rapid release may cause gastric irritation owing to the formation of a high drug concentration in localized areas.

- Both hard gelatin capsules and tablets may become lodged in the esophagus, resulting high localized concentration of certain drugs (e.g. doxycycline, potassium chloride, indomethacin) may cause damage.
- The requirement for specialized manufacturing equipment.
- Potential stability problems associated with capsules containing liquids.
- Problems regarding the weight variation and content uniformity may be associated with capsule formulations.

Classification of Capsules

Several categories of capsules may be distinguished:

1. Hard capsules
2. Soft capsules
3. Gastro-resistant capsules
4. Modified-release capsules
5. Cachets

Materials and Manufacture of Capsules

Capsules are primarily (but not exclusively) manufactured using gelatin; however, the suitability of other materials, e.g. hydroxy-propylmethylcellulose and starch, has been investigated as suitable replacements. Gelatin is prepared by the hydrolysis of collagen obtained from animal connective tissue, bone, skin, and sinew. Gelatin can vary in its chemical and physical properties, depending on the source of the collagen and the manner of extraction. There are two basic types of gelatin.

Type A, which is produced by an acid hydrolysis, is manufactured mainly from pork skin. **Type B gelatin,** produced by alkaline hydrolysis, is manufactured mainly from animal bones.

Commonly, various soluble synthetic dyes (coal tar dyes) and insoluble pigments

are used to change the color of the capsule shell. Commonly used pigments are the iron oxides. Colorants not only play a role in identifying the product, but may also play a role in improving patient compliance. Titanium dioxide may be included to render the shell opaque. Opaque capsules may be employed to provide protection against light or to conceal the contents. When preservatives are employed, parabens are often used. In general, information on capsules is printed before filling. Empty capsules can be handled faster than filled capsules and, moreover there is no danger of any loss of active ingredients, when empty stells are used for printing.

Hard Shell Sizes and Shapes

For human use, empty gelatin capsules are manufactured in eight sizes, ranging from 000 (the largest) to 5 (the smallest). The volumes and approximate capacities for the traditional eight sizes are listed in Table 5.12.

Table 5.12: Approximate capacities of capsules		
Human sizes	Capacity (ml)	Fill weight at 0.8 g/ml density
5	0.12	0.10
4	0.20	0.19
3	0.27	0.24
2	0.37	0.30
1	0.48	0.40
0	0.67	0.54
00	0.95	0.76
000	1.36	1.10

Description and Manufacture of Hard Gelatin Capsules

Hard gelatin capsules are composed of two halves, termed as the cap and the body. During manufacture of the dosage form, the formulation is filled into the body (using a range of different mechanical techniques) and the cap is pushed into place. The two halves of the capsule are joined, the cap overlapping with the body. Due to the tight fit between the two halves, separation of the cap and body does not normally occur under normal storage conditions or in clinical use.

Sealing of hard gelatin capsules may also be performed using two further methods:

1. *Gelatin band sealing*: In this method, a dilute solution of gelatin is applied to the center of the capsule (between the two halves) which, once dried, produces a hermetic seal.

2. *Hydroalcoholic solvent seal*: A hydroalcoholic solution (1:1 water/ethanol) is applied to the center of the capsule (between the two halves). This softens the capsule and, following heating to 45°C, the interface fuses to produce a seal.

Steps involved in the manufacturing of hard gelatin capsules

The various stages of this are as follows:

1. **Preparation of the gelatin solution:** Initially a concentrated solution of gelatin is prepared (35–40% w/w) in demineralised hot water with stirring. Following dissolution of the polymer, a vacuum is then applied to the mixing vessel to remove entrapped air.

2. **Incorporation of other constituents of the capsule:** Other excipients may be included within the heated gelatin solution, e.g. colorants, wetting agents/lubricants.

3. **Control of the viscosity of the gelatin solution:** Following the inclusion of all components within the heated gelatin solution, the viscosity of the solution is then modified (reduced). Control of the viscosity is important as this regulates the thickness of the capsule. As the viscosity is lowered, the capsule thickness will decrease.

4. **Dip-coating the gelatin solution on to metal pins (moulds):** The machine used to manufacture capsules consists of two sets of bars, each containing a series of pins (aligned in columnar formation) that have been lubricated prior to use.

❖ The pins (one set for the production of the cap and one for the body of the capsule) are dipped into a pan that contains the heated gelatin solution (maintained at 35–45°C).

❖ Following adsorption of the gelatin solution on to the surface of the pins, the bar containing the pins is removed and rotated.

❖ The reduction in the temperature of the gelatin and the rotating action cause the gelatin to gel on the surface of the pins in a uniform manner.

❖ The pins are then advanced through a series of air driers in which air of the required humidity is passed across the surface of the gelatin film.

❖ Following this, the (hardened) capsules are removed from the pins and cut to the appropriate size prior to joining the two halves of the final capsule.

Formulation Considerations for Hard Gelatin Capsules

The contnat for hard gelatin capsules may be formulated either as a powder (or granule) containing the required drug or as a liquid into which the drug is either dispersed or dissolved. The formulation considerations for both of these strategies are individually described below.

Powders

In general, powder formulations for inclusion within hard gelatin capsules should exhibit the following properties:

1. Powder to be filled should be homogeneous

2. Good flow properties. Filling of the capsules requires the reproducible flow of the powder from the powder bed, through the filling apparatus and into the capsule. Flow properties of the powder may be assessed by the following points:

❖ *Angle of repose*: Typically the flow properties of the powders are assessed by angle of repose. If the measured angle exceeds 50, the flow properties of the powder are poor. Typically, an angle of repose is 25, indicative of a powder that would be expected to exhibit suitable flow for manufacturing process. Powder that exhibit high angles of repose will require the addition of a glidant to reduce particle–particle cohesion.

❖ *Torque rheometry*: Torque rheometry is a rheological technique in which a stress is applied to the powder bed (by means of a mixing head) and the subsequent deformation (rate of shear) of the powder bed is determined. Powder beds that should demonstrate high cohesion will require greater shearing stresses to initiate and maintain flow.

❖ *Tap density*: Tap density measures the volume occupied by the powder bed. The ratio of the density of the powder bed before and after shaking is referred to as a Hausner ratio. Generally, a Hausner ratio of 1.2 is acceptable whereas, when the Hausner ratio exceeds 1.6, the powder may be problematic to fill into capsules due to the unnecessarily high cohesive interactions between the particles.

❖ *Compatibility*: Compatibility between the formulation components and the capsule. In particular, the following excipients are used for the formulation of powder fills as described in Table 5.13.

Liquids/semisolids fill for hard gelatin capsules

Liquids are essential part of the capsule contant. Liquids that are water soluble or volatile and ethyl alcohol cannot be included as major constituents of the capsule content since they can migrate into the hydrophilic gelatin shell and evaporate from the surface.

Liquids/semisolids fill for hard gelatin capsules may be subdivided into following categories:

• Lipophilic liquids/oils containing dissolved or dispersed therapeutic agent. Examples of the types of liquids that are commonly used in this category include vegetable oils (e.g. sunflower, arachis, olive) and fatty acid esters (e.g. glyceryl monostearate).

• Water-miscible liquids containing dissolved/dispersed therapeutic agent. Examples of the types of liquids that are commonly used in this category include polyethylene glycols (PEGs) that are solid at room temperature and liquid polyoxyethylene-polyoxypropylene block co-polymers.

To stabilize the liquid fill formulations for hard gelatin capsules, other excipients will be required, e.g. surface-active agents, viscositymodifying agents and stabilizers (e.g. antioxidants, colors).

Soft Gelatin Capsules

Soft gelatin capsules (sometimes referred to as softgels) are made from a more flexible, plasticized gelatin film than hard gelatin capsules.

Advantages and Disadvantages of Soft Gelatin Capsules

Several advantages of soft gelatin capsules derive from the fact that the encapsulation process requires that the drug be a liquid or at least dissolved, solubilized, or suspended in a liquid vehicle.

Advantages

1. Since the liquid filling into capsules is regulated by a positive-displacement pump, a much higher degree of reproducibility is achieved than powder or granule feed in the manufacture of tablets and hard gelatin capsules.

2. A higher degree of homogeneity is possible in liquid systems than can be achieved in

Tablet excipients	Comments	Examples
Diluents	Increase the working mass of the powder bed and thereby enhance the reproducibility of the filling process. In addition, the diluents may offer additional properties, most notably their flow properties and their ability to undergo compression.	Lactose (monohydrate), maize starch, microcrystalline cellulose.
Lubricants/glidants	Lubricants are used to reduce the interaction of the powders with the metal dossator and/or other metal components of the filling machine, whereas glidants are used to lower the interparticle attraction, thereby reducing clumping and aiding powder flow.	Magnesium stearate (and other stearates) as a lubricant, colloidal silicon dioxide as a glidant.
Disintegrants	Disintegrants are employed (as before) to break up the powder mass following release into the stomach.	Maize starch, microcrystalline cellulose, sodium starch glycolate, crospovidone, croscarmellose.
Surface-active agents	Surface-active agents increase the wetting properties of the powder, thereby improve the solubility of poorly soluble therapeutic agent.	Sodium lauryl sulfate, tween and span.
Viscosity-modifying agents	Stabilize the suspended therapeutic agent, modify the viscosity of the formulation to optimize filling of the capsule.	Natural hydrocolloids (gelatin, acacia), cellulose derivatives (methyl and ethyl cellulose).
Stabilizers	Stabilize the suspended therapeutic agent	Antioxidants (ascorbic acid, tocopherol), preservatives (methyl and propyl paraben), colors (FD&C approved colors).

Table 5.13: Excipients used for the formulation of powder fill

powder blends. A content uniformity of <3% has been reported for soft gelatin capsules manufactured in a rotary die process.

3. Another advantage that derives from the liquid nature of the fill is rapid release of the contents with potentially enhanced bioavailability.

4. Soft gelatin capsules are hermetically sealed as a natural consequence of the manufacturing process. Thus, this dosage form is suited for liquids and volatile drugs. Many drugs subject to atmospheric oxidation may also be formulated satisfactorily in this dosage form.

5. Soft gelatin capsules are available in a wide variety of sizes and shapes. They may be packed in tube form (ophthalmics, ointments) or bead form (various cosmetics) are also possible.

Disadvantages

1. Additional quality control measures may be required.

2. Soft gelatin capsules are not an economic dosage form, particularly when compared with direct compression tablets.

3. There is a more intimate contact between the shell and its liquid contents than exists

with dry-filled hard gelatin capsules, which increases the possibility of interactions. For instance, chloral hydrate formulated with an oily vehicle exerts a proteolytic effect on the gelatin shell.

4. Drugs can migrate from an oily vehicle into the shell, and this has been related to their water solubility and the partition coefficient between water and the non-polar solvent.

Formulation of Soft Gelatin Capsules

The various components of the soft gelatin capsule shell are as follows: (1) gelatin, (2) plasticizing agents, (3) water, (4) miscellaneous excipients.

Gelatin: Typically type B (alkali-processed) gelatin is used; however, type A (acid-processed) may also be employed for the manufacture of soft gelatin capsules.

Plasticizing agents: The mechanical properties of the soft gelatin capsule are controlled by the inclusion (and concentration) of plasticizers. For this purpose polyhydric alcohols, principally glycerol or sorbitol or mixtures of these, are used. The concentration of plasticizer is generally 20–30% w/w of the wet mass.

Water: Water is required both during the manufacturing process (to facilitate manufacture) and in the finished product to ensure that the capsule is flexible. A final capsule water content of 5–8% w/w. If the capsule is over dried a brittle product will result.

Miscellaneous excipients: As is the case for hard gelatin capsules, soft gelatin capsules may be colored or opaque, the chosen color(s)/opacifiers being added during the manufacturing process. Titanium dioxide is primarily used as an opacifier for capsules. In addition, if required, flavoring agents may be added to the capsule shell.

Manufacture of Soft Gelatin Capsules

In this method, the wet mass formulation is initially prepared containing gelatin, plasticizer(s), water and other excipients, as required. Following this, the gelatin solution is fed on to two drums via a spreader box, at this stage ribbons of gelatin are produced. The two sets of ribbons are then fed between two rotary dies (generally lubricated with mineral oil) to form pockets whilst, simultaneously, a metered volume of the capsule fill material is dispensed into the pocket. The two halves of capsule (containing the fill material) are sealed by the application of heat (37 to 40°C) and pressure, detached from the gelatin ribbon and collected. Following collection, the capsules are washed to remove any lubricant (mineral oil) from the surface of the capsule.

Compendial Standards and Regulatory Requirements for Capsules

As is the case for tablets, several requirements and specifications are set for capsules in the USP (Table 5.14). These specifications ensure the stability, quality, and release of drugs from capsules.

Examples of Capsule Formulations

Example 1: Sustained release matrix capsule dosage form		
Formula	Quantity%	Use
Pseudoephedrine HCl	24	Active
Hydropropylcellulose (Klucel HXF)	15	Binder
MCC	20	Filler
Pregelatinized starch	20	Filler
Dicalcium phosphate	20	Filler
Magnesium stearate	1	Lubricant

Method

1. Blend everything except magnesium stearate in a V-shaped blender for 10 min.
2. Fill the blend into size 0 gelatin capsules using an automatic capsule filling machine with dosator piston force of 200 N.

Table 5.14: USP-recommended tests and specifications for quality control and quality assurance of capsules

Test	Specification
Containers' permeability and sealing	There are specifications listed in the pharmacopeia prescribing the type of container suitable for the repackaging or dispensing of each official capsule and tablet. Depending on the item, the container might be required to be tight, well-closed, and light resistant.
Disintegration	The compendial disintegration test for hard and soft gelatin capsules follows the same procedure and uses the same apparatus as described in this chapter under the head Tablets. The capsules are placed in the basket-rack assembly, which is repeatedly immersed 30 times per minute into a thermostatically controlled fluid at 37°C and observed over the time described in the individual monograph. To fully satisfy the test, the capsules disintegrate completely into a soft mass with no firm core and only some fragments of the gelatin shell.
Dissolution	The compendial dissolution test for capsules uses the same apparatus, dissolution medium, and test as that for uncoated and plain coated tablets. However, in instances in which the capsule shells interfere with the analysis, the contents of a specified number of capsules can be removed and the empty capsule shells dissolved in the dissolution medium before proceeding with the sampling and chemical analysis.
Stability	Stability testing of capsules is performed to determine the intrinsic stability of the active drug molecule and the influence of environmental factors such as temperature, humidity, light, formulation components, and the container and closure system. The accelerated stability tests help to determine the appropriate conditions for storage and the product's anticipated shelf life.
Moisture	The USP requires determination of the moisture-permeation characteristics of single-unit and unit dose containers to assure their suitability for packaging capsules. The degree and rate of moisture penetration is determined by packaging the dosage unit together with a color-revealing desiccant pellet, exposing the packaged unit to known relative humidity over a specified time, observing the desiccant pellet for color change (indicating absorption of moisture) and comparing the pre- and post-weight of the packaged unit.
Weight variation	The uniformity of dosage units may be demonstrated by determining weight variation or content uniformity. The weight variation method is as follows. **Hard capsules**: Ten capsules are individually weighed and the contents removed. The emptied shells are individually weighed and the net weight of the contents calculated by subtraction. From the results of an assay performed as directed in the individual monograph, the content of active ingredient in each of the capsules is determined. **Soft capsules**: The gross weight of 10 intact capsules is determined individually. Then each capsule is cut open with scissors or a sharp blade, and the contents are removed by washing with a suitable solvent. The solvent is allowed to evaporate at room temperature over a period of about 30 min, with precautions taken to avoid uptake or loss of moisture. The individual shells are weighed and the net contents calculated. From the results of the assay directed in the individual monograph, the content of active ingredient in each of the capsules is determined.
Content uniformity	Unless otherwise stated in the monograph for an individual capsule, the amount of active ingredient, determined by assay, is within the range of 85 to 115% of the label claim for 9 of 10 dosage units assayed, with no unit outside the range of 70 to 125% of label claim. Additional tests are prescribed when two or three dosage units are outside of the desired range but within the stated extremes.

Storage: Stored in an airtight container and in a cool place.

Use: Nasal decongestant.

Example 2: Liquid filled formula for sealed hard gelatin capsules		
Formula	**Quantity %**	**Use**
Acetaminophen	500 mg	Active
Glycerol esters of saturated fatty acids	300 mg	Carrier

1. Drug is mixed into the melted carrier and kept at a constant temperature of 40°C.

2. Capsules are moistened with a 50:50 water and ethanol mixture sprayed on to the joint and capillary action draws the liquid into the space between the body and the cap.

3. Excess fluid is removed by suction because the melting point of gelatin is lowered by the presence of water.

4. The product is maintained at a constant temperature of 40°C while filling.

5. A homogeneous suspension is maintained in the product hopper.

6. The required volumes of liquid are accurately dosed into capsules.

7. The machine ejects a filled capsule body when the cap is missing.

8. Application of gentle heat of approximately 45°C completes the melting over a period of about 1 min, and the two gelatin layers are fused together to form a complete 360° seal.

9. The gelatin setting or hardening process is completed while the product returns to room temperature. This process is best carried out on trays.

Storage: Stored in an airtight container and in a cool place.

Use: Analgesic and antipyretic.

Example 3: Phenytoin sodium capsule	
Ingredients	**Quantity**
Phenytoin sodium	50 mg
Lactose	100 mg

Method

1. As phenytoin sodium and lactose are both hygroscopic in nature, it is advisable to double-wrap both powders, using an inner wrapper of waxed paper.

2. Weigh and mix the ingredients; pass through a no. 250 sieve and remix.

3. Fill the capsules by apply a thin ring of acacia mucilage or water near the rim of the capsule body, using a very finely tipped camels hair brush. Put on the cap with a slight twisting motion and make sure that it is fully pressed down. If an excess of liquid is used the capsule will soften and distort.

4. Leave to dry for about 15 min. Then roll or tap each to loosen the contents and fill the cap. Finally clean the outsides by rolling between sheets of cellulose tissue.

Storage: Capsule should be kept in an airtight container.

Use: Antiepileptic and anticonvulsant.

CACHETS

Cachets are solid preparations consisting of a hard shell containing a single dose of one or more active substances. The cachet shell is made of unleavened bread usually from rice flour and consists of 2 prefabricated flat cylindrical sections. Before administration, the cachets are immersed in water for a few seconds, placed on the tongue and swallowed with a draught of water. Cachets are of two types: wet seal and dry seal. In **wet seal cachets,** two halves seal together with little water and in **dry seal cachet,** the upper half slightly larger than lower half. The powdered drug is filled in lower half and the upper half is fitted over it.

Advantages and Disadvantages of Cachet

Advantages

1. They can be prepared easily
2. They can disintegrate easily
3. They are available in unit dosage form
4. Being available in solid dosage form are more stable than liquids and semisolid preparation.

Disadvantages

1. They must be soften before swelling
2. Promote the growth of microorganism, as the shells are composed of rice starch.
3. They cannot protect the enclosed drugs from light and moisture.
4. They are not suitable for filling liquid and semisolids.

Example 1: Powdered rhubarb cachet BP	
Ingredients	Quantity
Powdered rhubarb	0.5 gm
Heavy magnesium carbonate	0.5 gm

Method

1. Check that the machine is clean and open it ready for use.
2. Weigh and mix the ingredients; pass through a no. 250 sieve and remix.
3. Weigh 1 gm of the mixture and form its bulk decide the appropriate size of cachet to use.
4. Fit six half-cachets into the center plate of the machine and cover their flanges with the correct side plate. Fit the other halves into the remaining plate and confirm that they fit firmly and will not fall out when the plate is turned over to bring the haves together. If none of the haves of the halves will fit tightly, it is possible that the wrong size plate has been used to cover the flanges. Storage under very dry condition causes shrinkage and since the shells are hygroscopic, the size varies slightly with atmospheric humidity.
5. Weigh the powders for each cachet on to papers prepared and arranged as for the making of divided powders.
6. Chose the correct funnel and thimble for the size of cachet.
7. Place the funnel over the first hole; carefully tip the powder in and try to keep it from the sides as far as possible.
8. Press down gently with thimble; heavy pressure causes the powder to put out of the funnel. After the removal of the thimble, the surface of the powder should be convex. Gently remove the funnel.
9. Fill the rest of the cachets. Lift the covering plate and check that the flanges are clean.
10. Moisten the roller by passing it through a cachet of plastic foam. Dampen with water, in a tray. Remove excess water from the role it over a piece of white dummy paper. Dampen the empty halves of the cachets and turn the plate over the filled haves and press it down firmly to ensure the good seal. Raise it again and the complete cachets will be lifted. Press them out gently without touching the flanges and leave them dry.
11. Test the sealing and reject any that are open or have badly cricked edges, due to under or over wetting respectively.

Storage: Cachets should be kept in an airtight container.

Use: As a laxative.

PASTILLES

Pastilles are a type of candy or medicinal pill made of a thick liquid that has been solidified and is meant to be consumed by light chewing and allowing it to dissolve in the mouth. They are also used to describe certain forms of incense. A pastille is also known as a "troche", or a medicated lozenge that dissolves like candy. Pastille bases consist of principally of a mixture of gelatin and glycerol or a mixture of both.

Advantages and Disadvantages of Pastilles

Advantages

1. They can be prepared easily
2. They are available in suitable flavor base, help to mask the bitter and unpleasant taste of medicaments
3. They are available in unit dosage form
4. Pastilles are placed in the mouth where they slowly dissolve and thus produce sustained therapeutic action
5. Being available in solid dosage form are more stable than liquids and semisolid preparation.

Disadvantages

1. Heat liable drugs are difficult to dispense
2. They are not suitable; where there are immediate action was intended.

Production

Pastilles are made by pouring a thick liquids into a powdered, sugared or waxed mold and then allowing the liquid to set and dry. The substances contained in the dried liquid are slowly released when chewed and allowed to dissolve in the mouth. The substances are then absorbed by the mucous membranes of the oral cavity or in the lower gastrointestinal tracts. Various substances, including medicaments and other excipients can be put into pastille forms. Due to the oily nature of these active substances (essential oils, tinctures and extracts), pastilles are usually based on a mixtures of starch and gum arabic, which emulsifies the substance and binds them in a hydrocolloidal matrix. The starch and gum also reduces the rate in which the pastille dissolves and moderates the amount of active substances delivered at an item. Gum arabic also hardens the pastilles and makes them more sturdy in storage and transport.

Storage: Pastiles are dispensed in flat boxes made of metal. They should be stored in a cool and dry place.

Example 1: Gelatin pastilles	
Ingredients	**Quantity**
Gelatine	200 g
Glycerol	400 g
Sodium benzoate	2 g
Citric acid monohydrate	20 g
Sucrose	50 g
Lemon oil	1 ml
Amaranth solution	20 ml
Purified water, freshly boiled and cooled sufficient to produce	1000 ml

Method: Soak the gelatin in 300 g of purified water until softened, add the glycerol, heat on a water bath until the gelatin has dissolved and the mass weighs 850 g separately dissolve the sucrose, the citric acid monohydrate and the sodium benzoate in 60 ml of purified water, add the solution to mass, add the lemon oil and the amaranth solution and sufficient purified water to produce 1000 g strain and allow to cool. The rate at which the pastille basis dissolves may be reduced by replacing part of the gelatin in above formula with agar the product will be opalescent. Care should be taken to minimize microbial contamination during the preparation of pastille basis.

Storage: Keep in a dry and cool place.

Use: As directed.

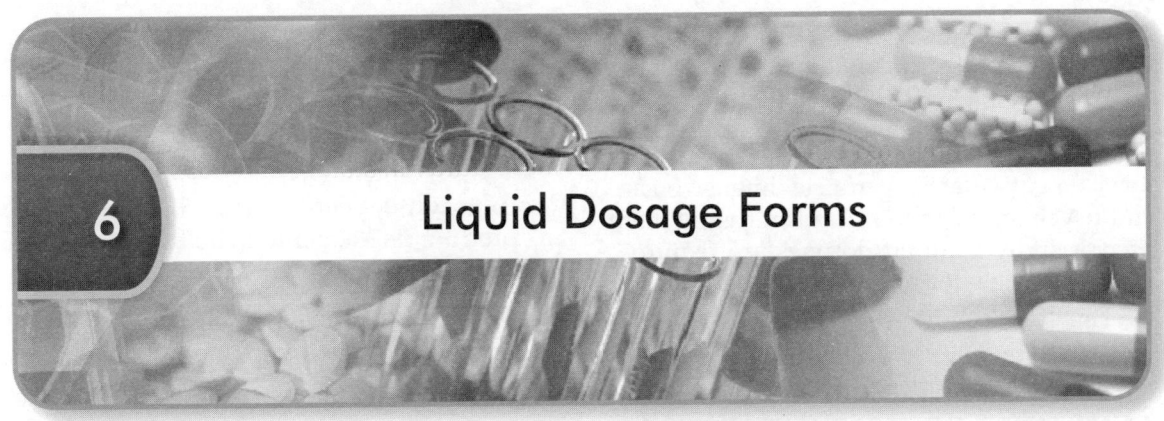

6 Liquid Dosage Forms

INTRODUCTION

The effectiveness of a pharmaceutical agent depends on its form and route of administration; therefore, it is important to understand the various forms in which drugs are dispensed. Liquid dosage forms are one of the oldest dosage forms used in the treatment of patients and afford rapid and high absorption of medicinal products. Therefore, the compounding of liquid dosage forms retains an important place in therapeutics today. They are particularly useful for individuals who have difficulty in swallowing solid dosage forms (e.g. pediatric, geriatric, intensive care and psychiatric patients), and in cases where precise, individualised dosages are required. Liquid dosage forms prepared by dissolving the active ingredient(s) in an aqueous or non- aqueous solvent, including solutions, suspensions, and emulsions.

ADVANTAGES AND DISADVANTAGES OF LIQUID DOSAGE FORMS

Advantages

1. The active agent is homogeneously dispersed throughout the product.
2. The active agent is in solution and does not need to undergo dissolution; therefore, the therapeutic response is generally faster than solid dosage form like tablet or capsule.
3. The dose of the active agent is easily and conveniently adjusted by measuring a different volume.
4. Solutions may be swallowed by patients, who have difficulty taking tablets or capsules, as might be the case with pediatric or geriatric patients.
5. Drugs such as potassium chloride that may cause ulceration to the mucosa in a tablet formulation avoid this side effect when present in solution.
6. Bitter and unpleasant drugs can be formulated in sweetened, colored and flavored vehicles.
7. Hygroscopic and deliquescent medicaments which are not suitably dispensed in solid dosage forms can easily be given in liquid dosage forms.

Disadvantages

1. The active ingredients, when present in solution, are usually more susceptible to chemical degradation, particularly hydrolysis, than when they are in a solid dosage form.
2. As a consequence of item 1, the solution product has a limited shelf life than the solid formulation.
3. Drug substance having unpleasant taste or smell is difficult to mask in solutions.
4. Liquid dosage forms are heavier and take up more shelf space than corresponding solid dosage forms. If the container breaks, the product is invariably lost.
5. Liquid dosage forms may require special storage facilities in very cold or very hot conditions. In one case, the drug might need to be kept refrigerated, and in another case the patient may need to protect the drug from freezing.
6. The delivery of the dose depends upon the patient, measuring the proper volume. This can be a significant issue for vision-impaired patients, patients with arthritis, or patients unable to read the numbers on an oral dosing syringe or medicine cup.
7. Solutions are often susceptible to microbial contamination, and therefore, preservatives are frequently incorporated into the formulation. Some patients may be allergic to certain preservatives.
8. Two incompatible drugs cannot be dispensed together as it is possible in case of solid dosage forms.

CLASSIFICATION OF LIQUID DOSAGE FORM

Liquid preparations are typically classified on the basis of their physical properties. Method of preparation, use, and ingredient types or concentrations are enlisted in Table 6.1.

Table 6.1: Classification of liquid dosage forms

Type	Product illustration	Description and labeling requirements
1.	**Monophasic liquid dosage form for oral use**: Oral solutions are administered to the gastrointestinal tract to provide systemic absorption of the therapeutic agent. Due to the resilience of the gastrointestinal environment, oral solutions may be formulated over a broad pH range. There are three principal types of solution formulations that are administered orally— oral solutions, oral syrups and oral elixirs. In addition, other solution formulations are employed for a local effect, e.g. mouthwashes and gargles.	
Syrup	Syrup	Syrups are highly concentrated (66.7%w/w according to BP and IP and 85% w/v as per USP), aqueous solutions of sugar or a sugar substitute that traditionally contain a flavoring agent, e.g. cherry syrup, cocoa syrup, orange syrup, raspberry syrup. Therapeutic agents either may be directly incorporated into these systems or may be added as the syrup is being prepared. Labels of liquid dosage forms must contain information's like drug content, alcohol content (if present), storage conditions, batch no., Mfg. Lic. No., date of manufacturing, date of expiry and name and address of the manufacturer.
Elixir	Banophen ALLERGY Elixir	An elixir is a clear, hydroalcoholic solution that is formulated for oral use. The concentration of alcohol required in the elixir is unique to each formulation and is sufficient to ensure that all of the other components within the formulation remain in solution. For this purpose, other polyol cosolvents may be incorporated into the formulation. The presence of alcohol in elixirs presents a possible problem in pediatric formulations and indeed for those adults who wish to avoid alcohol. Labels of elixirs should contain all requirements as discussed in syrups but one most important point here is the amount of alcohol content should be mentioned on the label and all other necessary requirements of liquid dosage forms.
Linctuses	Actifed DM COUGH LINCTUS Linctuses	Linctuses are viscous preparations that contain the therapeutic agent dissolved in a vehicle composed of a high percentage of sucrose and, if required, other sweetening agents. These formulations are administered orally and are primarily employed for the treatment of cough, due to their soothing actions on the inflamed mucous membranes. Linctuses may also be formulated as sugar-free alternatives in which sucrose is replaced by sorbitol and the required concentration of sweetening agent. Labels must contain all necessary requirements of liquid dosage forms.

contd...

Table 6.1: Classification of liquid dosage forms (*contd.*)

Type	Product illustration	Description and labeling requirements
Aromatic water	Aromatic water	Aromatic waters are saturated solutions of volatile oils or other aromatic substances in water, usually employed for their flavoring rather than their medicinal properties. Aromatic waters contain a small amount of ethanol. Aromatic waters are normally prepared by diluting a concentrated, ethanolic solution of the aromatic substance with water. The label states: (1) the date after which the aromatic water is not intended to be used; (2) the conditions under which the aromatic water should be stored.
Fluid extract	Fluid extract	Fluid extracts are concentrated alcoholic solutions of animal or vegetable drugs obtained by removal of active constituent by extraction (maceration, percolation). Infusions are prepared by extracting the drug using 25% alcohol, but without the application of heat. Traditionally, these preparations are then diluted 1:10 in the final product. Tinctures are alcoholic extracts of drugs but are relatively weak compared with extracts. Labels of fluid extracts should contain all requirements as discussed in elixirs.

2. **Monophasic liquid dosage form for external use:** Monophasic liquid dosage forms for external use are aqueous, oily or alcoholic liquid preparations intended for external application. It must bear the directions like for external use only and all other necessary requirements of liquid dosage forms.

Type	Product illustration	Description and labeling requirements
Lotions	Lotion applicator	Lotions are the aqueous, oily or alcoholic liquid preparations or suspensions, intended for external application without friction. They are usually applied on the affected parts with the help of some absorbent materials such as cottons. It must bear the directions like for external use only. Keep out of the children and apply without rubbing and other necessary requirements of liquid dosage forms.
Liniments	Liniment to be applied with friction	Liniments are usually alcoholic and oily liquid preparations or emulsions intended for external use with friction. They are applied on the skin with rubbing and should never be applied on the broken skin. They are supplied in the fluted bottles. In addition to these, they must bear the directions like external use only, apply with gentle rubbing, not to apply on the broken skin and keep out of the reach of the children and other necessary requirements of liquid dosage forms.

contd...

Table 6.1: Classification of liquid dosage forms (*contd.*)

Type	Product illustration	Description and labeling requirements
Collodions	Collodion	Collodions are fluid preparations for the external use. They contain volatile vehicle which evaporate on the applications to the skin, leaving a flexible, protective covering on the affected site. The preparation is applied with either brush or rod.
Tincture		Tinctures are alcoholic or hydroalcoholic solutions prepared from vegetable materials or chemical substances by dissolution or extraction. Labels of tincture should contain all requirements as discussed in elixirs.
Spirit	Chloroform spirit	They are hydroalcoholic solutions of aromatic or volatile substances. Labels of spirits should contain all requirements as discussed in elixirs.

3. **Monophasic liquid dosage form for special use**: These are monophasic liquid dosage preparations consisting of aqueous solutions used to cleanse, deodorize, soothe or medicate wounds, body orifices or cavities after applying them. It must bear the directions like for external use only and all other necessary requirements of liquid dosage forms.

Type	Product illustration	Description and labeling requirements
Gargles, mouth-washes	How to use of gargel	Mouthwashes/gargles are designed for the treatment of infection and inflammation of the oral cavity. Formulations designed for this purpose employ water as the vehicle, although a cosolvent, e.g. alcohol, may be employed to solubilize the active agent. Labels on the bottles must bear the directions like for external use only, dilution ratio with warm water and all other necessary requirements of liquid dosage forms.
Nasal sprays and nasal drops	Inflamed nose	These are formulated as small-volume solutions in an aqueous vehicle, oils being no longer used for nasal administration. Because the buffering capacity of nasal mucus is low, formulation at a pH of 6.8 is necessary. Nasal drops should also be made isotonic with nasal secretions using sodium chloride, and viscosity can also be modified using cellulose derivatives if necessary. Labels on the bottles must bear the directions like for external use only, for the use only in nose and number of drops to be instilled at a time. It should contain other necessary requirements of liquid dosage forms.

contd...

Type	Product illustration	Description and labeling requirements
	Table 6.1: Classification of liquid dosage forms (*contd.*)	
Douches	Various types of container used to dispense douches.	Douches are aqueous solutions used to cleanse, deodorize, soothe or medicate wounds, body orifices or cavities after applying them in low pressure. Labels on the bottles must bear the directions like for external use only, dilution ratio with warm water, quantity of powder or number of tablets to be dissolved in the specified quantity of water and other necessary requirements of liquid dosage forms.
Eyedrops	Use of eyedrops	Eyedrops are sterile aqueous or oily solutions or suspensions for instillation into the eye. They may contain excipients, to adjust tonicity or viscosity, to adjust or stabilize the pH, to increase the solubility of the active substances, to stabilize the preparation or to provide adequate antimicrobial properties. Eyedrops are supplied in small volumes, not more than 15 ml so to avoid repeated use of the same preparation for long time. Labels on the bottles must bear the directions like for external use only, do not touch the dropper with the eye, avoid contamination during use, and discard after one month of opening the container and other necessary requirements of liquid dosage forms.
Eardrops	Use of eardrops	Ear preparations are liquid, semi-solid or solid preparations intended for instillation, for spraying, for insufflation, for application to the auditory meatus or as an ear wash. Ear preparations usually contain one or more active substances in a suitable vehicle and stabilizers like tonicity modifier, preservatives, antioxidants may present to stabilize the preparation or to provide adequate antimicrobial properties. The excipients do not adversely affect the intended medicinal action of the preparation or, at the concentrations used, cause toxicity or undue local irritation. Ear preparations are supplied in multi-dose or single-dose containers, provided, if necessary, with a suitable administration device which may be designed to avoid the introduction of contaminants. Eardrops are supplied in containers of glass or suitable plastic that are fitted with an integral dropper or with a screw cap of suitable materials incorporating a dropper and rubber or plastic teat. Alternatively, such a cap assembly is supplied separately. The label states: (1) the names and concentrations of the active ingredients; (2) that the ear drops are intended for external use only.

contd...

Table 6.1: Classification of liquid dosage forms (*contd.*)

Type	Product illustration	Description and labeling requirements
Inhalations	 Use of an inhaler	Inhalations are liquid solutions or suspensions preparations consisting of volatile substances. They are used to relieve congestion and inflammation of the respiratory tract. They are supplied in a fluted glass bottle which should be airtight. Labels on the bottles must bear the directions like for external use only, store in a cool place, for nasal inhalation, quantity required to be added in the hot water and other necessary requirements of liquid dosage forms.
Enemas	 Route for enema administration	Enemas are pharmaceutical solutions that are administered rectally and are employed to ensure clearance of the bowel, usually by softening the faces or by increasing the amount of water in the large bowel (osmotic laxatives). Enemas may be aqueous or oil-based solutions and, in some formulations, the vehicle is the agent that promotes bowel evacuation, e.g. arachis oil retention enema. Aqueous formulations usually contain salts (e.g. phosphates) to alter the osmolality within the rectum, thereby increasing the movement of fluid to the rectal contents. Viscosity-enhancing agents, e.g. glycerol, may be included to aid retention of the formulation within the rectum and to reduce the incidence of seepage. Labels on the bottles must bear the directions like for external use only, store in a cool place, lubricate the nozzle before administration, warm the solution up to 37°C along with other necessary requirements of liquid dosage forms.

4. **Monophasic liquid dosage form for parenteral use**: They are introduced into body compartment. One has to be very careful about their sterility, isotonicity and clarity. Labels must bear the necessary directions of liquid dosage forms for internal use in addition to the route of administration.

Parenteral solution	 Parental route	Parenteral solutions are sterile drug solutions intended for administration by injection under or through one or more layers of skin or mucous membrane. They should be sterile, isotonic and clear solutions. Labels must bear the necessary directions of liquid dosage forms for internal use in addition to the route of administration. These must be depicted clearly on the label with a dose to be administered at a time, if multi-dose container is used.

contd...

Type	Product illustration	Description and labeling requirements
Table 6.1: Classification of liquid dosage forms (*contd.*)		
Biphasic liquid dosage form (emulsions) liquid in liquid.		
Emulsions	Oil Droplets / Water / Oil in water emulsion	Emulsions are thermodynamically unstable system consisting of two immiscible liquid phases, one of which is dispersed as globules in the other liquid phase with the help of emulsifying agents. In pharmaceutical emulsions, one phase is usually water and the other are non-aqueous, i.e. lipids or oils. There are two types of emulsions depending on the existence of the phase, viz. internal or external. They may be oil in water, in these types of emulsions, oil is internal phase dispersed in water which is external phase. These types of preparation are usually used for external application. Labels on the bottles must bear the directions like shake well before use and other necessary requirements of liquid dosage forms depending on its application , i.e. intended for external or internal use.
Biphasic liquid dosage form (suspensions) solid in liquid.		
Suspensions	Suspensions	Suspensions are referred as solid–liquid dispersions. They are heterogeneous preparations in which poorly soluble drugs in finer particle size are distributed in the vehicle. Labels on the bottles must bear the directions like shake well before use and all other necessary requirements of liquid dosage forms depending on its application, i.e. intended for external or internal use.

DESIGN AND FORMULATION OF LIQUID DOSAGE FORM

Design of liquid preparation involves the combination of ingredients with therapeutically active agents to enhance the acceptability or effectiveness of the product. The formulation of pharmaceutical liquids requires several considerations—drug concentration; drug solubility; vehicle selection; physical and chemical stability; preservation; and appropriate additives such as buffers, solubilizers, sweetening agents, viscosity-controlling agents, colors, and flavors. Solubility is of paramount importance when developing oral solutions. The drug and other dissolved substances should remain solubilized throughout the shelf life of the product. Several physicochemical properties, including molecular weight, volume, density, hydrogen bond donors and hydrogen bond acceptors affect the solubility of the therapeutic agents. Furthermore, the properties of the solid state, e.g. crystal habit, crystalline/amorphous properties, will also affect the solubility of the therapeutic agent. The solubilities of therapeutic agents that are either acids or bases (representing the vast majority of drug substances) are pH-dependent.

EXCIPIENTS USED IN LIQUID DOSAGE FORMS

Excipients in pharmaceutical formulations are physiologically inert compounds that are included in the formulation to facilitate the administration of the dosage form, e.g. pourability, palatability, to protect the formulation from issues regarding physical and chemical stability and to enhance the solubility of the therapeutic agent. Pharmaceutical solutions commonly contain a wide range of excipients, the details of which are provided below.

Vehicles

Water is the most common vehicle for the liquid preparations. Other than water, there are some aromatic waters, elixirs and syrups which form the vehicles for other oral preparations. Other vehicles are also employed for dispensing many other preparations like liquid for external use and parenteral solutions. Uses and properties of different vehicles are given in Table 6.2.

Stabilizers

Stabilizers are the materials which stabilize the pharmaceutical preparations if they are to be kept for longer period of time. As the

Table 6.2: Vehicles used for liquid dosage forms		
Components and additives	**Examples**	**Comments**
Vehicle	Purified water USP	It is prepared by distillation, ion exchange methods or by reverse osmosis. The solid residue (obtained after evaporation) is less than 1 mg per 100 ml of evaporated sample.
		It must not be used for the preparation of parenteral formulations.
	Water for injection	It is prepared by triple distillation. It should be deionised, sterile, pyrogen free, clear and colorless.
	Sterile water for injection	It is prepared by triple distillation. It should be deionised, sterile, pyrogen free, clear and colorless. They must be suitable packaged in single dose containers not exceeding 100 ml. No bacteriostatic agent added.
	Bacteriostatic water for injection	They are sterile water for injection containing one or more suitable bacteriostatic agents.
	Corn oil, cottonseed oil, peanut oil and seasome oil	They must be clear, light or pale yellow and odorless.
	Glycerol	Glycerol (also termed glycerin) is an odorless, sweet liquid that is miscible with water
	Alcohol USP	Alcohol USP contains between 94.9 and 96.0% v/v ethyl alcohol (ethanol) and is commonly used as a cosolvent, both as a single cosolvent and with other cosolvents, e.g. glycerol.
	Propylene glycol USP	Propylene glycol USP is an odorless, colorless, viscous liquid. It is used in pharmaceutical preparations as a cosolvent, generally as a replacement for glycerin.
	PEG	Lower-molecular-weight grades (PEG 200, PEG 400) are preferred as cosolvents in pharmaceutical solutions.
	Aromatic waters	They are aqueous saturated solution of volatile oils or substances.

time passes, there are chances of some factors which might affect the stability of preparations like microbial growth, oxidation, change in pH, etc. to avoid these types of changes during the shelf life of the formulation, stabilizers like preservatives, antioxidants and buffer are to be added.

Preservatives

Preservatives are included in pharmaceutical solutions to control the microbial growth. Ideally, preservatives should exhibit the following properties:

- Possess a broad-spectrum of antimicrobial activity encompassing gram-positive and gram-negative bacteria and fungi.
- Chemically and physically stable over the shelf life of the product.
- Have low toxicity.
- Compatible with the ingredients in the dosage form.
- Free of taste and odor.

Antioxidants

Antioxidants are included in pharmaceutical solutions to enhance the stability of therapeutic agents that are susceptible to oxidation.

- The ideal antioxidant should be stable and effective over a wide pH range, soluble in its oxidized state, colorless, non-toxic, nonvolatile, non-irritating, effective in low concentration, thermostable and compatible with container, closures and formulation ingredients.
- Antioxidants that are commonly used for aqueous formulations include sodium sulfite, sodium metabisulfite, sodium formaldehyde sulfoxylate and ascorbic acid.
- Antioxidants that are used for oily formulations include propyl gallate, butylated hydroxyl toluene, butylated hydroxyl anisole and alpha tocopherol.

Buffers

Buffers are used to adjust the pH of a formulation. pH is an important factor in determining the rate of hydrolysis. The solubility of weakly acidic and basic drugs is markedly influenced by the pH. Pharmaceutical buffer should exihibit following properties:

- The buffer must have adequate capacity of maintaning pH in the desired pH range.
- The buffer must be biologically safe for intended use.
- The buffer should be non-toxic, non-irritating, effective in low concentration, and compatible with formulation ingredients.

Viscosity-enhancing Agents

The viscosity of the formulation must be sufficiently controlled in order to ensure the accurate measurement of the volume to be dispensed. The viscosity of pharmaceutical solutions may be easily increased (and controlled) by the addition of non-ionic or ionic hydrophilic polymers. Examples of both of these categories are shown below.

1. Non-ionic (neutral) polymers cellulose derivatives, e.g. methylcellulose, hydroxyethylcellulose, hydroxypropylcellulose, polyvinylpyrrolidone
2. Ionic polymers, e.g. sodium carboxymethylcellulose (anionic), sodium alginate (anionic). These agents must be tested for their incompatibilities with drug and other additives in the formulation.

Sweetening Agents

Sweeteners are indispensable components of many liquid oral dosage forms, especially those containing bitter or other unacceptable tastes. The use of sweetening agents must be done on the basis of their physical and chemical properties, relative sweetness and toxic effects.

Flavoring Agents

Unfortunately, the vast majority of drugs in solution are unpalatable and, therefore, the addition of flavors is often required to mask the taste of the drug substance. Taste-masking using flavors is a difficult task; however, there are some empirical approaches that may be taken to produce a palatable formulation. The four basic taste sensations are salty, sweet, bitter and sour. It has been proposed that certain flavors should be used to mask these specific taste sensations.

Coloring Agents

Colors are pharmaceutical ingredients that impart the preferred color to the formulation.

When used in combination with flavors, the selected color should 'match' the flavor of the formulation, e.g. green with mint-flavored solutions, red for strawberry-flavored formulations. Although the inclusion of colors is not a prerequisite for all pharmaceutical solutions, certain categories of solution (e.g. mouthwashes/gargles) are normally colored. The commonly used stabilizers for liquid preparations are listed in Table 6.3.

Function	Agent	Concentration (%)
Preservatives	Benzalkonium chloride	0.01
	Benzyl alcohol chlorobutanol	2.0–0.5
	Chlorocresol	0.1–0.3
	Cresol	0.3–0.5
	Methyl paraben	0.18
	Propyl paraben	0.02
	Phenol	0.5
	Phenylmercuric nitrate	0.002
	Thimerosal	0.01
Antioxidants	Ascorbic acid	0.02–0.1
	Butyl hydroxyanisole	0.005–0.02
	Butyl hydroxytoluene	0.005–0.02
	Sodium bisulfite	0.1–0.15
	Sodium formaldehyde sulfoxylate,	0.1–0.15
	Thiourea	0.005
	Tocopherol	0.05–0.075
Chelating agents	Ethylenediamine tetra-acetic acid	0.01–0.075
Buffering agents	Salts acetic acid Salt citric acid	1–2 1–3
Tonicity agents	Acid salts of phosphoric acid dextrose sodium chloride	0.9 0.8–2 5
Sweetener	Sucrose	65
	Fructose	65
	Glucose	65–80
	Sorbitol	25–30
	Saccharin,	1–2
Flavors	Allyl benzoate (cherry)	3000 ppm
	Allyl caproate (pineapple)	1000 ppm
	Allyl cyclohexylbutyrate (pineapple)	1000 ppm
	Allyl cyclohexylcaproate (peach/apricot)	1500 ppm
	Allyl cyclohexylvalerate (apple)	600 ppm
	Allyl phenoxyacetate (honey/pineapple)	2000 ppm
	Anethol (anise)	3000 ppm

Table 6.3: Pharmaceutical additives used in liquid oral preparations

GENERAL METHOD FOR THE PREPARATIONS OF LIQUID DOSAGE FORMS

The following general method should be used in the preparation of a solution:

1. Calculate the quantities required for each ingredient in the formula to produce the required final volume.
2. Weigh all solids ingredients.
3. Identify the soluble solids and calculate the quantity of vehicle required to dissolve the solids. If more than one solid is to be dissolved, they are dissolved one by one, in order of solubility (i.e. the least soluble first). Remember that the solubility of the soluble solids will be dependent on the vehicle used.
4. Transfer the appropriate amount of vehicle to a glass beaker.
5. If necessary, transfer the solid to a glass mortar and use the glass pestle to reduce particle size to aid dissolution.
6. Transfer the solid to the beaker and stir to aid dissolution. If a mortar and pestle have been used to reduce particle size, ensure that the mortar is rinsed with a little vehicle to ensure complete transfer of the powders.
7. When all the solid(s) has/have dissolved, transfer the solution to the conical measure that will be used to hold the final solution.
8. Rinse out the beaker in which the solution was made with a portion of the vehicle and transfer the rinsing to the conical measure.
9. Add any remaining liquid ingredients to the conical measure and stir.
10. Make up to final volume with remaining vehicle.
11. Transfer to a suitable container, label and dispense to the patient.

GENERAL LABELING REQUIREMENTS OF LIQUID DOSAGE FORM

The following requirements are applicable to medicines manufactured or prepared in accordance with medicines legislation. They are not intended to apply to repackaging and assembly activities. These critical items of information, which should be located together on the pack and appear in the same field of view, are— name, strength, route of administration, dosage and warnings.

- The common name of the product.
- A statement of the active ingredients expressed qualitatively and quantitatively per dosage unit or for a given volume or weight.
- Route of administration.
- Instructions for use, including any special warnings.
- The pharmaceutical form.
- The contents of the container by weight, volume or by number of doses.
- Excipients of known effect. For injectable, topical (including inhalation products) and ophthalmic medicines, all excipients.
- Keep out of reach and sight of children.
- The expiry date expressed in unambiguous terms.
- Any special storage precautions.
- The manufacturer's ML number, where appropriate.
- The manufacturer's name and address.
- The batch number.
- For external use only (for liquids intended for topical application).
- Shake well before use (for biphasic liquid dosage forms).
- Statutory warnings required for particular actives, e.g. aspirin, paracetamol.
- For small containers, certain details may be omitted, but the label should contain, as a minimum, including following information: common name of the product, its therapeutic use, content of active principles, manufacturing license no. date of manufacturing, date of expiry and warning if any other details may be included in packaging inserts.

PACKAGING REQUIREMENTS OF LIQUID DOSAGE FORM

A brief overview of the main considerations for the packaging of solutions will be given here. When selecting packaging for extemporaneously prepared solutions, consideration should be given to the route or method of administration. Liquid preparations that are intended for the oral route should be packed in plain (smooth) amber bottles. External preparations and preparations that are not intended to be taken internally (e.g. mouthwashes) should be packaged in fluted amber bottles (i.e. amber bottles with vertical ridges or grooves). This will enable simple identification, by both sight and touch, of preparations that are not to be taken via the oral route. Pharmaceutical bottles come in a variety of different sizes and it is important to choose a suitably sized container to match the volume of preparation to be dispensed. Obviously, it is important not to use a container that is too large for the volume of preparation to be dispensed for both cost and appearance issues (Table 6.4).

Syrups

Syrups are concentrated solutions of sugar such as sucrose in water or other aqueous liquid.

Simple syrup: When water is used alone for making syrup.

Medicated syrup: When the aqueous preparation contains some added medicinal substance.

Flavored syrup: Which contains aromatic or pleasantly flavored substances and is intended to be used as a vehicle or flavor for prescriptions.

Important Characteristics of Syrup

- Syrup exerted an osmotic pressure due to that the growth of bacteria, fungi and moulds was inhibited.
- If sucrose concentration is not proper, i.e. 66.7%w/w, it is prone to microbial growth, which requires addition of preservatives.
- The choice of syrup vehicle must be performed with due consideration to the physicochemical properties of the therapeutic agent. For example, cherry syrup and orange syrup are acidic and therefore the solubility of acidic drugs may be lowered and may result in precipitation of the drug substance.
- A saturated solution of sucrose may lead to crystallization of a part of the sucrose under conditions of changing temperature.

Table 6.4: Summary of packaging for pharmaceutical solutions			
Site of administration	Container	Typical sizes	Pharmaceutical products
Oral liquids	Amber flat medical bottle.	50 ml, 100 ml, 150 ml, 200 ml, 300 ml, 500 ml	Draughts, elixirs, linctuses, mixtures, spirits, syrups, pediatric drops.
	Amber round medical bottle with dropper top.	10 ml	Pediatric drops
External liquids	Amber fluted medical bottle.	50 ml, 100 ml, 200 ml	Applications collodions, enemas and douches, gargles and mouthwashes, liniments, lotions
	Amber fluted medical bottle with dropper top	10 ml	Eardrops, nose drops

- Syrups possess remarkable masking properties for bitter and saline drugs.

- Sucrose also retards oxidation because it is partly hydrolyzed into the reducing sugars glucose and fructose.

Invert Syrup

- It is prepared by hydrolyzing sucrose with hydrochloric acid and neutralizing the solution with Ca or Na carbonate.

- The sucrose in the 66.7% w/w solution must be at least 95% inverted.

- The invert syrup, when mixed in suitable proportions with syrup, prevents the deposition of crystals of sucrose under most conditions of storage.

Preparation of Syrups

Syrups should be carefully prepared in clean equipment to prevent contamination. Three methods may be used to prepare syrups.

1. Solution with Heat

- This is the usual method of making syrups:
  - ❖ In the absence of volatile agents or thermoliable substance.
  - ❖ When it is desirable to make the syrup rapidly.

- The sucrose is added to the purified water or aqueous solution and heated until dissolved, then strained and sufficient purified water added to make the desired weight or volume.

- Excessive heating in the preparation of syrups must be avoided to prevent inversion of sucrose, with increased tendency to fermentation. Syrups cannot be sterilized by autoclaving without caramelization (yellow color).

- The specific gravity of syrup is an important property to identify its concentration. Syrup has a specific gravity of about 1.313,

which means that each 100 ml of syrup weighs 131.3 g.

2. Agitation without Heat

- This process is used in those cases where heat would cause loss of valuable volatile constituents.

- The syrup is prepared by adding sucrose to the aqueous solution in a bottle of about twice the size required for the syrup. This permits active agitation and rapid solution.

- The stoppering of the bottle is important, as it prevents contamination and loss during the process.

3. Addition of a Medicating Liquid to Syrup

- This method is resorted in those cases in which fluid extracts, tinctures, or other liquids are added to syrup to medicate it.

- Syrups made in this way usually develop precipitates since alcohol is often an ingredient of the liquids, thus, used and the resinous and oily substances dissolved by the alcohol precipitate when mixed with syrup.

- A modification of this process consists of mixing the fluid extract or tincture with the water, allowing the mixture to stand to permit the separation of insoluble constituents, filtering and then dissolving the sucrose in the filtrate.

This procedure is not permissible when the precipitated ingredients are the valuable medicinal agents.

Percolation

- In this procedure, purified water or an aqueous solution is permitted to pass slowly through a bed of crystalline sucrose, thus dissolving it and forming a syrup a pledget of cotton is placed in the neck of the percolator.

- If necessary, a portion of the liquid is repassed through the percolator to dissolve all of the sucrose.

Preservation

- The USP suggests that syrups must be kept at a temperature not above 25°C.
- Preservatives such as glycerin, methyl paraben, benzoic acid and sodium benzoate may be added to prevent bacterial and mold growth, particularly when the concentration of sucrose in the syrup is low.
- The concentration of preservative is proportional to the free water.
- The official syrups should be preserved in well-dried bottles and stored in a cool dark place.

Labeling

Labels must contain information's like drug content, alcohol content (if present), storage conditions, batch no., Mfg. Lic. no., date of manufacturing, date of expiry and name and address of the manufacturer and also comply with other general requirements for labeling of oral liquids.

Example 1: Codeine phosphate syrup (IP, 1966)

Ingredients	Quantity
Codeine phosphate	5 g
Chloroform spirit	25 ml
Purified water	15 ml
Syrup sufficient to produce	1000 ml

Method

1. Dissolve the codeine phosphate in the purified water.
2. Add the 750 ml of syrup and chloroform spirit.
3. Mix and add sufficient syrup to produce 1000 ml.

Storage: Codeine phosphate syrup in well-closed container protected from light.

Use: Analgesic, antitussive.

Example 2: Chocolate syrup

Ingredients	Quantity
Chocolate	180 gm
Sucrose	600 gm
Liquid glucose	180 gm
Glycerin	50 ml
Sodium chloride	2 gm
Vanillin	0.2 gm
Sodium benzoate	1 gm
Purified water q.s	1000 ml

Method

1. Mix chocolate and sucrose, and to this mixture gradually add a solution of liquid glucose, glycerin, sodium chloride, vanillin, and sodium benzoate in 325 ml of hot purified water.
2. Bring the entire mixture boil, and maintain at boiling temperature for 3 minutes.
3. Allow to cool to room temperature, and add sufficient purified water to make the product measure 1000 ml.

Packaging and storage: Preserve in airtight containers, and avoid exposure to excessive heat.

Use: Vehicle and pharmaceutical aid.

Example 3: Cherry syrup

Ingredients	Quantity
Cherry juice	475 ml
Sucrose	800 gm
Alcohol	20 ml
Purified water q.s	100 ml

Method

1. Dissolve sucrose in cherry juice by gently heating on a steam bath, cool, and remove the foam and floating solids.
2. Add alcohol and sufficient purified water to make 1000 ml and mix.

Packaging and storage: Preserve in airtight, light-resistant containers, and prevent exposure to excessive heat.

Use: Pharmaceutical aid.

Example 4: Ferrous sulfate syrup	
Ingredients	**Quantity**
Ferrous sulfate	40.0 g
Citric acid	2.1 g
Peppermint spirit	2 ml
Sucrose	825 g
Purified water	To make 1000 ml

Method

1. Dissolve the ferrous sulfate, citric acid, peppermint spirit, and 200 g of the sucrose in 450 ml of purified water and filter the solution until clear.
2. Dissolve the remainder of the sucrose in the clear filtrate and add purified water to make 1000 ml.
3. Mix, and filter if necessary through a pledge of cotton.

Packaging and storage: Preserve in airtight, light-resistant containers, and prevent exposure to excessive heat.

Use: Iron supplement.

Example 5: Amantadine hydrochloride syrup	
Ingredients	**Quantity**
Amantadine hydrochloride	10.0 g
Citric acid	2.1 g
Artificial raspberry flavor	2 ml
Methylparaben	825 g
Propylparaben	0.5 g
Sorbitol solution	To make 1000 ml

Method: Dissolve the amantadine hydrochloride, the citric acid, flavor and preservative in the sorbitol solution. In some syrups, the high quantity of sucrose is sufficient to preserve them. Others require the addition of preservatives.

Packaging and storage: Preserve in airtight, light-resistant containers, and prevent exposure to excessive heat.

Use: Antiviral.

Elixirs

- Elixirs are clear, pleasantly flavored, sweetened hydroalcoholic liquids intended for oral use.
- They are used as flavors and vehicles.
- The main ingredients in elixirs are ethanol and water, but glycerin, sorbitol, propylene glycol, flavoring agents, preservatives, and syrups are often used in the preparation of the final product.
- Elixirs contain ethyl alcohol, however, the alcoholic content will vary greatly, from elixir containing only a small quantity to those that contain a considerable portion as a necessary aid to solubility.
- An elixir may contain water and alcohol soluble ingredients.

Incompatibility of Elixirs

- Alcohol precipitates water soluble substances, e.g. tragacanth, acacia agar and many inorganic salts from aqueous solutions.
- If an aqueous solution is added to an elixir, a partial precipitation of ingredients may occur. This is due to the reduced alcoholic content of the final preparation.

Non-medicated Elixirs

When there is no therapeutically active component in the elixir. It is used as a solvent or vehicle for the preparation of medicated elixirs— aromatic elixirs (USP), isoalcoholic elixirs (NF) or compound benaldehyde elixirs (NF).

Medicated Elixirs

- When there is presence of therapeutically active components in the elixir.
- *Antihistaminic elixirs*: Used against allergy, chlarphenivamine maleate elixirs (USP), diphenhydramine HCl elixirs.
- *Sedative and hypotonic elixirs*: Sedatives induce drowsiness and hypotonics induce sleep, pediatric chloral hydrate elixirs.
- *Expectorant*: Used as productive cough (cough with sputum), terpin hydrate elixirs.

- *Miscellaneous*: Acetaminophen (paracetamol) elixirs which are used as analgesic.

Preparation

When preparing an elixir, it is important to pay attention to the solubility and the solubility strength of each ingredient. Here is an example of a method to prepare an elixir:

1. Dissolve water-soluble ingredients in a part of water.
2. Add and solubilize sugar in this aqueous solution (sugar decreases the solubilizing properties of water).
3. Dissolve alcohol-soluble ingredients in alcohol.
4. Add the aqueous phase to the alcoholic phase.
5. Add clarifying agents like talc if needed.
6. Filter if needed.
7. Make to volume with water.

Labeling

The label states: (1) the date after which the oral liquid is not intended to be used; (2) the conditions under which the oral liquid should be stored with other general requirements for labeling of oral liquids.

Example 6: Elixir of vitriol (aromatic sulfuric acid)	
Ingredients	**Quantity**
Strong ginger tincture	50 ml
Cinnamon oil	1.5 ml
Sulfuric acid	70 ml
Alcohol (90%)	To 1000 ml

Method

1. Mix the sulfuric acid gradually with 600 ml of the alcohol (90%) and cool.
2. Dissolve the cinnamon oil and add the strong ginger tincture and sufficient of alcohol (90%) to produce the required volume.

Storage: Preserve in a well-closed container and avoid prolong exposure to excessive heat.

Use: Pharmaceutical aid and carminative.

Example 7: Terpin hydrate elixir (IP, 1966)	
Ingredients	**Quantity**
Terpin hydrate	50 g
Orange oil	0.2 ml
Glycerin	400 ml
Alcohol	425 ml
Syrup	100 ml
Purified water q.s	1000 ml

Method

1. Dissolve the terpin hydrate in alcohol.
2. Add successively the orange oil, glycerin, syrup and sufficiently purified water to the product measure 1000 ml.
3. Mix well and filter if necessary.

Storage: Preserve the terpin hydrate elixir in airtight container.

Use: Expectorant.

Example 8: Cascara elixir (BP, 1980)	
Ingredients	**Quantity**
Cascara in coarse powder	1000 g
Liquorice, unpeeled in coarse powder	125 g
Light magnesium oxide	50 g
Coriander oil	0.15 ml
Anise oil	0.2 ml
Ethanol (90%)	12.5 ml
Saccharin sodium	1 g
Glycerol	300 ml
Water	a sufficient quantity

Method

1. Mix the cascara, the liqourice and the light magnesium oxide.
2. Moisten with 1250 ml of boiling water, still thoroughly.
3. Macerate in well-covered vessel for 24 hours, pack moderately tightly in a

percolator, and percolate with boiling water until exhausted.

4. Evaporate the percolate to about 650 ml on a water bath.

5. Dissolve the coriander oil and anise oil in the ethanol (90%); dissolve the saccharin sodium in 12 ml of the water; mix the two solutions with the glycerol.

6. Add the concentrated percolate and sufficient water to produce 1000 ml, and shake thoroughly and allowed to stand for not less than 12 hours; filter, if necessary.

Storage: Preserve in a well-closed container and avoid prolong exposure to excessive heat.

Use: Expectorant.

Example 9: Pediatric chloral elixir (BP, 1980)	
Ingredients	Quantity
Chloral hydrate	40 g
Water	20 ml
Black currant syrup	200 ml
Syrup sufficient to produce	1000 ml

Method

1. Dissolve the chloral hydrate in the water.
2. Add the black currant syrup and sufficient syrup to produce 1000 ml and mix.

Storage: Preserve in a well-closed container and avoid prolong exposure to excessive heat.

Use: Sedative.

Example 10: Ephedrine hydrochloride elixir (BP, 1980)	
Ingredients	Quantity
Ephedrine hydrochloride	3 g
Water	60 ml
Glycerol	200 ml
Compound tartrazine solution	10 ml
Ethanol (90%)	100 ml
Chloroform spirit	40 ml
Lemon spirit	0.2 ml
Invert syrup	200 ml
Syrup sufficient to produce	1000 ml

Method

1. Dissolve the ephedrine hydrochloride in the water.

2. Add the glycerol, the compound tartrazine solution, the ethanol(90%). The chloroform spirit, the lemon spirit, the invert syrup, and sufficient syrup to produce 1000 ml.

3. Mix properly.

Storage: Preserve in a well-closed container and avoid prolong exposure to excessive heat

Use: Bronchodilator.

Example 11: Pediatric paracetamol elixir (BP, 1980)	
Ingredients	Quantity
Paracetamol	24 g
Ethanol(96%)	100 ml
Propylene glycol	100 ml
Chloroform	20 ml
Concentrated raspberry juice	25 ml
Invert syrup	275 ml
Amaranth solution	2 ml
Glycerol sufficient to produce	100 ml

Method: Dissolve the paracetamol in a mixture of the ethanol (96%) propylene glycol and the chloroform spirit; dilute the concentrated raspberry juice with the invert syrup and add the amaranth solution and sufficient glycerol to produce 1000 ml mix.

Storage: Pediatric paracetamol elixir should be protected from light.

Use: Analgesic and antipyretic.

Example 12: Phenobarbitone elixir (BP, 1980)	
Ingredients	Quantity
Phenobarbitone	3 g
Ethanol (90%)	400 ml
Compound orange spirit	24 ml
Glycerol	400 ml
Compound tartrazine solution	10 ml
Water sufficient to produce	1000 ml

Method

1. Dissolve the phenobarbitone in the ethanol (90%), add the compound orange spirit, the glycerol, the compound tartrazine solution and sufficient water to produce 1000 ml.
2. Add 25 g of purified talc, previously sterilized. Shake, allow standing for few hours, shaking occasionally; filtering.

Storage: Preserve in a well-closed container and avoid prolong exposure to excessive heat.

Use: Antiepileptic.

Example 13: Piperazine citrate elixir (BP, 1980)	
Ingredients	Quantity
Piperazine citrate	187.5 g
Green S and tartrazine solution	15 ml
Glycerol	100 ml
Syrup	500 ml
Peppermint syrup	5 ml
Water sufficient to produce	1000 ml

Method

1. Dissolve the piperazine citrate in 300 ml of the water.
2. Add the greens and green tartrazine solution, the glycerol, the syrup, the peppermint spirit, and sufficient to produce 1000 ml.
3. Mix.

Storage: Piperazine citrate elixir should be protected from light and stored at a temperature not exceeding 25°C.

Use: Anthelmintics.

Linctuses

Linctuses are viscous solutions of one or more medicaments, usually containing large amounts of sucrose. They are intended for use in the treatment of cough, being sipped and swallowed orally without the addition of water. They may contain suitable antimicrobial preservatives.

Dilutions of Linctuses

If a dose is prescribed which is less than or not a multiple of 5 ml, the linctus should be suitably diluted to achieve a dose volume that is a multiple of 5 ml, using the specified diluents. Diluted linctus should be used within two weeks of preparation or such other period as may be prescribed and the date after which they should not be used is stated on the label.

Labeling

Comply with the general requirements for labeling of oral liquids.

Example 14: Codeine linctus, pediatric BPC	
Ingredients	Quantity
Codeine phosphate	3 g
Lemon syrup	200 ml
Benzoic acid solution	20 ml
Chloroform spirit	20 ml
Water	20 ml
Compound tartrazine solution	10 ml
Syrup, to	1000 ml

Method

1. Very carefully calibrate a 250 ml wide mouthed conical flask at 200 ml.
2. Weigh the codine phosphate and have it checked; transfer it to the flask.
3. Measure 4 ml of water with a pipette, use part to rinse the scale pan, taking care to drain the pan well and the rest to the flask. A pipette allows better control of rinsing than a measure and therefore, there is less risk of spoilage.
4. Dissolve the solid, using gentle heat if required.
5. To the solution, cooled if necessary, add the coloring and preservative solution, agitating after each addition. Preferably use pipette because of the difficulty of rinsing measures with syrup. If measures are used, drain well.

6. Add the lemon syrup, rinse the measure with syrup, and drain well.

Storage: Should be protected from light.

Use: Antitussive.

Example 15: Methadone linctus	
Ingredients	**Quantity**
Methadone hydrochloride	400 ml
Water	120 ml
Compound tartrazine solution	8 ml
Glycerol	250 ml
Tolu syrup	q.s to produce 1000 ml

Method

1. Dissolve the methadone hydrochloride in the water, and the compound tartrazine solution, the glycerol and the sufficient tolu syrup to produce 1000 ml.

2. Mix well.

Storage: Stored in an airtight container and should be protected from light.

Use: Analgesic.

Example 16: Noscapine linctus	
Ingredients	**Quantity**
Noscapine	3 gm
Citric acid monohydrate	10 gm
Purified water, freshly boiled and colled	100 ml
Compound tartrazine solution	3 ml
Chloroform spirit	75 ml
Syrup	q.s to produce 1000 ml

Method

1. Add the noscapine and the citric acid monohydrate to the purified water, previously heated to about 50°C, and stir until dissolved, cool.

2. Add 800 ml of syrup, the compound tartrazine solution, the chloroform spirit, and sufficient syrup to produce 1000 ml; mix.

Storage: Stored in an airtight container.

Use: Antitussive.

Example 17: Opiate squill linctus	
Ingredients	**Quantity**
Squill oxymel	300 ml
Camphorated opium tincture	300 ml
Tolu syrup	300 ml

Method: Mix alternatively, dispense 0.1 g of xanthan gum 0.5 g of powdered tragacanth in the camphorated opium tincture, add the squill oxymel and the tolu syrup and mix. If xanthan gum is used, a high-speed stirrer is required in order to dispense the material.

Storage: Stored in an airtight container and should be protected from light.

Use: Expectorant.

Aromatic Water

- Aromatic waters (medicated waters) are clear, saturated aqueous solution of volatile oils or other aromatic or volatile substances.
- They are used principally as flavored or perfumed vehicles.
- Volatile oils solutions represent an incompatibility problem of salting out. This occurs after the incorporation of a very soluble salt in their solution.
- Aromatic water will deteriorate with time therefore:
  - ❖ Should be made in small quantities.
  - ❖ Protected from intense light and excessive heat by storing in airtight, light-resistant containers.
- If they become cloudy or otherwise deteriorate; they should be discarded. Deterioration may be due to volatilization, decomposition or mould growth.

Production

There are 2 official methods of preparation:

1. **Distillation process** (e.g. stronger rose water Nf):

Advantage: Most satisfactory method.

Disadvantage: Slow and expensive.

❖ The drug should be coarsely ground and mixed with sufficient quantity of purified water in the distillation unit.

❖ After distillation, any excess oil in the distillate is removed by filtration.

❖ Drug should not be exposed to the action of direct heat during distillation; otherwise, the odor of the carbonized substance will be noticeable in the distilled aromatic water.

❖ If the volatile principle in the water are present in small quantities, the distillate is returned several times to the still with fresh portions of drug.

2. **Solution Process** (e.g. peppermint water): Aromatic water may be prepared by shaking volatile substance with purified water. The mixture is set aside for 12 hours and filtered. Talc (inert) may be used to increase the surface of the volatile substance, insure more rapid saturation of the water and act as a filter aid.

Labeling

The label states: (1) the date after which the aromatic water is not intended to be used; (2) the conditions under which the aromatic water should be stored.

Example 18: Chloroform water	
Ingredients	Quantity
Chloroform	2.5 ml
Purified water sufficient to produce	1000 ml

Method: Dissolve the chloroform in the purified water by shaking.

Storage: Preserve chloroform water in a well-filled, well-closed container in a cool place.

Use: Pharmaceutical aid.

Infusion

Infusions are dilute solutions containing the readily soluble constituents of crude drugs. Fresh infusions are prepared by macerating the drugs for a short period of time with either cold or boiling water. They are usually prepared by diluting one volume of a concentrated infusion to ten volumes with water. For dispensing purposes, infusions should be used within 12 hours of their preparation.

Labeling

The label states: (1) the time after which the infusion is not intended to be used; (2) the conditions under which the infusion should be stored.

Example 19: Concentrated compound gentian infusion	
Ingredients	Quantity
Gentian, cut small and bruised	125 gm
Dried bitter-orange peel, cut small	125 gm
Dried lemon peel, cut small	125 gm
Ethanol 25 %	1200 ml

Method: Macerate the gentian, the dried bitter-orange peel, and the dried lemon peel in a covered vessel for 48 hours with 1000 ml of ethanol (25%); press out the liquid to the pressed marc, add 200 ml of the ethanol (25%), macerate for 24 hours, press, and add the liquid to the product of the first pressing, allow to stand for not less than 14 days; filter.

Storage: Preserve the infusion in a tightly closed container protected from light and store in a cool place.

Use: Hepatoprotective.

Example 20: Concentrated orange peel infusion	
Ingredients	Quantity
Dried bitter-orange peel, cut small	500 gm
Ethanol 25 %	1350 ml

Method: Macerate the dried bitter orange peel in a covered vessel for 48 hours with 1000 ml of ethanol 25%; press out the liquid to the pressed marc, add 350 ml of the ethanol (25%), macerate for 24 hours, press, and add the liquid to the product of the first pressing, allow standing for not less than 14 days; filtering.

Storage: Preserve the infusion in a tightly closed container protected from light and store in a cool place.

Use: Carminative and pharmaceutical aid.

Example 21: Concentrated senega infusion	
Ingredients	**Quantity**
Senega root, in course powder	500 gm
Dilute ammonia solution	q.s
Ethanol 25 %	q.s

Method: Extract the senega by percolation with ethanol 25%, reserve the first 750 ml of percolate, continue percolation until a further 1000 ml has been collected, evaporate to a syrupy consistence, dissolve the residue in a reserved portion, gradually add dilute ammonia solution until the product is faintly alkaline, dilute to 1000 ml with ethanol 24%, and mix, allow to stand for not less than 14 days; filter.

Storage: Preserve the infusion in a tightly closed container protected from light and store in a cool place.

Use: Stimulant and expectorant.

Example 22: Concentrated compound chirata infusion	
Ingredients	**Quantity**
Chirata cut small	1000 g
Dried orange peel thinly sliced	100 g
Lemon peel thinly sliced	200 g
Alcohol (25%)	1200 ml

Method: Macerate the chirata, the dried orange peel and the lemon peel with 800 ml of alcohol (25%) in a covered vessel for 48 hours.

1. Press out the liquid.

2. Add 400 ml of alcohol (25%) in resultant liquid.
3. Add the liquid to the product of first pressing.
4. Set aside for not less than 14 days
5. Filter if necessary.

Storage: Preserve the infusion in a tightly closed container protected from light and store in a cool place.

Use: Bitter and tonic.

Fluid Extracts

Fluid extracts are liquid preparations of vegetable drugs, contain alcohol as solvent or as preservative, or both, so made that each ml contains the therapeutic constituents of 1 gm of the standard drug. USP states that pharmacopoeial fluid extracts are made by percolation.

Extracts are defined as concentrated preparations of vegetable or animal drugs obtained by removal of the active constituents of crude drugs with suitable menstrum. Three forms of extracts are recognized: semisolids or liquids of syrupy consistency and dry powders. Most extracts are prepared by extracting the drug by percolation. The percolate is concentrated generally by distillation under reduced pressure.

Labeling

Labels must contain alcohol content, storage conditions, and also comply with other general requirements for labeling of liquids.

Example 23: Cascara liquid extract	
Ingredients	**Quantity**
Cascara, in coarse powder	1000 g
Ethanol (90%)	250 ml
Purified water, sufficient to produce	1000 ml

Method: Exhaust the cascara with purified water by percolation, evaporate the percolate to about 600 ml, add the ethanol (90%), previously mixed with 150 ml of purified water, and, if necessary, sufficient purified water to produce

1000 ml. Allow to stand for not less than 4 weeks; filter.

Storage: Preserve the extract in a tightly closed container protected from light and store in a cool place.

Use: Laxative.

Example 24: Ipecacuanha liquid extract	
Ingredients	Quantity
Ipecacuanha, in fine powder	1000 g
Ethanol (80%)	A sufficient quantity

Method: Exhaust the ipecacuanha by percolation with ethanol (80%), reserving the first 750 ml of the percolate. Remove the ethanol from the remainder of the percolate by evaporation under reduced pressure at a temperature not exceeding 60°C and dissolve the residual extract in the reserved portion. Determine the proportion of alkaloids in the liquid thus obtained by the assay described below. To the remainder of the liquid, add sufficient ethanol (80%) to produce an ipecacuanha liquid extract of the required strength. Allow to stand for not less than 24 hours; filter.

Storage: Preserve the extract in a tightly closed container protected from light and store in a cool place.

Use: Expectorant.

Example 25: Belladonna liquid extract (IP, 1966)	
Ingredients	Quantity
Belladonna herb in moderately coarse powder	1000 g
Alcohol (80%) q.s	Of each a sufficient quantity

Method

1. Percolate the belladonna herb in moderately coarse powder with alcohol (80%) until exhausted and reserve the first 400 ml.
2. Recover the alcohol from the remainder of the percolate and evaporate the residue to a soft extract under reduced pressure.
3. Dissolve the extract in the reserved liquid.
4. Determine the proportion of alkaloids in the liquid.
5. To the remainder of liquid, add sufficient alcohol (80%) to produce a belladonna liquid extract of the required strength.
6. Set aside for 12 hours and filter, if necessary.

Storage: Preserve belladonna liquid extract in a small wide mouthed, well-closed container and store in cool place.

Use: Parasympatholytic.

Example 26: Belladonna liquid extract (IP, 1966)	
Ingredients	Quantity
Belladonna herb in moderately coarse powder	100 g
Alcohol (70%)	Of each a sufficient quantity

Method

1. Percolate the belladonna herb in moderately coarse powder with alcohol (70%) until exhausted and reserve the first 400 ml.
2. Recover the alcohol from the remainder of the percolate and evaporate the residue to a soft extract under reduced pressure.
3. Dissolve the extract in the reserved liquid.
4. Determine the proportion of alkaloids in the liquid.
5. To the remainder of liquid add sufficient alcohol (70%) to produce a belladonna tincture of the required strength.
6. Set aside for 24 hours and filter, if necessary.

Storage: Preserve belladonna liquid extract in a small wide-mouthed, well-closed container and store in cool place.

Use: Parasympatholytic.

Example 27: Cinchona extracts (IP, 1966)	
Ingredients	Quantity
Cinchona in moderately fine powder	1000 g
Calcium hydroxide	A sufficient quantity
Glycerin	A sufficient quantity
Alcohol (90%)	A sufficient quantity

Method

1. Treat the cinchona powder with calcium hydroxide.
2. Exhaust with 90% alcohol by percolation.
3. Remove the alcohol from the percolate.
4. Add 100 ml glycerin and evaporate to the consistence of a soft extract.
5. Evaporate the extract and dilute it with sufficient glycerin to produce an extract of the required strength.

Storage: Preserve cinchona extract in small, wide-mouthed, well-closed containers in cool place.

Use: Antimalarial.

Solutions

A solution is a liquid preparation that contains one or more chemical substances dissolved in water. The solute usually is non-volatile. Solutions are used for the specific therapeutic effect of the solute, either internally or externally.

Preparation of solution. There are three methods for the preparation of solution.

1. **Simple solution.** Solutions of this type are prepared by dissolving the solute in a suitable solvent. The solvent may contain other ingredients. Calcium hydroxide topical solution, sodium phosphate oral solution and strong iodine solution are examples.
2. **Solution by chemical reaction.** These solutions are prepared by reacting two or more solutes with each other in a suitable solvent e.g. calcium carbonate and lactic acid used to prepare calcium lactate mixture.
3. **Solution by extraction.** Plant or animal products are prepared by suitable extraction process. Preparations of this type may be classified as solutions but more often, are classified as extractives. Extractives will be discussed separately.

Labeling

Stored in an airtight container and also comply with other general requirements for labeling of liquids.

Example 28: Lugol's solution (aqueous iodine solution) (IP, 1966)	
Ingredients	Quantity
Iodine	50 g
Potassium iodide	100 g
Purified water sufficient to produce	1000 ml

Method: Dissolve the potassium iodide and iodine in 100 ml of purified water. Add sufficient purified water to produce the required volume.

Storage: Preserve aqueous iodine solution in a well-closed container that is resistance to iodine.

Use: Local anti-infective.

Example 29: Benzoic acid solution	
Ingredients	Quantity
Benzoic acid	50 g
Propylene glycol	750 ml
Purified water, freshly boiled and cooled sufficient to produce	1000 ml

Method: Dissolve benzoic acid in propylene glycol and add sufficient purified water in small quantity and with constant stirring, to produce 1000 ml.

Storage: Preserve benzoic acid solution in a well-closed container.

Use: Local anti-infective.

Example 30: Eusol	
Ingredients	**Quantity**
Chlorinated lime	12.5 g
Boric acid in powder	12.5 g
Purified water, freshly boiled and cooled sufficient to produce	1000 ml

Method: Reduce the chlorinated lime to fine powder, triturate it with sufficient of the purified water to form a paste and then add a further portion of purified water. Add boric acid shake well, add sufficient purified water to produce the required volume, allow to stand and filter.

Storage: Chlorinated lime and boric acid solution should be kept in a well-filled, well-closed container protected from light. It should not be stored at a temperature not exceeding 20°C. The solution deteriorates on storage and should be used within two weeks of its preparation.

Use: Antiseptic

Example 31: Chloroxylenol solution	
Ingredients	**Quantity**
Chloroxylenol	50.0 g
Potassium hydroxide	13.6 g
Oleic acid	7.5 g
Castor oil	63 g
Terpineol	100 ml
Ethanol (96%)	200 ml
Purified water, freshly boiled and cooled sufficient to produce	1000 ml

Method: Dissolve potassium hydroxide in 15 ml of purified water, add a solution of the castor oil in 63 ml of the ethanol, mix, allow to stand for one hour or until a small portion of the mixture remains clear when diluted with

nineteen times its volume of purified water and then add oleic acid. Mix the terpineol with a solution of the chloroxylenol in the remainder of the ethanol pour it into the soap solution and add sufficient of the purified water to produce the required volume.

Storage Chloroxylenol solution should be kept in a well-closed container.

Use: Antiseptic.

Example 32: Aqueous iodine solution lugols solution	
Ingredients	**Quantity**
Iodine	50 g
Potassium iodide	100 g
Purified water to produce	1000 ml

Method: Dissolve the potassium iodide and the iodine in 100 ml of purified water and add sufficient purified water to produce 1000 ml.

Storage: Aqueous iodine solution should be kept in well-closed containers the material of which are resistant to iodine.

Use: Antiseptic.

Example 33: Coal tar solution	
Ingredients	**Quantity**
Coal tar	200 g
Polysorbate 80	50 g
Ethanol (96%) sufficient to produce	1000 ml

Method: Mix the coal tar, warmed if necessary to render it fluid, with the polysorbate 80, pour this mixture in a thin stream into 800 ml of ethanol in a closed vessel fitted with an agitator; continue agitation throughout the addition of the mixture and for one hour thereafter. Allow the mixture to stand for not less than 24 hours, decant and filter the supernatant liquid, wash the vessel and filter with ethanol combine the filtrate and washings, and add sufficient ethanol to produce 1000 ml.

Storage: Coal tar solution should be kept in a well-closed container.

Use: Antipsoriatics.

Example 34: Strong coal tar solution	
Ingredients	Quantity
Coal tar	400 g
Polysorbate 80	50 g
Ethanol (96%) sufficient to produce	1000 ml

Method: Mix the coal tar, warmed if necessary to render it fluid, with the polysorbate 80, pour this mixture in a thin stream into 700 ml of ethanol in a closed vessel fitted with an agitator; continue agitation throughout the addition of the mixture and for one hour thereafter. Allow the mixture to stand for not less than 24 hours, decant and filter the supernatant liquid, wash the vessel and filter with ethanol combine the filtrate and washings, and add sufficient ethanol to produce 1000 ml.

Storage: Strong coal tar solutissson should be kept in a well-closed container.

Use: Antipsoriatics.

Example 35: Strychnine hydrochloride solution (IP, 1966)	
Ingredients	Quantity
Strychnine hydrochloride	10 g
Alcohol (90%)	250 ml
Purified water sufficient to produce	1000 ml

Method
1. Mix the alcohol (90%) with an equal volume of purified water.
2. Dissolve the strychnine hydrochloride in the mixture.
3. Add sufficient purified water to produce the required volume.
4. Mix the content.

Storage: Preserve the strychnine hydrochloride solution in well-closed container in cool place.

Use: CNS stimulant.

Glycerins

- Glycerins or glycerites are solutions or mixtures of medicinal substances in not less than 50% by weight of glycerin.
- Most of the glycerins are extremely viscous.
- Glycerin is a valuable pharmaceutical solvent forming permanent and concentrated solutions not otherwise obtainable.
- Glycerin is used as the sole solvent for the preparation of antipyrine and benzocaine otic solution USP. As noted under otic solutions, glycerin alone is used to aid in the removal of cerumen.
- Glycerins are hygroscopic and should be stored in tightly closed containers.

Labeling

Stored in an airtight container and also comply with other general requirements for labeling of liquids.

Example 36: Borax glycerin	
Ingredients	Quantity
Borex	120 g
Glycerin	880 g

Method
1. Powder the borax.
2. Triturates with glycerin.
3. Warm gently with constant stirring until. solution is effected.
4. Filter if necessary.

Storage: Preserve the borax glycerin in a well-closed container.

Use: Bacteriostatic.

Example 37: Phenol glycerin (IP, 1966)	
Ingredients	Quantity
Phenol	160 g
Glycerin	840 g

Method

1. Mix the phenol and glycerin.
2. Warm gently, if necessary, until solution is affected.

Storage: Preserve phenol glycerin in a well-closed container.

Use: Local analgesic, antiseptic.

Example 38: Tannic acid glycerin (IP, 1966)	
Ingredients	**Quantity**
Tannic acid	200 g
Sodium citrate	10 g
Dried sodium sulfite	2 g
Glycerin	788 g

Method

1. Rub the tannic acid, dried sodium sulfite and sodium citrate in a porcelain dish with about half of the glycerin until a smooth mixture is produced.
2. Add the remainder of the glycerin and mix well.
3. Heat the mixture on a sand bath to a temperature between 115 to 120°C with occasional stirring until solution is complete.

Storage: Preserve tannic acid glycerin in a tight container.

Use: Astringent.

Lotions

- Lotions are liquid or semiliquid preparation containing one or more medicaments, intended to be applied on the unbroken skin without friction.
- The addition of alcohol to aqueous lotions increases the rapidity of evaporation from the surface to which they are applied, their cooling effect being consequently accentuated.
- Most lotions are oil-in-water emulsions using a substance such as cetosteryl alcohol to keep the emulsion together, but water-in-oil lotions are also formulated.

- Lotions are usually applied to skin with bare hands, a clean cloth, cotton wool or gauze; creams and gels usually only with one's fingers or palms.
- Many lotions, especially hand creams and face cream are formulated not as a medicine delivery system, but simply to smooth and soften the skin.
- Lotions can be used for the delivery to the skin of medications such as antibiotics, antiseptics, antifungals, corticosteroids, anti-acne agents, soothing, smoothing, moisturizing or protective agents (such as calamine).

Dilutions of Lotions

Care should be taken in diluting lotions, particularly to prevent microbial contamination. The appropriate diluents should be used and heating should be avoided during mixing.

Labeling

Comply with the general requirements for labeling in addition the label on the container states: (1) that the preparation is intended for external use only; (2) that the contents should be shaken before use.

Example 39: Calamine lotion (IP, 1966)	
Ingredients	**Quantity**
Calamine	150 g
Zinc oxide	50 g
Bentonite	30 g
Sodium citrate	5 g
Liquified phenol	5 ml
Glycerin	50 ml
Rose water of commerce sufficient to produce	1000 ml

Method

1. Triturate the calamine, zinc oxide and the bentonite with solution of the sodium citrate in about 700 ml of rose water.

2. Add the liquified phenol, glycerin and sufficient rose water to produce 1000 ml.

Storage: Preserve calamine lotion in a well-closed container.

Use: Protective.

Example 40: Oily calamine lotion	
Ingredients	Quantity
Calamine	50 gm
Oleic acid	5 ml
Wool fat	10 gm
Arachis oil	500 ml
Calcium hydroxide solution	q.s to produce 1000 ml

Method: Melt together the oleic acid, the wool fat, and the arachis oil, triturate the calamine with the mixture, transfer to a suitable container, add the calcium hydroxide solution and shake vigorously.

Storage: Preserve calamine lotion in a well-closed container.

Use: Protective.

Example 41: Salicylic acid lotion	
Ingredients	Quantity
Salicylic acid	20 gm
Castor oil	10 ml
Ethanol 96 %	q.s to produce 1000 ml

Method: Dissolve the salicylic acid in a portion of ethanol 96%, add the castor oil and sufficient ethanol 96% to produce 1000 ml and mix.

Storage: Preserve salicylic acid lotion in a well-closed container.

Use: Keratolytic.

Liniments

- Are solutions or mixtures of various substances in oil, alcoholic solutions of soaps, or emulsions.

- They are intended for external application and should be so labeled.

- They are applied with rubbing to the affected area, the oil or soap base providing for ease of application and massage.

- Alcoholic liniments are used generally for their rubefacient and counterirritant effects. Such liniments penetrate the skin more readily than do those with an oil base.

- The oily liniments are milder in their action and may function solely as protective coatings.

- Liniments should not be applied to skin that are bruised or broken.

- Liniments should be dispensed in containers, easily distinguishable by touch from those in use for medicines intended for internal administration, and, in addition to any prescribed directions, should always be plainly labeled "Not to be Taken" or "Poison."

Labeling

Comply with the general requirements for labeling in addition the label on the container states: (1) that the preparation is intended for external use only; (2) that the contents should be shaken before use.

Example 42: Ammoniated camphor liniment (IP, 1966)	
Ingredients	Quantity
Camphor	125 g
Eucalyptus oil	5 ml
Ammonia solution strong	250 ml
Alcohol (90%) sufficient to produce	1000 ml

Method

1. Dissolve the camphor and the eucalyptus oil in 600 ml of alcohol (90%).

2. Add the ammonia solution strong gradually with frequent shaking.

3. Volume makeup with alcohol (90%) to produce required alcoholic strength.

Storage: Preserve ammoniated camphor liniment in a well-closed glass stoppered bottle.

Use: Antipruritic, counterirritant.

Example 43: Soap Liniment (IP, 1966)	
Ingredients	**Quantity**
Soft soap	80 g
Camphor	40 g
Lemongrass oil	15 ml
Purified water	170 ml
Alcohol (90%) sufficient to produce	1000 ml

Method

1. Dissolve the soft soap, camphor and lemon grass oil in 600 ml of alcohol (90%).
2. Add the purified water and sufficient alcohol (90%) to produce the required volume.
3. Set aside for a week and filter.

Storage: Preserve soap liniment in well-closed container.

Use: Detergent.

Example 44: Turpentine liniment	
Ingredients	**Quantity**
Soft soap	75 gm
Camphor	50 gm
Turpentine oil	650 ml
Water freshly boiled and cooled	225 ml

Method

1. Triturate the camphor with soft soap until thoroughly mixed and gradually add the turpentine oil, triturating well after each addition.
2. Transfer the mixture to a bottle with the aid of the purified water and shake thoroughly until a creamy emulsion is formed.

Storage: Preserve soap liniment in well-closed container.

Use: Detergent.

Example 45: White liniment	
Ingredients	**Quantity**
Oleic acid	85 ml
Turpentine oil	250 ml
Dilute ammonia solution	45 ml
Ammonium chloride	12.5 gm
Water	625 ml

Method

1. Mix the oleic acid with the turpentine oil.
2. Diluted the dilute ammonia solution with 45 ml of water, previously warmed.
3. Add to the oily solution, and shake to form an emulsion.
4. Separately dissolve the ammonium chloride in the remained of the water, and add to the emulsion.
5. Mix.

Storage: Preserve liniment in well-closed container.

Use: Stimulant.

Collodions

- Collodions are liquid preparations containing pyroxylin (a nitrocellulose) in a mixture of ethyl ether and ethanol.
- They are applied to the skin by means of a soft brush or other suitable applicator and when the ether and ethanol have evaporated, leave a film of pyroxylin on the surface.
- The official medicated collodion, salicylic acid collodion USP, contains 10 % w/v of salicylic acid in flexible collodion USP and is used as a keratolytic agent in the treatment of corns and warts.
- Collodion is made flexible by the addition of castor oil and camphor.

Labeling

The label states: (1) that the collodion is intended for external use only; (2) the date after which the collodion is not intended to be used; (3) the conditions under which the collodion should be stored; (4) the directions for using the collodion; (5) any special precautions associated with the use of the collodion. Collodions should be stored remote from fire.

Example 46: Flexible collodions	
Ingredients	Quantity
Colophony	25 g
Castor oil	25 g
Collodions	sufficient to produce 1000 ml

Method: Mix the ingredients and stir until the colophony has dissolved; allow any deposit to settle and decant the clear liquid.

Storage: Flexible collodion should be kept in well-closed container and temperature not exceeding 25°C, remote from fire.

Use: Flexible collodion is a protective application to the skin. When collodion is prescribed or demanded, flexible collodion should be supplied.

Tincture

Tinctures are defined as alcoholic or hydroalcoholic solutions prepared from vegetable materials or from chemical substances. USP specifically describes two general processes for preparing tinctures, one by percolation and the other by maceration. Tinctures will detoriate with time and should, therefore, be made in small quantities and protected from intense light, excessive heat and stored in airtight, light-resistance containers.

Labeling

Labels must contain alcohol content, stored in an airtight container and also comply with other general requirements for labeling of liquids.

Example 47: Compound cardamom tincture (IP 1966)	
Ingredients	Quantity
Cardamom seeds in moderately coarse powder	14 g
Caraway in moderately coarse powder	14 g
Cinnamon in moderately coarse powder	28 g
Amaranth	5 g
Glycerin	50 ml
Alcohol (45%) sufficient to produce	1000 ml

Method

1. Moisten the mixed powder with sufficient quantity of alcohol (45% v/v).
2. Prepare 900 ml of tincture by percolation.
3. Add the glycerin, amaranth and sufficient alcohol (45% v/v) to produce 1000 ml.
4. Filter if necessary.

Storage: Preserve the tincture in a well-filled, well-closed container in a cool place.

Use: Carminative

Example 48: Weak iodine solution (iodine tincture) (IP, 1966)	
Ingredients	Quantity
Iodine	20 g
Potassium iodide	25 g
Alcohol (50%) sufficient to produce	1000 ml

Method: Dissolve the potassium iodide and iodine in sufficient alcohol (50% v/v) to produce the required volume.

Storage: Preserve aqueous iodine solution in a well-closed container that is resistance to iodine.

Use: Antiseptic

Example 49: Camphored opium tincture (IP, 1966)	
Ingredients	Quantity
Opium tincture	50 ml
Benzoic acid	5 g
Camphor	3 g
Anise oil	3 ml
Alcohol (60%) sufficient to produce	1000 ml

Method

1. Dissolve the benzoic acid, camphor and anise oil in 900 ml of alcohol (60% v/v).
2. Add opium tincture into the above formulation.
3. Make-up the volume with alcohol (60% v/v) to produce required volume.
4. Filter it, if necessary.

Storage: Preserve camphored opium tincture in a tightly closed container protected from light and store in a cool place.

Use: Hypnotic, sedative.

Spirits

- Alcoholic or hydroalcoholic solutions of volatile substances. The active ingredient may be gas, liquid or solid.
- Spirits may be used internally for their medicinal value, by inhalation but is mostly used as flavoring agents.
- Spirits should be stored in tight, light-resistant containers and in a cool place.
- Spirits are preparation of high alcoholic strength and when diluted with aqueous solutions or liquids of low alcoholic content turbidity may occur.

Preparation of spirits

There are four methods for the preparation of spirits:

1. **Simple solution:** This is the method by which majority of spirits are prepared. The formula and procedure given for aromatic ammonia spirit illustrate this method of preparation.

2. **Solution with maceration:** In this method, crude drugs are macerated in purified water to extract water soluble matter. Macerated crude drugs are added to a prescribed quantity of alcohol. The volatile oil is added to the macerated liquid.

3. **Chemical reaction:** No official spirits are prepared by this process. Ethyl nitrite is made by the action of sodium nitrite on a mixture of alcohol and sulfuric acid in the cold.

4. **Distillation:** Brandy and whisky are made by distillation. Whisky is derived from the fermented mash of malt and the brandy from the fermented juice of ripe grapes.

Labeling

Labels must contain information's like drug content, alcohol content, storage conditions, stored in an airtight container and also comply with other general requirements for labeling of liquids.

Example 50: Aromatic ammonia spirit	
Ingredients	Quantity
Nutmeg oil	3 ml
Lemon oil	5 ml
Ethanol	750 ml
Ammonium bicarbonate	25 g
Strong ammonium solution	67.5 ml
Purified water to produce	1000 ml

Method: Distil a mixture of lemon oil, nutmeg oil, ethanol and 375 ml of purified water, reserve the first 875 ml of the distillate, distill the further 55 ml, and add ammonium bicarbonate and strong ammonia solution. Heat on water bath to 60°C in a sealed bottle of not less than 120 ml capacity until solution is complete, cool, filter through adsorbent cotton, mix the filtrate with reserved distillate, and add sufficient purified water to produce 1000 ml and mix.

Storage: Preserve aromatic spirit of ammonia in a well-filled, well-closed container in a cool place.

Use: Respiratory stimulant.

Example 51: Benzaldehyde spirit	
Ingredients	Quantity
Benzaldehyde	10 ml
Ethanol	800 ml
Purified water to produce	1000 ml

Method: Dissolve the benzaldehyde in ethanol and sufficient purified water to produce 1000 ml.

Storage: Benzaldehyde spirit is kept in well-filled container, protected from light.

Use: Antispasmodic

Example 52: Aromatic spirit of ammonia (IP, 1966)	
Ingredients	Quantity
Ammonium bicarbonate	25 g
Ammonia solution strong	70 ml
Lemon oil	5 ml
Nutmeg oil	3 ml
Alcohol (90%)	750 ml
Purified water sufficient to produce	1000 ml

Method

1. Place the lemon oil, the nutmeg oil and the alcohol (90%) with 375 ml of purified water in still.
2. Distill 875 ml then distill and separately collect an additional 35 ml.
3. Place the latter together with ammonium bicarbonate and the ammonium solution in a bottle of more than 120 ml capacity.
4. Securely close the bottle and gently warm it in a water bath to 60°C, shaking from time to time until all the salt has dissolved.

5. Filter the resulting solution, when cold through cotton wool and gradually mix the filtrate with the portion first distilled.
6. Add sufficient purified water to produce the required volume.

Storage: Preserve aromatic spirit of ammonia in a well-filled, well-closed container in a cool place.

Use: Stimulant.

Gargles

- Gargles are aqueous solutions frequently containing antiseptics, antibiotics and/or anesthetics used for treating the pharynx (throat) and nasopharynx by forcing air from the lungs through the gargle, which is held in the throat; subsequently, the gargle is expectorated.
- Many gargles must be diluted with water prior to use. Although mouthwashes are considered as a separate class of pharmaceuticals but many are used as gargles, either as it is or diluted with water.
- The product should be labeled so that it cannot be mistaken for preparations intended for internal administration.

Labeling

The label states: (1) the directions for dilution of the gargles, if appropriate; (2) the date after which the gargles is not intended to be used; (3) the conditions under which it should be stored.

Example 53: Potassium chlorate and phenol gargel BPC	
Ingredients	Quantity
Potassium chlorate	34.3 gm
Planet blue V	15.6 ml
Liquified phenol	15.6 ml
Water	1000 ml

Method

1. Dissolve the potassium chlorate in about 150 ml of warm water.

2. Cool before adding the liquified phenol. Remember that liquified phenol is very caustic; if measurement in a pipette is ever necessary the mouth must not be used.
3. Add the dye solution, filter, if necessary, and make-up to volume.

Storage: Gargle should be stored in a cool, dry, well-ventilated area in tightly sealed containers.

Use: Antiseptic and expectorant.

Example 54: Phenol gargle BPC	
Ingredients	Quantity
Phenol glycerin	50 ml
Amaranth solution	10.4 ml
Purified water q.s	1000 ml

Method

1. Since all the ingredients are water soluble, hence this is prepared by simple solution method.
2. Dissolve phenol glycerin with amaranth solution and add purified water to produce 1000 ml.

Storage: Phenol gargle should be stored in a cool, dry, well-ventilated area in tightly sealed containers.

Use: Antiseptic.

Mouthwashes

Mouthwashes are the aqueous solutions of one or more medicaments. They are intended, usually after dilution with warm water, for use in contact with the mucous membranes of oral cavity. They may contain alcohol, glycerin, synthetic sweeteners and surface active agents as hexidine and cetylpyridinium chloride. They may be effective in reducing bacterial concentrations and odors in the mouth for short period of time.

Labeling

The label states: (1) the directions for dilution of the mouthwash, if appropriate; (2) that large quantities of the mouthwash should not be swallowed; (3) the date after which the mouthwash is not intended to be used; (4) the conditions under which it should be stored.

Example 55: Compound sodium chloride mouthwash	
Ingredients	Quantity
Sodium bicarbonate	10 g
Sodium chloride	15 g
Concentrated peppermint emulsion	25 ml
Double strength chloroform water	500 ml
Water, freshly boiled and cooled sufficient to produce	1000 ml

Method

1. Since all the ingredients are water soluble, hence this is prepared by simple solution method.
2. Dissolve all the components in purified water to produce 1000 ml.

Storage: Compound sodium chloride mouthwash should be stored in a cool, dry, well-ventilated area in tightly sealed containers.

Use: Antiseptic.

Nasal Solutions

Nasal preparations are liquid, semisolid or solid preparations intended for administration to the nasal cavities to obtain a systemic or local effect.

They contain one or more active substances. Nasal preparations are as far as possible non-irritating and do not adversely affect the functions of the nasal mucosa and its cilia. Aqueous nasal preparations are usually isotonic and may contain excipients, e.g. to adjust the viscosity of the preparation, to adjust or stabilize the pH, to increase the solubility of the active substance, or to stabilize the preparation. Nasal preparations are supplied in multidose or single-dose containers, provided, if necessary, with a suitable administration device, which may be designed to avoid the introduction of contaminants.

Labeling

The label state: (1) the name and quantity of the active ingredient; (2) the name and quantity of any added substance; (3) that the preparation is for intranasal administration; (4) the date after which the preparation is not intended to be used; (5) the conditions under which the preparation should be stored.

Example 56: Epinephrine nasal-drops BPC	
Ingredients	Quantity
Epinephrine hydrochloride	5 gm
Chlorbutol	15 ml
Sodium chloride	8.5 gm
Water q.s	1000 ml

Method

1. Transfer the medicament to a glass mortar, rinsing the scale pan thoroughly, make 20 ml.
2. Grind the crystal with water; add more water and regrind. Allow undisclosed crystals to settle and pour the supernatant into a 1 liter conical flask, using a spatula to stop liquid from running down the outside of the mortar. Rinse the spatula into the solution. Add more water to the mortar regrind and decant, repeating these procedures until all the solid has dissolved and the mortar is free from color.
3. Confirm that no undisclosed crystals remain by turning the flask so that the solution drains from each part of the sides and bottom in turn. If necessary, stir until solution is complete from the beginning of the solution.
4. Dissolve the salts in the warm solution.
5. Cool, filter through a clean sintered glass filter and make-up to volume through the filter.

Storage: Epinephrine nasal-drops should be stored in a cool, dry and airtight container.

Use: Nasal decongestant.

Douches

- Douche is an aqueous solution, which is directed against a part or into a cavity of the body.
- It functions as a cleansing or antiseptic agent.
- Eye douches are used to remove foreign particles and discharges from the eyes. It is directed gently at an oblique angle and is allowed to run from the inner to the outer corner of the eye.
- Pharyngeal douches are used to prepare the interior of the throat for an operation and to cleanse it in supportive conditions. Similarly, there are nasal and vaginal douches.
- Douches most frequently dispensed in the form of a powder with directions for dissolving in a specified quantity of water.

Labeling

The label state: (1) the names and concentrations of the active ingredients; (2) that the preparation should not be swallowed; (3) the directions for using the douches.

Example 57: Potassium permanganate solution	
Ingredients	Quantity
Potassium permanganate	0.1 gm
Water, to	100 ml

Method

1. Transfer the medicament to a glass mortar, rinsing the scale pan thoroughly.
2. Grind the crystal with water; add more water and regrind. Allow undisclosed crystals to settle and pour the supernatant into a 1 liter conical flask, using a spatula to stop liquid from running down the outside of the mortar. Rinse the spatula

into the solution. Add more water to the mortar regrind and decant, repeating these procedures until all the solid has dissolved and the mortar is free from color.

3. Confirm that no undisclosed crystals remain by turning the flask so that the solution drains from each part of the sides and bottom in turn. If necessary, stir until solution is complete from the beginning of the solution.

4. Filter through a clean sintered glass filter and make up to volume through the filter.

Storage: This douche should be stored in a cool, dry and airtight container protected from light.

Use: Antiseptic.

Eyedrops

- Eyedrops are sterile solutions or suspensions of one or more medications intended for instillation into the conjunctival sac for diagnostic or therapeutic purposes.

- Eyedrops are prepared using methods designed to ensure their sterility and to avoid the introduction of contaminants and growth of micro-organisms.

- Aqueous preparations supplied in containers intended for use on more than one occasion contain suitable antimicrobial preservatives at appropriate concentrations except when the preparation itself has adequate antimicrobial properties.

- Eyedrops may contain added substances, e.g. to adjust the tonicity or viscosity, to adjust or stabilize the pH, to increase the solubility of the medicaments, or to stabilize the preparation.

- Eyedrops for use in surgical procedures do not contain added antimicrobial preservatives or buffering agents and are supplied in containers intended for use on occasion only.

- Eyedrops which are suspensions may show sediment which readily disperses when shaken; the suspension remains sufficiently dispersed to enable the correct dose to be removed from the container.

Containers

Containers for eyedrops are made from materials which do not cause deterioration of the product. They may be of glass or other suitable material. The compatibility of plastics or rubber is confirmed before use. If eyedrops without antimicrobial preservatives are prescribed, they should be supplied wherever possible in containers intended for use on one occasion only. Containers holding sufficient of the preparation for instillation into one eye on one occasion may be of suitable plastic and are shaped to facilitate administration without contamination. The packaging of such products is such as to maintain sterility of the contents and the applicator up to the time of use. Alternatively, such eyedrops may be supplied in suitable glass containers. Any remainder of eyedrops intended for use on one occasion should be discarded. Eyedrops intended for use on more than one occasion may be supplied in glass or other suitable containers which permit the withdrawal of successive doses of the preparation. Unless otherwise justified and authorized such containers hold not more than 10 ml.

Labeling

The label states: (1) the names and percentages of the active ingredients, (2) the date after which the eyedrops are not intended to be used, (3) the conditions under which the eyedrops should be stored.

For multi-dose containers, the label states that care should be taken to avoid contamination of the contents during use. Single-dose containers that because of their size bear only an indication of the active ingredient and the strength of the preparation.

Example 58: Atropine sulfate	
Ingredients	Quantity
Atropine sulfate	1 gm
Phenylmercuric nitrate solution	50 ml
Water, to	100 ml

Method

1. Weigh the medicament and dissolve it in the bactericidal solution in a small conical flask. Cool, if necessary, transfer to a 10 ml measure, rinse the flask, and adjust to volume with purified water.
2. Filter using 0.8 μm polypropylene membrane filter.
3. Sterilize by autoclaving at 115°C for 30 minutes. No lag time is necessary, if the bottle is put into the autoclave before the water is heated. When eyedrops are sterilized by this method, it is particularly important to allow the pressure to fall slowly to atmospheric temperature after sterilization, to avoid bursting the teat.
4. Clearly examine the contents for particulate matter and confirm visually that there has been no change in volume due to a faulty closure.
5. Fit a cap and allow to dry. Polish the bottle. Check the labels and fit them symmetrically over the unribbed panels.

Storage: This eyedrops must be stored in an airtight container and placed in a cool and dry place.

Use: Mydriatics.

Example 59: Physostigmine sulfate	
Ingredients	Quantity
Physostigmine sulfate	0.5 gm
Sodium metabisulfite	0.2 gm
Benzalkonium chloride solution	0.02 ml
Water, to	100 ml

Method

1. Weigh the medicament, mix the sodium metabisulfite and preservative solutions, dissolve the medicament in the mixture, rinse the flask, and adjust to volume with purified water.
2. Filter through membrane filter. With forceps remove the teat from the storage solution (containing 0.4 % w/v of sodium metabisulfite and 0.04 % v/v of benzalkonium chloride solution). Rinse for several times in fresh membrane filtered solution to remove particles acquired during storage. Dry as completely as in cellulose film discs and expel contained liquid. Fit into the cap, insert the dropper, without touching the latter with the fingers, and screw the cap on to the bottle.
3. Use a simple electric heater steamer and remember to keep it closed throughout the sterilization period.
4. Clearly examine the contents for particulate matter and confirm visually that there has been no change in volume due to a faulty closure.
5. Fit a cap and allow to dry. Polish the bottle. Check the labels and fit them symmetrically over the unribbed panels.

Storage: This eyedrop must be stored in an airtight container and placed in a cool and dry place.

Use: Miosis.

Eardrops

Eardrops are aqueous or oily solutions of one or more medicaments intended for instillation into the ear for therapeutic purposes.

- The main classes of drugs used for topical administration to the ear include local anesthetics, e.g. benzocaine; antibiotics, neomycin and anti-inflammatory agents, cortisone.

- These preparations include the main types of solvents used, namely glycerin or water.

- The viscous glycerin vehicle permits the drug to remain in the ear for a long time.

- Anhydrous glycerin, being hygroscopic, tends to remove moisture from surrounding tissues, thus reducing swelling.

- Viscous liquids like glycerin or propylene glycol either are used alone or in combination with a surfactant to aid in the removal of cerumen (ear wax).

- In order to provide sufficient time for aqueous preparations to act, it is necessary for the patient to remain on his side for a few minutes so the drops do not run out of the ear.

Labeling

The label states: (1) the names and concentrations of the active ingredients, (2) that the ear drops are intended for external use only.

Containers

Eardrops should be supplied in containers of glass or suitable plastic which are fitted with an integral dropper or with a gap of suitable materials incorporating a suitable dropper tube and rubber or plastic teat. Alternatively, such a cap assembly is supplied separately. Ear preparations are supplied in multi-dose or single-dose containers, provided, if necessary, with a suitable administration device which may be designed to avoid the introduction of contaminants.

Example 60: Aluminum acetate eardrops	
Ingredients	Quantity
Aluminum sulfate	225 g
Acetic acid (33%)	250 ml
Tartaric acid	45 g
Calcium carbonate	100 g
Purified water	750 ml

Method: Dissolve the aluminum sulfate in 600 ml of the purified water, add the acetic acid and then the calcium carbonate mixed with the remainder of the purified water and allow to stand for not less than 24 hours in a cool place, stirring occasionally. Filter and add the tartaric acid to the filtrate and mix.

Storage: Aluminum acetate ear drops should be kept in a well-filled container and stored at a temperature not exceeding 25°C.

Use: Otic sterile solution.

Example 61: Hydrogen peroxide eardrops	
Ingredients	Quantity
Hydrogen peroxide solution (6%)	25 ml
Purified water sufficient to produce	100 ml

Method: Dissolve the hydrogen peroxide in 100 ml of the purified water, and allow to stand for not less than 24 hours in a cool place, stirring occasionally. Filter, if necessary.

Storage: Hydrogen peroxide eardrops should be kept in an airtight, well-filled container and stored in a cool and dry place.

Use: Cleansing solution.

Example 62: Sodium bicarbonate eardrops	
Ingredients	Quantity
Sodium bicarbonate	5 g
Glycerol	30 ml
Purified water, freshly boiled and cooled sufficient to produce	100 ml

Method: Dissolve sodium bicarbonate in about 60 ml of purified water, add the glycerol and sufficient purified water to produce 100 ml mix. Sodium bicarbonate eardrops should be prepared in shorter time span.

Storage: Sodium bicarbonate eardrops should be kept in an airtight container and stored in a cool and dry place.

Use: Wax softening agent.

Inhalation

Inhalations are solutions or suspensions of one or more medicaments which may contain an inert suspensed diffusing agent. They are intended to release volatile constituents for inhalation either when placed on a pad or when added to hot water.

Labeling

The label on the container states: (1) the names and concentrations of the active ingredients, (2) that the inhalation is not to be taken by mouth, (3) the date after which the inhalation is not intended to be used, (4) the conditions under which the inhalation should be stored.

Example 63: Benzoin inhalation	
Ingredients	Quantity
Sumatra benzoin,crushed	100 gm
Prepared storax	50 gm
Ethanol 96%	q.s to produce 1000 ml

Method: Macerate the crushed sumatra benzoin and the prepared storax with 750 ml of the ethanol 96% for 24 hours, filter and pass sufficient ethanol 96% through the filter to produce a filterate of 1000 ml. In making benzoin inhalation, the ethanol 96% may be replaced by industrial methylated spirit provided that the law and the statutory regulations governing the use was observed.

Storage: Sumatra benzoin inhaler should be kept in a light-resistant, airtight container stored in a cool and dry place.

Use: Expectorant.

Example 64: Menthol and benzoin inhalation	
Ingredients	Quantity
Menthol	20 gm
Benzoin inhalation	q.s to produce 1000 ml

Method: Dissolve the menthol in a portion of the benzoin inhalation, add sefficient benzoin inhalation to produce 1000 ml, and mix.

Storage: Menthol inhaler should be kept in a light-resistant, airtight container and stored in a cool place.

Use: Germicidal and soothing activity for cough treatment.

Example 65: Menthol and eucalyptus inhalation	
Ingredients	Quantity
Menthol	20 gm
Eucalyptus oil	100 ml
Light magnesium carbonate	70 gm
Water 0.05–0.075	1000 ml

Method: Dissolve the menthol in the eucalyptus oil, add the light magnesium carbonate, and sufficient water to produce 1000 ml.

Storage: This inhaler should be kept in a light-resistant, airtight container and stored in a cool place.

Use: Germicidal and soothing activity for cough treatment.

Throat Spray

- Throat sprays are solutions of drugs in aqueous vehicles and are applied to the mucous membrane of the nose and throat by means of an atomizer nebulizer.
- The spray device should produce relatively coarse droplets, if the action of the drug is to be restricted to the upper respiratory tract. Fine droplets tend to penetrate further into the respiratory tract than is desirable.

Labeling

The label on the container states: (1) the names and concentrations of the active ingredients, (2) the date after which the spray is not intended to be used, (3) the conditions under which the spray should be stored.

Example 66: Adrenaline and atropine spray, BPC	
Ingredients	Quantity
Adrenaline acid tartrate	8 g
Atropine methonitrate	1 g

contd...

Example 66: Adrenaline and atropine spray, BPC (*contd.*)	
Papaverine hydrochloride	8 g
Sodium metabisulfite	1 g
Chlorbutol	5 g
Propylene glycol	50 ml
Purified water boiled and cooled, to	1000 ml

Method

1. Using a conical flask plugged with non-absorbent cotton wool, boil about 150 ml of purified water for about 10 minutes, to remove oxygen and destroy vegetative bacteria and mould spores. Cool and use pan for the triturates.

2. Mix the three solutions and dissolve the papaverine salt in the mixture.

3. If a 5 mg weight is not available, weigh the chlorbutol on an analytical balance. Dissolve it in the propylene glycol and add the solution to the mixtures of salts.

4. Filter, if necessary, and adjust to volume through the filter.

Storage: This spray should be kept in a light-resistant, airtight container and stored in a cool place.

Use: It is useful in cases of chronic asthma and hay fever.

Enema

- These preparations are rectal injections employed to:
  - ❖ Evacuate the bowel (evacuation enemas).
  - ❖ Influence the general system by absorption (retention enemas), e.g. nutritive, sedative or stimulating properties.
  - ❖ Affect locally the site of disease (e.g. anthelmintic property).
  - ❖ They may contain radiopaque substances for roentgenographic examination of the lower bowel.
- Retention enemas are used in small quantities (about 30 ml) and are thus called retention microenema.

- Starch enema may be used either by itself or as a vehicle for other forms of medication.

Labeling

The label states: (1) the names and concentrations of the active ingredients, (2) that the preparation should not be swallowed, (3) the date after which the enema is not intended to be used, (4) the conditions under which the enema should be stored, (5) the directions for using the enema.

Example 67: Paraldehyde enema	
Ingredients	**Quantity**
Paraldehyde	0.1 gm
Sodium chloride solution	100 ml

Method

1. Calibrate container at 110 ml.

2. Weigh the sodium chloride and dissolve it in a suitable volume of water that has been chilled in a refrigerator to aid solution of the paraldehyde.

3. If the solution requires filtration, pass it through a sintered glass using vacuum. The completed enema should not be filtered to avoid the contact of the drug to air.

4. Put the paraldehyde into the bottle, adjust the volume with vehicle and shake vigorously until solution is complete.

5. Paraldehyde attack cork and certain of the plastics used as liners for screw caps.

Storage: This enema should be kept in a light-resistant, airtight container and stored in a cool place.

Use: Hypnotic.

Example 68: Phosphate enema	
Ingredients	**Quantity**
Sodium acid phosphate	160 g
Sodium phosphate	60 g
Purified water sufficient to produce	1000 ml

A suitable antimicrobial preservative may be included.

Method

1. Weigh the sodium acid phosphate and sodium phosphate and dissolve it in a suitable volume of water.
2. If the solution requires filtration, pass it through a sintered glass using vacuum. The completed enema should not be filtered to avoid the contact of the drug to air.
3. Adjust the volume with vehicle and shake vigorously until solution is complete.

Storage: This enema should be kept in an airtight container and stored in a cool place.

Use: Laxative.

Paints

Paints are liquid preparations usually medicated with substances possessing antiseptic, caustic, soothing or stimulating properties. They are prepared with vehicles which render their consistence suitable for application to the skin or mucous surfaces by means of a brush. The character of the bases differs considerably, their selection depending upon the nature of the medicament to be applied, the duration of contact desired and the degree of absorption required. Paints intended to remain in contact with a specified surface are usually prepared with collodion, glycerin, glycerin and water, solution of egg albumen in alcohol, or solution of gutta-percha. Paints intended to be absorbed are prepared with oleic acid or fatty oils. Caustic substances when employed as paints are usually applied dissolved in distilled water and occasionally in alcoholic or ethereal vehicles. Resinous substances, such as benzoin, storax, balsam of tolu or sandarac, dissolved in ether, are employed as bases for medicated varnishes and used for application to the skin and raw mucous surfaces. Bottles fitted with glass stoppers are usually most suitable as containers for paints. Paints

containing chromic acid are applied by means of glass brushes.

Labeling

The label states: (1) the names and concentrations of the active ingredients, (2) the date after which the paint is not intended to be used, (3) the conditions under which the paint should be stored, (4) the directions for using the paint, (5) any special precautions associated with the use of the paint. Paints should be kept in airtight containers.

Example 69: Brilliant green and crystal violet paint	
Ingredients	Quantity
Brilliant green	5 g
Crystal violet	5 g
Ethanol (90%)	500 ml
Water to produce	1000 ml

Method: Dissolve the brilliant green and crystal violet in the ethanol (90%) and add sufficient water to produce 1000 ml.

Storage Paints should be kept in airtight containers.

Use: Antibacterial.

Example 70: Compound mastic paint	
Ingredients	Quantity
Mastic	400 g
Castor oil	12.5 g
Acetone	Sufficient quantity
Industrial methylated spirit	Sufficient quantity

Method: Dissolve the mastic in 450 ml of a mixture of equal volumes of acetone and industrial methylated spirit add the castor oil, add sufficient of a mixture of equal volumes of acetone and industrial methylated spirit to produce 1000 ml and filter.

Storage: Paints should be kept in airtight containers.

Use: Sealant over wounds.

Example 71: Coal tar paint	
Ingredients	**Quantity**
Coal tar	100 g
Acetone to produce	1000 ml

Method: Disperse the coal tar in 700 ml of acetone, allow to stand for one hour filter, if necessary, dilute with acetone to 100 ml.

Storage: Paints should be kept in airtight containers. The label on the container states that the preparation is flammable and that it should be kept away from naked flames.

Use: Antipsoriatic.

Example 72: Mandl's paint	
Ingredients	**Quantity**
Potassium iodide	25 g
Iodine	12.5 g
Alcohol 90%	40 ml
Water	25 ml
Peppermint oil	4 ml
Glycerol , to	1000 ml

Method

1. Put the water into a 50 ml conical measure; use a squat type to facilitate stirring.

2. Dissolve the potassium iodide; it dissolves very rapidly in water and need not be powered.

3. Add the iodine and stir until completely dissolved. Although iodine is only slightly soluble in water it is readily soluble in aqueous solutions of iodides.

4. In a 10 ml conical measure, dissolve 0.2 ml of peppermint oil in 2 ml of alcohol 90%. Using a pipette graduated in fiftieths of a ml, transfer 1.76 ml to the iodine solution and mix well.

5. Make up the volume with glycerol and mix thoroughly. If the iodine solution is not well mixed with the glycerol, the preparation is streaky.

Storage: Mandl's paints should be kept in airtight containers.

Use: Antiseptic.

Parenteral Preparations

Parenteral preparations are sterile preparations intended for administration by injection, infusion or implantation into the human or animal body. Parenteral preparations may require the use of excipients, e.g. to make the preparation isotonic with respect to blood, to adjust the pH, to increase solubility, to prevent deterioration of the active substances or to provide adequate antimicrobial properties, but not to adversely affect the intended medicinal action of the preparation or, at the concentrations used, to cause toxicity or undue local irritation. Containers for parenteral preparations are made as far as possible from materials that are sufficiently transparent to permit the visual inspection of the contents, except for implants and in other justified and authorized cases.

Labeling

Where appropriate the label states the strength of the parenteral preparation in terms of the amount of active ingredient in a suitable dose-volume. The label also states: (1) the name of any added substance, (2) the date after which the parenteral preparation is not intended to be used, (3) the conditions under which the parenteral preparation should be stored. The label of a single-dose parenteral preparation states that any portion of the contents remaining should be discarded.

Example 73: Adrenaline tartrate injection (IP, 1966)	
Ingredients	**Quantity**
Adrenaline bitartrate	0.18 g
Sodium metabisulfite	0.1 g
Sodium chloride	0.8 g
Water for injection sufficient to produce	100 ml

Method

1. Dissolve the sodium metabisulfite in 10 ml of water for injection and dissolve the adrenaline bitartrate in this solution.
2. Dissolve the sodium chloride in 75 ml of water for injection.
3. Mix the two solutions and add the sufficient quantity of water for injection to produce the required volume.
4. Sterilize by heating in an autoclave.

Storage: Preserve adrenaline tartrate injection protected from light. It shall be made up only in single dose container of 0.5 or 1 ml capacity. The label on the container states the date of manufacturing and the date of expiry, the intervening period not to exceed one year.

Use: Bronchodilator.

Example 74: Digoxin injection (IP, 1966)	
Ingredients	**Quantity**
Digoxin	25 mg
Alcohol (80%)	12.5 ml
Propylene glycol	40 ml
Citric acid	75 mg
Sodium phosphate	0.45 mg
Water for injection, sufficient to produce	100 ml

Method

1. Dissolve the digoxin in the alcohol (80%).
2. Add propylene glycol, a solution of citric acid and the sodium phosphate in water for injection.
3. Volume make-up sufficient to produce 100 ml.
4. Distribute in ampoules and sterilize by heating in an autoclaving.

Storage: Preserve the digoxin injection, protect from light.

Use: Cardiotonic.

EMULSION

An emulsion is liquid preparation containing two immiscible liquids, one of which is dispersed as globules (dispersed phase or internal phase) in the other liquid (continuous phase or external phase). Droplet diameters vary enormously, but in pharmaceutical emulsions, they are typically polydispersed with diameters ranging from approximately 0.1 to 50 µm. Emulsions are conveniently classified as oil-in-water (o/w) or water-in-oil (w/o), depending on whether the continuous phase is aqueous or oily. Figure 6.1 shows a photomicrograph of a simple o/w system. Multiple emulsions, which are prepared from oil and water by the re-emulsification of an existing emulsion so as to provide two dispersed phases, are also of pharmaceutical interest. Multiple emulsions of the oil-in-water-in-oil (o/w/o) type are w/o emulsions in which the water globules themselves contain dispersed oil globules; conversely, water-in-oil-in-water (w/o/w) emulsions are those where the internal and external aqueous phases are separated by the oil.

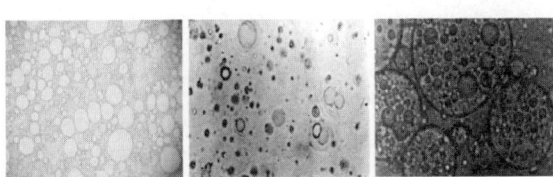

Fig. 6.1: Photomicrographs of typical emulsions. (A) A liquid paraffin-in-water emulsion; (B) A liquid paraffin–water cream stabilized; (C) A multiple w/o/w emulsion. Water droplets can clearly be seen within the larger oil droplets

Types of Pharmaceutical Emulsions

Emulsions are generally classified as oil-in-water (o/w), water-in-oil (w/o), micro-emulsions and multiple emulsion o/w/o or w/o/w.

Oil-in-water (o/w): In which, oil is the dispersed or internal phase and water is the dispresion or internal phase. Such emulsions are generally preferred for oral use. However, o/w emulsions are also useful for products intended for external application, e.g. creams, lotions and liniments.

Water-in-oil (w/o emulsion): In which, water is the dispersed and oil is the dispersion medium. They are mostly used externally as creams, ointments, and lotions.

Microemulsion: Microemulsions contain dispersed phase having diameters less than 0.1 micrometer. Droplets of such dimensions unable to refract light and therefore microemulsion appear as transprent solutions. Microemulsions have been used for the preparation of both external and internal formulations. Microemulsions exhibits better absorption and bioavailability than conventional emulsion.

Multiple emulsions: In which, the oil-in-water or water-in-oil emulsions are further dispersed in either oil or water. If o/w emulsion is dispersed as fine droplets in oil, then the emulsion is defined as oil-in-water-in-oil (o/w/o).

w/o/w emulsions consist of droplets of water dispersed in the oil phase of an oil-in-water emulsion. Multiple emulsions have been proposed as potential candidates for sustained release dosage forms. Multiple emulsions can be prepared in two phases.

Primary and secondary emulsions (Fig. 6.2)
- Primary emulsion containing one internal phase, e.g. oil-in-water emulsion (o/w) and water-in-oil emulsion (w/o).
- Secondary emulsion or multiple emulsion contains two internal phase, for instance, o/w/o or w/o/w. It can be used to delay release or to increase the stability of the active compounds.

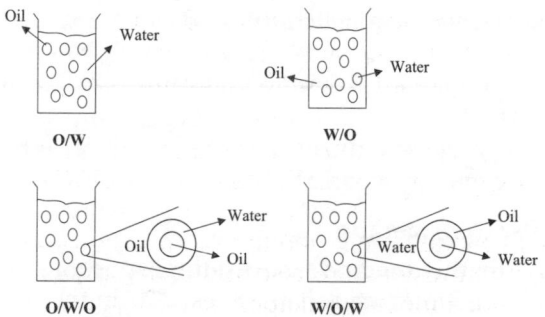

Fig. 6.2: Primary and secondary emulsions

Properties of Emulsions

The characteristics of an acceptable pharmaceutical emulsion include the following:

- Physical stability (no phase separation).
- The flow properties of the emulsion/ cream should enable the formulation to be easily removed from the container.
- Furthermore, if the formulation is designed for external or topical application, the formulation must be easily spread over the affected area.
- The formulation must be aesthetically and texturally pleasing.
- If the emulsion is designed for oral application, the flavor must be suitable whereas if emulsions are to be externally applied, they must have the correct 'feel'.

Advantages and Disadvantages of Pharmaceutical Emulsions

Advantages

- Pharmaceutical emulsions may be used to deliver drugs that exhibit a low aqueous solubility. Some drugs are more readily absorbed when administered as an emulsion than as other oral formulations.
- Pharmaceutical emulsions may be used to mask the taste of therapeutic agents, in which the drug is dissolved in the internal phase of an o/w emulsion. The external phase may then be formulated to contain the appropriate sweetening and flavoring agents.
- Emulsions may be commonly used to administer oils that may have a therapeutic effect. For example, the cathartic effect of oils, e.g. liquid paraffin, is enhanced following administration to the patient as droplets within an o/w emulsion. The taste of the oil may be masked using sweetening and flavoring agents.
- If the therapeutic agent is irritant when applied topically, the irritancy may be reduced by formulation of the drug within the internal phase of an o/w emulsion.
- Pharmaceutical emulsions may be employed to administer drugs to patients who have difficulty in swallowing solid dosage forms.

- Emulsions are employed for total parenteral nutrition.

Disadvantages

- Pharmaceutical emulsions are thermodynamically unstable and therefore must be formulated to stabilize the emulsion from separation of the two phases. This is by no means straight forward.
- Pharmaceutical emulsions may be difficult to manufacture.

Theories of Emulsification

In case of two immiscible liquids as shown in Fig. 6.3, when mixed together and kept aside, they tend to aggregate and separate out.

This phenomenon is because of cohesive force between the molecules of each separate liquid which exceeds adhesive force between two liquids. This is manifested as interfacial energy or tension at boundary between the liquids.

Therefore, to prevent the coalescence and separation, emulsifying agents have been used.

Table 6.5 enlists the types of emulsifier, their mode of emulsification with examples.

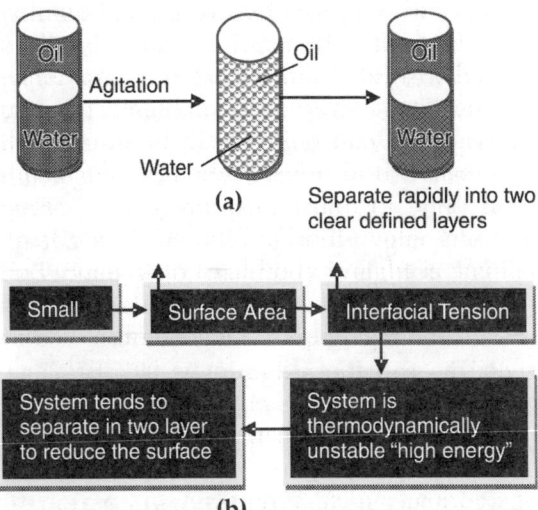

Fig. 6.3: (a) Typical representation of biphasic immiscible liquid system. (b) Schematic representation of interfacial phenomenon of an emulsion

Methods of Emulsion Preparation

In the small scale extemporaneous preparation of an emulsion, the following three methods are used. However, the selection of the method depends on the nature of the emulsion components and the equipment available.

Dry Gum Method

1. This method is also referred to as the 4:2:1 method because for every four parts (volumes) of oil, two parts of water and one part of gum is added in preparing the initial or primary emulsion in a dry porcelain mortar.
2. The gum is added slowly to the oil first with continuous trituration. After the oil and the gum have been mixed, the two parts of water are added all at once, and the mixture is triturated rapidly and continuously until a creamy white emulsion that produces a crackling sound to the movement of the pestle forms.
3. Other liquid formulative ingredients that are soluble in or miscible with the external phase may then be added to the primary emulsion with mixing.
4. Preservatives, stabilizers, colorants, and flavoring agents are usually dissolved in a suitable volume of water (assuming water is the external phase) and added as a solution to the primary emulsion.
5. The emulsion is transferred to a graduated cylinder and made to volume with water previously swirled about in the mortar to remove the last portion of the emulsion. An electric mixer or blender may also be used for making the primary emulsion.

Wet Gum Method

1. In this method, the same proportions of oil, water, and gum are used as in the dry gum method, but the order of mixing is different.
2. Mucilage of the gum is prepared by triturating the gum with twice its weight in water in a mortar.

Table 6.5: Types of emulsifying agents and their mode of emulsification			
Types of emulsifier	**Theories of emulsification**	**Class**	**Examples**
Surface active agents	• Reduction of the interfacial tension. • Form coherent monolayer to prevent the coalescence of two droplet when they approach each other. • Provide surface charge which cause repulsion between adjust particles. • Combination of surface-active agents is used most frequently. The combination should form film that is closely packed and condensed.	Anionic (anionic SAA are mainly used for external uses). Cationic (cationic SAA are used for external used. They have, also, good antimicrobial activity). Non-ionic (non-ionic SAA are stable over wide range of pH. They are not affected by change in pH or addition of electrolytes. They are less toxic and main function to provide steric repulsion).	Sodium lauryl sulfate Benzalkonium chloride, cetrimide Tween and span
Multimolecular adsorption	• Hydrophilic colloids form multimolecular adsorption at the oil/water interface. They have low effect on the surface tension. • Their main function as emulsion stabilizers is by making coherent multi-molecular film. This film is strong and resists the coalescence. They have, also, an auxiliary effect by increasing the viscosity of dispersion medium. • Most of the hydrophilic colloids form oil-in-water emulsions. • Some of them can provide electrostatic repulsion like acacia, which contains arabic acid and proteins (COOH and NH_3)	Polysaccharides Amphoterics Synthetic and semisynthetic polymers	Agar, acacia, gaur gum, tragacanth. Gelatin Carbomer resins, cellulose ether, carboxymethyl chitin, PEG.
Solid particle adsorption	• Finely divided solid particles are adsorbed at the surface of emulsion droplet to stabilize them. Those particles are wetted by both oil and water (but not dissolved) and the concentration of these particles form a particulate film that prevent the coalescence.	Finely divided solids	Bentonite, kaolin, magnesium aluminum silicate, silica, aluminum hydroxide.

contd...

Table 6.5: Types of emulsifying agents and their mode of emulsification (*contd.*)

Types of emulsifier	Theories of emulsification	Class	Examples
	• Particles that are wetted preferentially by water from o/w emulsion, whereas those wetted more by oil form w/o emulsion. • Note that they are very rare to use and can affect rheology of the final product. • Size of the particle is very important, larger particles can lead to coalescence.		
Natural emulsifying agents	• *Egg yolk*: It contains phospholipids and cholesterol. The main drawback is that spoils quickly; therefore, it cannot be used in industry. It is used for extemporaneous preparation. • *Wool fat*: Anhydrous lanolin, it is used to prepare w/o emulsion for external uses. • *Starch*: It forms starch mucilage and it is restricted for enemas preparation. • *Cholesterol*: It has stabilizing action; therefore, another emulsifier should be included.	Polysaccharides, lipids and protein. They are primarily used to increase the viscosity of dispersion medium and also form multilayers formation arround the dispersed phase due to its lyophilic behaviors.	Egg yolk, cool, fat, gelation, cholesterol, phospholipids.

3. The oil is then added slowly in portions and the mixture is triturated to emulsify the oil.
4. After all of the oil has been added, the mixture is thoroughly mixed for several minutes to ensure uniformity.
5. Then the other formulative ingredients are added and the emulsion is transferred to a graduated cylinder and made to volume with water.

Bottle Method
1. In this method, powder gum is placed in a dry bottle, two parts of oil are then added, and the mixture is thoroughly shaken in the capped container.
2. A volume of water approximately equal to the oil is then added in portions, the mixture being thoroughly shaken after each addition.

3. When all the water has been added, the primary emulsion thus formed may be diluted to the proper volume with water or an aqueous solution containing other formulative agents.
4. The method is useful for the extemporaneous preparation of emulsions from volatile oils or oleaginous substances of low viscosities.

The ratio of oily phase to aqueous phase to gum in a primary emulsion

Type of oil	Oil	Aqueous	Gum
Fixed	4	2	1
Mineral	3	2	1
Volatile	2	2	1

General Method of Preparation of an Emulsion Using the Dry Gum Method

It is relatively easy for an emulsion to crack, resulting in a failed product. Remember that the key points opposite are critical when preparing emulsions. The preparation of an emulsion has two main components:

1. Preparation of a concentrate called the primary emulsion
2. Dilution of the concentrate.

Preparation of the Primary Emulsion

- Measure the oil accurately in a dry measure. Transfer the oil into a large dry porcelain mortar, allowing all the oil to drain out.

- Measure the quantity of aqueous vehicle required for the primary emulsion. Place this within easy reach.

- Weigh the emulsifying agent and place on the oil in the mortar. Mix lightly with the pestle, just sufficient to disperse any lumps. *Caution*: Over mixing generates heat, which may denature the emulsifying agent and result in a poor product.

- Add the entire required aqueous vehicle in one addition. Then mix vigorously, using the pestle with a shearing action in one direction.

- When the product becomes white and produces a clicking sound, the primary emulsion has been formed. The product should be a thick, white cream. Increased degree of whiteness indicates a better-quality product. Oil globules or slicks should not be apparent.

Dilution of the Primary Emulsion

- Dilute the primary emulsion drop by drop with very small volumes of the remaining aqueous vehicle. Mix carefully with the pestle in one direction.

- Transfer emulsion to a measure, with rinsing. Add other liquid ingredients if necessary and make up to the final volume.

Tests to Identify the Type of Emulsion

There are several tests that may be performed to identify the type of emulsion that has formed:

- **Electrical conductivity:** o/w emulsions conduct electric current whereas w/o emulsions do not.

- **Dilution with water:** o/w emulsions may be diluted with water (as this is the composition of the external phase) whereas w/o emulsions cannot be diluted with water.

- **Use of dyes:** Oil-soluble dyes will stain the internal phase, if the emulsion is an o/w emulsion whereas water-soluble dyes will dye the internal phase of a w/o emulsion.

- **Direction of creaming:** If the direction of creaming is upward, indicate o/w emulsion. If the emulsion cream is downward, it is w/o type.

- **Fluorescence test:** Many oils when exposed to UV light, give fluorescence. When a drop of emulsion exposed to UV light, if it exhibits dotted pattern fluorescence indicate oil is the internal or dispersed phase, i.e. o/w emulsion. If entire field fluorescence observed indicate oil in the external or dispersion phase, i.e. w/o emulsion.

Emulsion Instability

One of the goals of the pharmaceutical scientist is to formulate an emulsion that is physically stable, i.e. where the droplets of the internal phase remain discrete, retain their diameter and are homogeneously dispersed throughout the formulation. Fundamental to achieving this goal is the presence of the interfacial film (monomolecular or multilayered) at the interface between the droplet and the external phase. Emulsion instability may be either reversible or irreversible and is manifest in the following ways: (1) cracking (irreversible instability); (2) flocculation; (3) creaming; and (4) phase inversion. Table 6.6 enlists the emulsion instability and their trouble shooting.

Table 6.6: Types of emulsion instability and its troubleshooting

Emulsion instability	Definition	Possible reasons for problem	Troubleshooting	Can the emulsion be saved?
Creaming	Separation of the emulsion into two regions, one containing more of the disperse phase.	Lack of stability of the system. Product not homogeneous.	Production of an emulsion of small droplet size. Increase in the viscosity of the continuous phase. Reduction in the density difference between the two phases. Control of disperse phase concentration.	The emulsion will reform on shaking.
Cracking	The globules of the disperse phase coalesce and there is separation of the disperse phase into a separate layer.	Incompatible emulsifying agent. Decomposition of the emulsifying agent. Change of storage temperature. Incorrect selection of emulsifying agents. Microbial spoilage.	The presence of long, cohesive hydrocarbon. Chains projecting into the oil phase will prevent coalescence. Maintain storage temperature.	The emulsion will not reform on shaking.
Phase inversion	From oil-in-water to water-in-oil or from water-in-oil to oil-in-water.	Amount of disperse phase greater than 74%.	Proper selection emulsifier. Maintain the proper balance of dispersed and dispersion phase.	The emulsion will not reform on shaking.
Flocculation	The ability of emulsion droplets to flocculate.	Incorrect selection of emulsifying agents.	The presence of a high charge density on the dispersed droplets will reduce the incidence of flocculation.	The emulsion will reform on shaking.
Coalescence and ostwald ripening.	Coalescence, where dispersed phase droplets merge to form larger droplets, takes place in two distinct stages. Drainage of liquid films of continuous phase from between the oil droplets.	Reducing the energy of interaction between adjacent globules.	Reducing the energy of interaction between adjacent globules.	The emulsion will reform on shaking.

contd...

Table 6.6: Types of emulsion instability and its troubleshooting (*contd.*)

Emulsion instability	Definition	Possible reasons for problem	Troubleshooting	Can the emulsion be saved?
	As they approach to one another, they end with the rupture of the film when a critical thickness is reached.	A salting-out effect, by which high concentrations of electrolytes is acquired.	A salting-out effect, by which high concentrations of electrolytes is acquired.	
Oxidation	Many of the oils and fats used in emulsion formulation are of animal or vegetable origin and can be susceptible to oxidation by atmospheric oxygen or by the action of microorganisms.	Rancidity is manifested by the formation of degradation products of unpleasant odor and taste.	Oxidation of microbiological origin is controlled by the use of antimicrobial preservatives, and atmospheric oxidation by the use of reducing agents or, more usually, antioxidants.	No

Example 1: Cod liver oil emulsion

Ingredients	Official quantity
Cod liver oil	100 ml
Acacia powder	25 gm
Tragacanth powder	1.5 gm
Saccharin sodium	0.02 gm
Benzaldehyde spirit	0.5 ml
Chloroform	0.5 ml
Water, to	200 ml

Method

1. Mix the two gum and prepare the primary emulsion by the dry gum method.
2. Dilute carefully, transfer to a measure add the saccharin sodium solution, benzaldehyde spirit and chloroform water with constant stirring.
3. Make up the volume.

Storage: Store in airtight container and protect from light.

Use: Dietary supplement

Example 2: Cold cream

Ingredients	Official quantity
White beeswax	10 gm
Liquid paraffin	30 gm
Borax	0.5 gm
Water	9.5 gm

Method

1. Grate the beeswax, melt it with the liquid paraffin and raise the temperature to 70°C.
2. Dissolve the borax in the water and heat the solution to 70°C.
3. Gradually add the solution to the melted mixture and stir, preferably mechanically, until the cream has set. Stirring should be rapid initially but care must be taken to avoid aeration as the preparation starts to thicken.
4. Pack in a pot and close tightly to prevent dehydration.

Storage: Store in a wide mouth container and protect from direct sunlight.

Use: Moisturizer.

Example 3: Cream	
Ingredients	Official quantity
Ichthammol	5 gm
Sorbitan monostearate	2 gm
Macrogol 300	40 gm
Macrogol 1500	40 gm
Water, to	100 gm

Method

1. Melt the macrogols with the sorbitan easter at about 60°C.
2. Dissolve the ichthammol in the water and heat to the same temperature.
3. Add the solution to the melted mixture and stir until cold.

Storage: Stored in an airtight container and protect from direct sunlight of a child's reach.

Use: As antibacterial in scrapes and skin injuries.

Example 4: Liquid paraffin emulsion (IP, 1966)	
Ingredients	Quantity
Liquid paraffin	500 ml
Indian gum in powder	125 ml
Tragacanth in powder	5 g
Sodium benzoate	5 g
Vanillin	0.5 g
Glycerin	125 ml
Chloroform	2.5 ml
Purified water	1000 ml

Method

1. Triturate the liquid paraffin and chloroform with the Indian gum, tragacanth and vanillin.
2. Add one quantity 250 ml of purified water and triturate until a creamy emulsion is formed.

3. Add the glycerin and sodium benzoate dissolved in 50 ml of purified water.
4. Add sufficient purified water to produce 1000 ml.
5. Mix the emulsion and store.

Storage: Preserve in well-closed container protected from light.

Use: Laxative

Example 5: Liquid paraffin and magnesium hydroxide emulsion	
Ingredients	Quantity
Liquid paraffin	250 ml
Chloroform spirit	15 ml
Magnesium hydroxide mixture q.s	1000 ml

Method: Mix the chloroform spirit with 650 ml of the magnesium hydroxide mixture, add to the liquid paraffin, add sufficient magnesium hydroxide mixture to produce 1000 ml, and pass through a homogenizer.

Storage: Preserve in well-closed container protected from light.

Use: Laxative.

Example 6: Concentrated peppermint emulsion	
Ingredients	quantity
Peppermint oil	20 ml
Polysorbate 20	1 ml
Double strength chloroform water	500 ml
Purified water	Qs to produce 1000 ml

Method

1. Purified water, freshly boiled and cooled sufficient to produce 1000 ml.
2. Shake the peppermint oil with the polysorbate 20.
3. Gradually add, shaking well after each addition, the double strength chloroform

water and sufficient purified water to produce 1000 ml.

Containers: The general direction to supply emulsions in wide-necked bottles does not apply to concentrated peppermint emulsion.

Storage: Preserve in well-closed container protected from light.

Use: Used as a flavoring.

SUSPENSIONS

Pharmaceutical suspensions are commonly referred to as dispersions in which the therapeutic agent is dispersed in the external phase (the vehicle). The diameter of the disperse phase may range from 0.5 to 100 micrometer. Systems in which the particle size diameter falls below the above range are termed colloidal. Pharmaceutical suspensions are employed to deliver therapeutic agents of low (predominantly aqueous) solubility.

- Pharmaceutical suspensions may be employed for the administration of drugs by many potential routes.

- Pharmaceutical suspensions are physically unstable; this instability is apparent by the presence of a solid cake and the resultant inability to redisperse the therapeutic agent. This leads to problems regarding the administration of the correct dosage of the therapeutic agent.

- In addition to enhancing the aesthetic properties, the excipients used in pharmaceutical suspensions are included to optimize the physical stability of the formulation.

- A pharmaceutical suspension would be considered stable if, after agitation (shaking), the drug particles are homogeneously dispersed for a sufficient time to ensure that an accurate dose is removed for administration to the patient.

Properties of Suspensions

The characteristics of an acceptable pharmaceutical suspension include the following:

- A low rate of sedimentation.
- The disperse phase must be easily redispersed with gentle shaking.
- The flow properties of the suspension should enable the formulation to be easily removed from the container (e.g. bottle, injection vial).
- Aesthetically pleasing.

Advantages and Disadvantages of Pharmaceutical Suspensions

Advantages

- Pharmaceutical suspensions are a useful drug delivery system for therapeutic agents that have a low solubility.

- Pharmaceutical suspensions may be formulated to mask the taste of therapeutic agents.

- Pharmaceutical suspensions may be employed to administer drugs to patients who have difficulty swallowing solid-dosage forms.

- Pharmaceutical suspensions may be formulated to provide controlled drug delivery, e.g. as intramuscular injections.

Disadvantages

- Pharmaceutical suspensions are fundamentally unstable and therefore require formulation skill to ensure that the physical stability of the formulation is retained over the period of the shelf-life.

- The formulation of stable suspension formulations is difficult.

- Suspension being the liquid dosage form, susceptible for physical, chemical and microbical contamination.

- Rhelogical properties of suspension is often difficult to maintain in suspension with high concentation of indiffusible solids.

Formulation of Suspension

The formulation of a suspension possessing optimal physical stability depends on whether the particles in suspension are to be flocculated or to remain deflocculated. The approaches commonly used in the preparation of physically stable suspensions fall into two categories— the use of a structured vehicle to maintain deflocculated particles in suspension and the application of the principles of flocculation to produce flocs that, although they settle rapidly, are easily resuspended with a minimum of agitation. Table 6.7 enlists the differences between flocculated and deflocculated suspension.

Excipients Used in the Formulation of Suspensions for Oral Administration

During the preparation of physically stable pharmaceutical suspensions, a number of +formulation components are used to keep the solid particles in a state of suspension (suspending agents), whereas other components are part of the liquid vehicle itself and have other functions in the dosage form. Table 6.8 enlists the commonly used additive in suspension.

1. Components of the suspending system:
   - ❖ Wetting agents
   - ❖ Dispersants or deflocculating agents
   - ❖ Flocculating agents
   - ❖ Thickeners
2. Components of the suspending vehicle or external phase.
   - ❖ pH control agents and buffers
   - ❖ Osmotic agents
   - ❖ Coloring agents, flavors, and fragrances
   - ❖ Preservatives to control microbial growth

General Method for the Preparation of a Suspension Containing a Diffusible Solid

1. Finely powder any ingredient not previously in fine powder.
2. Mix the insoluble powders in a mortar in geometric dilution technique.
3. Add enough vehicle to produce a smooth paste.
4. Add any non-volatile solids ingredients, dissolved in part of the vehicle, and mix well.
5. Examine the suspension critically and if it contains foreign particles, filter through muslin. Before use rinse the muslin with a little vehicle to detach loose fibers.
6. Strained into tared bottle.
7. Add any volatile solid ingredient, previously dissolved in some of the vehicle, and mix well.
8. Add any liquid ingredient, rinse the measures and mix well after each addition.
9. Make up to final volume with vehicle.
10. Stir gently, transfer to a suitable container, ensuring that all the solid is transferred from the conical measure to the bottle, and label ready to be dispensed to the patient.

Table 6.7: Relative properties of flocculated and deflocculated particles in suspension

Deflocculated	Flocculated
Particles exist in suspension as individual entities.	Particles form loose aggregates or floccules.
Rate of sedimentation is slow.	Rate of sedimentation is high.
The sediment eventually becomes very closely packed and the resulting hard cake is difficult, if not impossible, to redisperse.	The sediment is loosely packed and easy to redisperse.
Even after settling, the supernatant remains cloudy.	After rapid settling, a clear boundary exists between the sediment and the supernatant.

Additives	Function	Agent
	Table 6.8: Pharmaceutical additives commonly used in suspension	
Suspending agents	These are commonly used to enhance the viscostly, physical stability and to affect the flow properties of oral suspensions.	Carboxymethylcellulose Xanthan gum Algin Magnesium aluminum silicate Hydroxyethylcellulose Guar gum Tragacanth gum
Flocculating agents	Surface-active agents, both ionic and non-ionic, can interact with the suspended particles and, in so doing, can affect the magnitude of the zeta potential.	Calcium Citrate salt Alum Sulfate and phosphate salt
Thickeners, protective colloids	Protective or hydrophilic colloids, such as gelatin, natural gums, and cellulosic derivatives, that are adsorbed on insoluble particles, increase the strength of the hydration layer formed around suspended particles.	*Cellulosics*: Sodium carboxymethyl-cellulose, microcrystalline, cellulose, hydroxyethylcellulose, sodium starch glycolate, and powdered cellulose. *Clays*: Attapulgite, bentonite, magnesium aluminum silicate, kaolin, silicon dioxides. *Gums*: Acacia, agar, algins, carrageenan, guar, pectin, tragacanth, xanthan. *Polymers*: Carbomers, polyvinyl alcohol, povidone, polyethylene oxide. *Sugars*: Dextrin, maltitol, sucrose. *Others*: aluminummonostearate, emulsifying waxes, gelatin.
Wetting agent	Surface-active agents decrease the contact angle of insoluble particles, enabling greater wetting by the vehicle. This, in turn, assists product homogeneity and decreases aggregation.	Sodium lauryl sulfate Polyoxylakyl phenyl ethers Polyoxysorbitan esters, sorbitan esters
Preservatives	Preservatives are chemical compounds that are added to formulations to protect them from microbial contamination.	Benzalkonium chloride Benzyl alcohol Chlorobutanol Chlorocresol Cresol Methylparaben Propylparaben Phenylmercuric nitrate thimerosal

contd...

Table 6.8: Pharmaceutical additives commonly used in suspension (*contd.*)

Additives	Function	Agent
Antioxidants	Antioxidants are compounds that are redox systems which exhibit higher oxidative potential than the therapeutic agent or, alternatively, are compounds that inhibit free radical-induced drug decomposition.	Ascorbic acid
		Butyl hydroxyanisole
		Butyl hydroxytoluene
		Sodium bisulfite
		Sodium formaldehyde sulfoxylate, thiourea
Chelating agents, buffering agents	Buffers are sometimes used to control the pH and therefore keep the ionic state constant	Tocopherol
		Ethylenediamine tetra-acetic acid
		Acetic acid salt, citric acid
Sweetener	Sweetening agents and flavors are used for taste-masking purposes.	Sucrose
		Fructose
		Glucose
		Sorbitol
		Saccharin
Flavors	Flavors are used to make products more palatable.	Allyl benzoate (cherry)
		Allyl caproate (pineapple)
		Allyl cyclohexylbutyrate (pineapple)
		Allyl cyclohexylcaproate (peach/apricot)
		Allyl cyclohexylvalerate (apple)
		Allyl phenoxyacetate (honey/pineapple)
		Anethol (anise)

General Method for the Preparation of a Suspension Containing an Indiffusible Solid

Oral indiffusible suspensions are prepared using the same basic principles as for oral diffusible suspensions. The main difference is that the preparation will require the addition of a suspending agent.

1. Check the solubility in the vehicle of all solids in the mixture.

2. Calculate the quantities of vehicle required to dissolve any soluble solid.

3. Weigh all solids on an electronic balance.

4. Dissolve all soluble solids in the vehicle in a small glass beaker.

5. Mix any insoluble indiffusible powder and the suspending agent (compound tragacanth powder 2 g/100 ml or as the mucilage 10–20 ml/150 ml of product) in a porcelain mortar.

6. Add a small quantity of the vehicle (which may or may not be a solution of the soluble ingredients) to the solids in the mortar and mix using a pestle to form a smooth paste.

7. Add further vehicle in small quantities, and continue mixing until the mixture in the mortar is a pourable consistency.

8. Transfer the contents of the mortar to a conical measure of suitable size.

9. Rinse out the mortar with more vehicles and add any rinsing to the conical measure.

10. Add remaining liquid ingredients to the mixture in the conical measure. (These are added now, as some may be volatile and therefore exposure whilst mixing needs to be reduced to prevent loss of the ingredient by evaporation.)

11. Make up to final volume with vehicle.

12. Stir gently, transfer to a suitable container, ensuring that the entire solid is transferred from the conical measure to the bottle, and label ready to be dispensed to the patient.

General Method for the Preparation of a Suspension Containing Precipitate Forming Liquids

1. Check the solubility in the vehicle of all solids in the mixture.

2. Calculate the quantities of vehicle required to dissolve any soluble solid.

3. Dissolve all soluble solids in the vehicle in a small glass beaker.

4. Finely powder any insoluble and mix intimately with the suspending agent (compound tragacanth powder 2 g/100 ml or as the mucilage 10–20 ml/150 ml of product) in a porcelain mortar.

5. Measure the precipitate forming liquid in a dry measure and pour into the suspension, stirring rapidly using a pestle to form a smooth paste.

6. Add further vehicle in small quantities, and continue mixing until the mixture in the mortar become of pourable consistency.

7. Transfer the contents of the mortar to a conical measure of suitable size.

8. Rinse out the mortar with more vehicles and add any rinsing to the conical measure.

9. Add remaining liquid ingredients to the mixture in the conical measure.

10. Make up to final volume with vehicle.

11. Stir gently, transfer to a suitable container, ensuring that the entire solid is transferred from the conical measure to the bottle, and label ready to be dispensed to the patient.

Type of Suspension Instability and its Trouble Shooting

Suspension instability may be either reversible or irreversible, which can be determined by measuring different stability parameters (Table 6.9).

Example 1: Paediatric chalk mixture BP	
Ingredients	Quantity
Chalk BP	20 g
Tragacanth BP	2 g
Concentrated cinnamon Water BP	4 ml
Syrup BP	100 ml
Double strength chloroform Water BP	500 ml
Potable water to	1000 ml

Method

1. Calculate the composition of a convenient quantity of double strength chloroform water BP, sufficient to satisfy the formula requirements but also enabling simple, accurate measurement of the concentrated component.

2. Weigh 200 mg tragacanth BP accurately on an electronic balance.

3. Weigh 2 g chalk BP accurately on an electronic balance.

4. Measure 10 ml syrup BP in a 10 ml conical measure.

Table 6.9: Types of suspension instability and its troubleshooting			
Stability parameters	**Range/ideal requirments**	**Comments**	**Troubleshooting**
Sedimentation volume: Sedimentation volume is the ratio of final volume of the sediment to the original volume of suspension. F = sedimentation volume $F= V_F/Vo$ V_F = Final volume of sediment Vo = Original volume of suspension	F=1 F<1 F>1	Suspension looks elegant and pharmaceutically acceptable. Indicates rapid setting of the dispersed phase. Indicates that the network of flocculation is loose and it encompasses a greater volume than original.	Not necessary Proper selection of structured vehicle depending on the charge carried by the flocculating agents, e.g. anionic electrolytes are stabilized by gums.
Dgree of flocculation: It is the ratio of the sedimentation volume of the folcculated suspention to the sedimentation volume of the suspention when deflocculated. $\beta = F/F_\infty$ β = Degree of flocculation F = Sedimentation volume of flocculated suspension. F_∞ = Sedimentation volume of the suspension.	β = less than 2 β = more than 2	Not preferable Pharmaceutically acceptable.	Controlled flocculation can be achived by the selection of suitable flocculating agent like salt of aluminum or phosphate according to the electrolytes present in suspension. Flocculation can also be controlled by proper wetting agents, e.g. sodium laurly sulfate.
Zeta potential: Zeta potential is the potential difference between diffusive layers and electrical neutral layers.	Zeta potential = + 50 mV/ -50 mV	Zeta potential from = 50 mV/-50 mV results deflocculated suspension tend to from compact cake on storage.	Zeta potential can be modified by the addition of suitable electrolyers or peptidizer.

contd...

Table 6.9: Types of suspension instability and its troubleshooting (*contd.*)

Stability parameters	Range/ideal requirments	Comments	Troubleshooting
	Zeta potential = + 10 mV/ -10 mV	Zeta potential from = 10 mV/-10 mV results flocculated suspention which can be redisperse on shaking. These types of suspension are pharmaceutically acceptable.	Zeta potential is decreased by the addition of electrolytes leads to the formation of floccules.
Stability parameters	**Range/ideal requirments**	**Comments**	**Troubleshooting**
Rheological consideration: This is an important characteristic in pharmaceutical suspension as it affects the rate of sedimentation, flow properties, stability, dispersibility, syringeability (for injectable) and spreadebility of the suspension.	Most of the pharmaceutical suspensions exhibit plastic or pseudoplastic behavior.	Rheological properties depend on the degree of flocculation and the selection of suspending agents. Suspensions exhibit plastic or pseudoplastic behavior is pharmaceutically acceptable as they tend to form gel on storage which will control rate of sedimentation. In contrast on shaking convert to solution which helps in its pourability.	Proper selection and combination of flocculating and suspending agent can improve the physical stability of suspension like setting, caking and dispersability.
Physical, chemical and biological degradation: Suspentions being liquid dosage form are susceptible for oxidation, hydrolysis and microbial contamination.	Pharmaceutical suspension should be physically, chemically and biologically stable.	Presence of water and gums makes suspension susceptible for microbial decomposition.	Presence of adequate stabilizers like antioxidants, preservatives, buffers, chelating agents, etc. can improve the stability of suspension.

5. Measure 0.4 ml concentrated cinnamon water BP using a 1 ml syringe.

6. Measure 50 ml of double strength chloroform water BP in a 50 ml conical measure.

7. Transfer the tragacanth BP to a porcelain mortar.

8. Add the chalk BP to the mortar using the 'doubling-up' technique to mix the two powders.

9. Add the syrup BP to the mortar and mix to form a smooth paste.

10. Add some of the double strength chloroform water BP to the paste and mix until pourable.

11. Transfer the contents to a 100 ml conical measure.

12. Rinse out the mortar with more double strength chloroform water BP or potable water and add the rinsing to the conical measure.

13. Add the concentrated cinnamon water BP to the mixture in the conical measure.

14. Make up to volume with any remaining double strength chloroform water BP and potable water.

15. Transfer to an amber flat medical bottle label and dispense.

Storage: Preserve in well-closed container.

Use: Antidiarrheal.

MIXTURES

Mixtures are liquid preparation containing one or more medicaments dissolved, suspended or dispersed in suitable vehicle; they are intended for oral administration. Suspended solids may slowly separate on standing but are easily redispersed. Mixtures may also be prepared by adding liquid components to granules or powder just before dispensing. The term draught has been applied to a mixture intended to be administered as a single dose. Mixtures may contain suitable antimicrobial preservatives.

Mixtures include those liquid preparations containing oleaginous, mucilaginous, albuminous, or saccharin substances, which are used internally, and cannot properly be classed with infusions, decoctions, syrups, tinctures, emulsions, etc., also pharmaceutical compounds in which insoluble substances, whether liquid or solid, are suspended in aqueous fluids.

As a rule, those preparations containing oily substances in suspension belong with emulsions, although compounds not easily classified, as will be seen below, are included under the elastic term mixture. Saturations are effervescing draughts prepared by neutralizing with a carbonate solutions of a vegetable acid, like citric and tartaric acids, the container being tightly corked to prevent the escape of carbonic acid gas.

Dilution of Mixtures

If a dose is prescribed which is less than or not a multiple of 5 ml, the mixture should be suitably diluted to achieve a dose volume that is multiple of 5 ml, using the diluents specified in the monograph in the case of mixtures supplied as granules are powder, the product should be constituted and used to prepare the dilution.

Containers, Labeling and Storage

Containers, usually glass or plastic bottles for oral liquids, hold the formulation and are in direct contact with the product. All containers must be clean before they are filled. For stability concerns, the container must not physically or chemically interact with the product so as to alter the strength, quality, or purity of the product beyond the official requirements. The manufacturer addressee all these concerns prior to the selection of a suitable container. The product is eventually shipped to pharmacies for dispensing. Frequently, the shipping container is larger than the volume needed by the patient. This necessitates repackaging into proper containers for the patient by the pharmacist. Today, we usually repackage liquids into plastic, light-resistant bottles. In all cases, the caps should be closed tightly to avoid the loss, or premature degradation, of the drug or any of the components. Table 6.10 enlists general requirements of container and labeling for liquid preparation.

Example 1: Gentian and acid mixture B.N.F (Mixture containing liquids only)	
Ingredients	**Quantity**
Dilute hydrochloric acid	0.5 ml
Concentrated compound gentian infusion	1 ml
Chloroform water double strength	5 ml
Water to	10 ml

Method

1. Pour the double strength chloroform water into 250 ml conical measure.

2. Measure the concentrated infusion in 25 ml conical measure, pour into the 250 ml

Table 6.10: A guide to containers, lables and suitability for liquid preparations				
Preparation	Container	Important labeling instruction	Protection	Performance
For external applications only	Amber fluted bottle with CRC	For external use only	L, S, M	+
Eardrop	Hexagonal amber fluted glass bottle with a rubber teat and dropper closure	For external use only	L, S, M, G	+
Elixrs	Plain amber medicine bottle with CRC	Take as directed by the physician	L, S, M	+
Emulsions	Plain amber medicine bottle with CRC	Shake before use bottle	L, S, M	+
Enemas	Amber fluted bottle with CRC	For rectal use only orally Warm to body before use	L, S, M, G	++
Gargles and mouthwashes	Amber fluted bottle with CRC	Not to be taken orally Do not swallow in large amounts	L,S,M	+
Inhalations	Amber fluted bottle with CRC	Not to be taken orally Shake the bottle	L,S,M,W,G	++
Linctures	Plain amber medicine bottle with CRC		L,S,M	+
Liniments and lotions	Amber fluted bottle with CRC	For external use only before use bottle. Avoid application on broken skin	L,S,M	+
Mixtures and suspentions	Plain amber medicine bottle with CRC	Shake before use bottle	L,S,M	+
Nasal drops	Hexagonal amber fluted glass bottle with a rubber teat and dropper closure	Not to be taken orally	L,S,M,W,G	++

Protection: L (protects from light, if approprite); **S** (protects from solvent loss/leakage); **M** (protects sterile products or those with microbial limits from microbial contamination); **W** (protects from water vapor, if appropriate); **G** (protects from reactive gases, if appropriate)

Performance: ++: Frequently a consideration, +: May be a consideration.

measure, stirring meanwhile, and rinse the small measure with water until no color left inside. It is important to stir well after every addition, since undesirable physical or chemical changes may occur, if undiluted ingredients remain in contact.

3. Measure the acid, have the volume checked, and transfer to the 250 ml measure.

4. If the preparation contains foreign particles, strain into another measure and rinse the strainer to displace absorbed solution.

5. Make up the volume with water; stir well and pour into the bottle check that the correct volume has been dispensed; and when sufficient experience has been gained, that the appearance of the product is correct.

Storage: Preserve in a well-closed container and avoid prolong exposure to excessive heat.

Use: Bitter tonic and hepatoprotective.

Example 2: Ferric ammonium citrate mixture B.N.F (Mixture containing soluble solid only)	
Ingredients	Quantity
Ferric ammonium citrate	0.5 ml
Chloroform water double strength	5 ml
Water to	10 ml

Method

1. Pour the double strength chloroform water and about 10 ml of water into 250 ml conical measure.
2. Weigh the medicament and add it, and the rinsing from the pan, to the flask. Stir until solution is complete.
3. Make almost to volume, examine critically for foreign matter and filter, if necessary. Adjust to volume through the filter.

Storage: Preserve in a well-closed container and avoid from direct sunlight.

Use: Iron supplements in anemia.

Example 3: Strong sodium salicylate mixture B.P.C (Mixture containing diffusible solid only)	
Ingredients	Quantity
Sodium salicylate	100 g
Sodium metabisulfite	1 g
Peppermint emulsion, concentrated	25 ml
Chloroform water double strength	500 ml
Water, to	1000 ml

Method: Dissolve the solids as for the previous exercise but weigh the sodium salicylate first because it will take longer to dissolve than the much smaller amount of sodium metasulfite; their solubilities are not very different.

1. Peppermint emulsion tends to separate on storage and should be shaken thoroughly before measurement.
2. Rinse the measure well and adjust the mixture to volume with water.

Storage: Preserve in an airtight container and place in a cool and dry place.

Use: Antiphlogistic

Example 4: Magnesium hydroxide mixture (Mixture containing diffusible solid only)	
Ingredients	Quantity
Magnesium sulfate	47.5 g
Sodium hydroxide	15 g
Light magnesium oxide	52.5 g
Chloroform	2.5 ml
Water, freshly boiled and cooled sufficient to produce	1000 ml

Method

1. Dissolve the sodium hydroxide in 150 ml of purified water, add the light magnesium oxide, mix to form a smooth cream, then add sufficient purified water to produce 2500 ml.
2. Pour this suspension in a thin stream into a solution of magnesium sulfate in 2500 ml of purified water, stirring continuously during the mixing.
3. Allow the precipitate to subside, remove the clear liquid, transfer the residue to a calico strainer, allow to drain and wash the precipitate with purified water until the washings give only a slight reaction for sulfates.
4. Mix the washed precipitate with purified water, dissolve the chloroform in the mixture, add sufficient purified water to produce 1000 ml.

Storage: Magnesium hydroxide mixture should not be kept in a cold place.

Use: As an antacid, 5 to 10 ml repeated in accordance with the needs of the patient. As a laxative, 25 to 50 ml.

Example 5: Aromatic chalk with opium mixture (Mixture containing in-diffusible solid only)	
Ingredients	**Quantity**
Chalk	32.5 g
Sucrose	65 g
Opium tincture	50 ml
Compound ammonium solution	50 ml
Compound cardamom tincture	100 ml
Catechu tincture	50 ml

Example 5: Aromatic chalk with opium mixture (Mixture containing in-diffusible solid only) (contd.)	
Ingredients	**Quantity**
Powdered tragacanth	2 g
Double strength chloroform water	500 ml
Water, freshly boiled and cooled sufficient to produce	1000 ml

It should be prepared as per the above direction.

Storage: Stored in well-filled, tight containers.

Usual dose range for an adult, 10 to 20 ml. For a child, under one year, 1 ml; one to five years, 2 to 5 ml. Used in hypocalcemia.

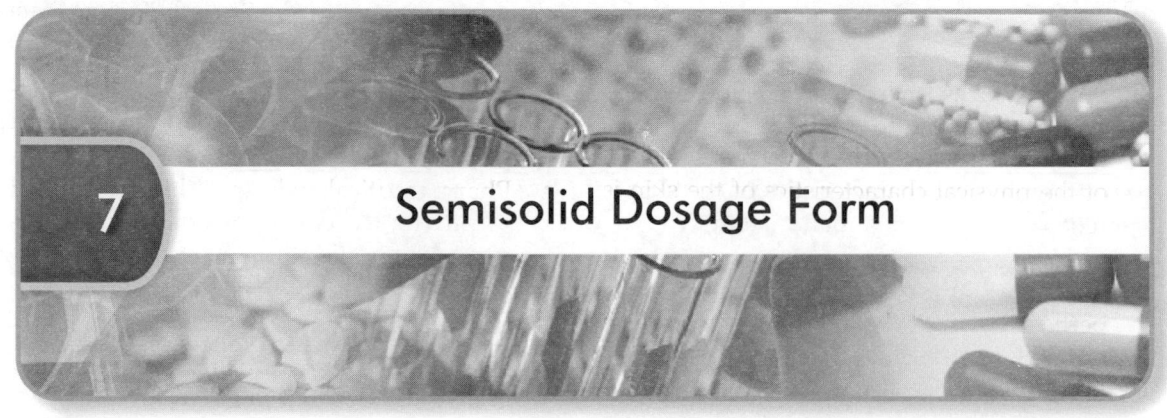

7   Semisolid Dosage Form

INTRODUCTION

Semisolids constitute a significant proportion of pharmaceutical dosage forms. They serve as carriers for drugs that are topically delivered through skin, cornea, rectal tissue, nasal mucosa, vagina, buccal tissue, urethral membrane, and external ear lining. Because of their specific rheological behavior, semisolids can adhere to the application surface for sufficiently long periods before they are washed off. This property helps prolong drug delivery at the application site. A semisolid dosage form is advantageous in terms of its easy application, rapid formulation, and ability to topically deliver a wide variety of drugmolecules.

ADVANTAGES AND DISADVANTAGES OF SEMISOLID PREPARATIONS

Advantages

- Pharmaceutical ointments may be easily spread on skin, being retained at the site of application as an occlusive layer, thereby preventing moisture loss from the skin. This is particularly useful whenever restoration of the physical characteristics of the skin is required (e.g. due to inflammation).

- Pharmaceutical ointments are associated with lubricating/emollient properties, properties that may be employed to reduce trauma of an affected site upon spreading.
- In general, pharmaceutical ointments persist at the site of application, enabling the duration of drug release to be greater than for many other topical dosage forms. The increased viscosity of pharmaceutical pastes ensures that a thick film of the dosage form is applied to the site of action, which shows excellent persistence. This property is particularly useful, if protection of an inflamed site is required, e.g. in eczema, psoriasis.
- The hydrophobicity and retention of pharmaceutical ointments are useful attributes whenever applied to mucosa, e.g. inflamed hemorrhoids, eyelids, where fluid flow/inflammation at these sites would normally serve to remove formulations (e.g. oil in water creams) by dilution.
- Due to the high solid contents, pharmaceutical pastes are often porous, allowing moisture loss from the applied site. Furthermore, pastes may act to absorb moisture and chemicals within the exudates.
- The opaque nature of pastes (due to the high solid contents) enables this formulation to be used as a sunblock.
- The chemical stability of therapeutic agents that are prone to hydrolysis will be dramatically enhanced by formulation within pharmaceutical ointments and pastes.
- Pharmaceutical gels may be formulated to provide excellent spreading properties and will provide a cooling effect due to solvent evaporation.

Disadvantages

- Pharmaceutical ointments are generally greasy and difficult to remove.
- Pharmaceutical pastes are generally applied as a thick layer at the required site and are therefore, considered to be cosmetically unacceptable.
- Staining of clothes is often associated with the use of pharmaceutical pastes and ointments.
- The viscosity of pharmaceutical ointments, and in particular pastes, may be problematic in ensuring spreading of the dosage form over the affected site.
- Pharmaceutical ointments may not be applied to exuding sites.
- Problems concerning drug release from pharmaceutical ointments may occur, if the drug has limited solubility in the ointment base.
- Pharmaceutical pastes are generally not applied to the hair due to difficulties associated with removal.
- Therapeutic agents that are prone to hydrolysis should not be formulated into aqueous gel.

Table 7.1. enlists the ideal properties of semisolid dosage form.

Table 7.1: Ideal properties of topical semisolid products	
Characteristics	Description
Physicochemical stability	No or little reversible change in properties such as color, odor, appearance, pH, and viscosity over the shelf-life of the product.
Chemical stability	Loss of potency with time should be within specified limits over the shelf-life of the product.

contd...

Table 7.1: Ideal properties of topical semisolid products (*contd.*)	
Microbiological stability	The product (including container-closure) should be within microbiological limits over the shelf-life of the product.
Aesthetic	The product (including container-closure) should be aesthetically appealing to the user, compatible with skin, and easy to apply and remove from the skin.
Skin toxicity	The product should not elicit any irritation or sensitization to the skin.
User-friendly	The product should be user-friendly and tamperproof.
Manufacturing/scale-up	The formulation and manufacturing should be simple and easy to scale-up from laboratory to large scale production.

CLASSIFICATION OF SEMISOLID DOSAGE FORM

Semisolid dosage forms include ointments, paste, gels, creams, plasters and poultices. Table 7.2 includes various types of semisolid dosage forms.

COMMONLY USED CATEGORIES AND USES OF TOPICAL PREPARATIONS

The major classes of agents that are delivered topically and act by chemical action include corticosteroids, antifungals, acne products, antibiotics, emollients, antiseptics, local anes-

Table 7.2: Classification of semisolid dosage forms		
Types	**Product illustration**	**Description**
Ointments	Ointments	Ointments are semisolid preparations usually consisting of solution or dispersion of one or more medicaments in suitable non-aqueous bases and are formulated so that the preparation is essentially immiscible with the skin secretion. They are used as emollients and intended to apply medicaments to the skin for protective, therapeutic purposes where a degree of occlusion is desired. They may contain suitable antimicrobial preservatives.
Creams	Creams	Creams are semisolid dosage forms containing one or more drug substances dissolved or dispersed in a suitable base. Creams are fluid compared to other semisolid dosage forms such as ointments and pastes, as the bases used in creams are generally oil-in-water emulsions. Occasionally, water-in-oil emulsions are also employed in the formulation of creams such as cold cream.
Pastes	Pastes	Pastes are defined as semisolid dosage forms that contain one or more drug substances intended for topical application. They differ from ointments in their consistency, as they contain larger amount of solids and consequently are thicker and stiffer. They can be made either of fatty bases, such as petrolatum and hydrophilic petrolatum or aqueous gels, such as celluloses. Pastes are well adsorbed into skin and absorb watery solutions, so that they can be used around oozing lesions. Pastes can be easily removed from skin, which is an important consideration when they are applied on traumatized skin.

contd...

Table 7.2: Classification of semisolid dosage forms (*contd.*)

Types	Product illustration	Description
Gels	Gel	Gels are semisolid systems containing either a suspension of small inorganic particles or large organic molecule. Gels can exist as a single phase system in which large organic molecules are dispersed in a liquid without any clear boundaries (e.g. carbomer or tragacanth in water) or as a two-phase system in which small particles are suspended in a liquid (e.g. aluminum hydroxide gel).
Poultices	Use of poultices	Poultices consist of a hydrophilic heat-retentive systems in which solid or liquid active substances are dispersed. They are usually spread thickly on a suitable dressing and heated before application to the skin.

thetics, and antineoplastic agents, in that order. Topical agents are used as protectives, adsorbents, emollients, and cleansing agents and act primarily through physical action.

The following is a brief explanation of each of these categories of drugs used in semisolid preparation with examples.

- **Protectives:** Shield exposed to skin surface and other membranes from harmful stimuli.
- **Absorbents:** Absorb moisture from skin and local wounds and thereby maintain dry conditions to discourage bacterial growth.
- **Demulcents:** Can alleviate irritation of mucous membranes or abraded tissues.
- **Emollients:** Fat or oily substances used to increase the moisture content of skin and other membranes and render them soft shiny and pliable.
- **Astringents:** Arrest blood hemorrhage by coagulating blood. These agents help wounds and cuts heal quickly.
- **Counter irritants:** Used to promote a secondary irritation that helps to counter an initial irritation.
- **Rubefacients:** Increase the skin temperature by increasing the circulation at the surface.

- **Caustics:** Destroy skin at the applied site (corrosive). They are useful in the treatment of warts, keratoses, and hyperplastic tissues.
- **Keratolytics:** Cause desquamation (peeling) of skin. These agents are useful in the treatment of eczema, acne, etc.

PERCUTANEOUS DRUG ABSORPTION

Semisolid dosage forms for dermatological drug therapy are intended to produce desired therapeutic action at specific sites in the epidermal tissue. A drug's ability to penetrate the skin's epidermis, dermis, and subcutaneous fat layers depends on the properties of the drug and the carrier base. Although some drugs are meant primarily for surface action on the skin, the target area for most dermatological disorders lies in the viable epidermis or upper dermis. Hence, a drug's diffusive penetration of the skin, percutaneous absorption, is an important aspect of drug therapy. The main portals of drug entry into the skin are the follicular region, the sweat ducts, or the unbroken stratum corneum between these appendages. A substance's particular route mainly depends on the physicochemical properties of the drug and the condition of the skin.

Factors Affecting the Drug Absorption

The factors that influence skin penetration are:

- **The physicochemical property of drug and the vehicle:** The release of drug from a vehicle and penetration to skin depend on the physiochemical activity of drug.

- **pH of the formulation**: pH of the formulation determine the degree of ionization of drug, as we know non-ionic drug absorbs better than ionized specis.

- **Hydration state of stratum corneum:** Increased water concentration in the skin layer apparently enhances the penetration of the steroid.

- **The temperature of skin and the concentration of the drug:** The rate of drug absorption directly proportional to the concentration of drugs at the site of administration and the temperature at the site of application.

- **The solubility of the drug:** The water or lipid partition coefficient influences the rate of transport. Lipid soluble drugs absorb better than water soluble drugs.

- **Molecular weight of drug**: Small molecules penetrate more rapidly than large molecules.

- **Viscosity of vehicle**: The rate of drug release from the base directly related to the viscosity of formulation.

- **Presence of penetration enhancer or surfactant**: Presence of surfactant or penetration enhancer like oleic acid improve the rate of drug absorption.

GENERAL LABELING REQUIREMENTS OF SEMISOLID DOSAGE FORM

The following requirements are applicable to medicines manufactured or prepared in accordance with medicines legislation. They are not intended to apply to repackaging. These critical information, which should be located together on the pack and appear in the same field of view, are: name, strength, route of administration, dosage and warnings. The label must contain following details.

- The common name of the product.
- Quantitative particulars are not required, as the product is official.
- 'For external use only' will need to be added to the label as the product is an ointment or other semisolid form for external use.
- The contents of the container by weight, volume or by number of doses.
- Directions to patient where necessary 'Apply as directed.'
- Keep out of reach and sight of children.
- The expiry date expressed in unambiguous terms.
- Any special storage precautions.
- The manufacturer's ML number, where appropriate.
- The manufacturer's name and address.
- The batch number.
- Statutory warnings required for particular actives.
- Date of expiry.

PREPARATION OF TOPICAL DOSAGE FORMS

Topical dosage forms generally contain the following ingredients:

- Base or body of the dosage form
- Medicinal agent (not always the case)
- Preservative and other additives.

However, the composition may vary slightly from one dosage form to another. The general methods of preparation of ointment will be described in the following section.

OINTMENTS

Ointments are semisolid preparations usually consisting of solution or dispersion of one or more medicaments in suitable non-aqueous bases. They are used as emollients and intended to apply medicaments to the skin for protective and therapeutic purposes. They have less solid contents than paste.

The objective of the ointment preparation and manufacturing process is to uniformly distribute the medicinal agent in an ointment base. The type of preparation or manufacturing method depends upon the type of base and the quantity of preparation. There are four different types of ointment bases and bases for other semisolid dosage forms, enlisted in Table 7.3.

Table 7.3: Types of bases for semisolid preparations			
Bases Ointment	**Comments**	**Characteristics**	**Examples**
Hydrocarbon bases	Hydrocarbon bases are also called oleaginous bases and contain petrolatum and/or modi-fied petrolatum waxes or paraffin oil to lower viscosity	Excellent retention on the skin-predominantly hydrophobic, and therefore difficult to remove from the skin by washing and difficult to apply to (spread over) wet surfaces (e.g. mucous membranes, wet skin) Only a low concentration (5%) of water may be incorporated into hydrocarbon bases (with careful mixing). Chemically inert Emollient and occlusive properties.	Hard paraffin; white/ yellow soft paraffin; liquid paraffin (mineral oil); and microcrystalline wax.
Absorption bases	These are hydrophilic anhydrous materials that form water-in-oil emulsions or hydrous bases that are already water-in-oil emulsions.	That can absorb additional quantities of water. Absorption bases are less greasy than hydrocarbon bases but offer emollient and occlusive properties.	Lanolin (wool fat); lanolin; alcohols (wool alcohols); and beeswax (white or yellow).
Water-miscible/ removable bases	These are water-miscible bases that are used to form oil in water emulsions for topical applications. They are able to accommodate large volumes of water, e.g. aqueous solutions of drug, excess moisture at the site of application, e.g. exudate from abrasions and wounds.	They are not occlusive. They may be easily washed from the skin and from clothing. Furthermore, they may be readily applied to (and removed from) hair. They are aesthetically pleasing.	Emulsifying ointment, cetrimide emulsifying ointment cetomacrogol emulsifying ointment (liquid paraffin 20% w/w; white soft paraffin 50% w/w; anionic, cationic or non-ionic emulsifying wax 30% w/w.).
Water-soluble bases	Water-soluble bases are composed entirely of water-soluble ingredients.	They are non-greasy and may be easily removed by washing. They are miscible with exudates from inflamed sites. They are generally compatible with the vast majority of therapeutic agents.	Blends of 60% w/w polyethylene glycol 400 (a liquid) and 40% w/w polyethylene glycol 4000 (a solid).

contd...

Table 7.3: Types of bases for semisolid preparations (*contd.*)

Bases	Comments	Characteristics	Examples
Paste			
Hydrocarbon bases	As discussed in ointment	As discussed in ointment	As discussed in ointment
Water soluble bases	As discussed in ointment	As discussed in ointment	As discussed in ointment
Water miscible base	As discussed in ointment	As discussed in ointment	As discussed in ointment
Cream			
Fatty bases	As discussed in ointment	As discussed in ointment	Hydrocarbon, hydrocarbon waxes, oleaginous substances and fatty bases.
Anionic emulsifier	Produce o/w emulsion	Water soluble, non-greasy	Sodium lauryl sulfate, various alkali soaps.
Cationic emulsifier	Produce o/w emulsion	Water soluble, non-greasy	Quaternary ammonium compound, benzalkonium chloride, benzethonium chloride, etc.
Non-ionic emulsifier	Produce o/w emulsion	Water soluble, non-greasy	Tween and span
Gels			
Natural and semisynthetic	2–3% produce desired gelling consistency.	Water miscible	Tragacanth, sodium alginate, pectin, starch and cellulose derivatives.
Synthetic	1–2% concentration produce desired consistency.	Water miscible and dry very quickly.	Polyvinyl alcohol.

Excipients Used in the Formulation of Semisolid Preparation

Other excipients may be included in ointments and pastes, including: (1) additional solvents, (2) preservatives, (3) antioxidants.

Additional Solvents

These are hydrophobic liquid components that may be added to ointment bases (predominantly hydrophobic or absorption bases). Examples of these include: (1) liquid silicone; (2) vegetable oils; and (3) organic esters.

Preservatives

Topically applied ointments and pastes are not sterile products; however, they are manufactured under clean conditions to minimise the microbial bioburden within the formulated product. Ointments/pastes that do not contain water, usually not require the addition of a preservative. However, if the product contains water, then a preservative will be required. Preservatives that may be used in formulations for external use include— phenol (0.2–0.5%), chlorocresol (0.075–0.12%), benzoic acid and salts (0.1–0.3%), methyl-parabens (methylparahydroxybenzoic acid) (0.02–0.3%), propylparabens (methylparahy-droxybenzoic acid) (0.02–0.3%) (and their mixtures) and benzyl alcohol (3.0%).

Antioxidants

In pharmaceutical ointments, antioxidants are used to prevent oxidative degradation. The types of antioxidants used for this pur-pose include—lipophilic antioxidants butyl-ated hydroxyanisole (0.005–0.02%), butylated hydroxytoluene (0.007–0.1%), propyl gallate (1%), hydrofilic antioxidants, e.g. sodium metabisulfate (0.01–0.1%) and sodium sulfite (0.1%).

General Method for Ointment Preparation

Once the appropriate base is selected, oint-ments are prepared by one of the following processes.

Incorporation by Lavigation

- The finely divided powdered drug material is lavigated thoroughly with a small quantity of base to produce a desired mass.
- The mass then is diluted geometrically with the remainder of the base.
- If the drug is water soluble, it can be dis-solved in water and the resulting solution incorporated into the vehicle using a small quantity of lanolin.
- Preparation of small quantities of oint-ments can be performed by mixing the dif-ferent components using a spatula on an ointment slab.
- On an industrial scale, ointment can be produced in a single batch. To mix such large quantities, commercial mixers such as hobart mixers and pony mixers are employed.

The incorporation of powders into an ointment base:

- Soluble solids should be added to the molten fatty bases at the lowest possible

temperature and the mixture stirred until cold.
- Insoluble solids should be incorporated using a glass tile and spatula. If there is more than one powder to be added, these should be mixed in a mortar using the 'doubling up' method.

The incorporation of liquids into an ointment base:

- Non-volatile, miscible liquids may be mixed with the molten fat in the evaporat-ing basin.
- Volatile or immiscible liquids, e.g. coal tar solutions, should be triturated with the ointment on the glass tile. A very small amount of the ointment should be placed on the glass tile and a 'well' made in the center. Then add small quantities of the liquid and fold into the base gently. If using coal tar or other volatile ingredients, these should not be weighed until immediately before use and the beaker in which it has been weighed should be covered with a watch glass to prevent evaporation.

Fusion

In the fusion method, the oil phase ingredients are combined and heated to about 75° C.

- In a separate beaker, the aqueous phase ingredients including emulsifier, are hea-ted together to slightly above 75°C.
- The aqueous phase then is added to the oil phase, slowly and with constant agitation.
- When the emulsion is formed, the mixture is allowed to cool, maintaining slow agita-tion.
- Ointments containing beeswax, paraffin, stearyl alcohol, and high molecular weight polyethylene glycols do not blend into solid state, and they need to be melted to mix uniformly.
- While preparing such ointments, generally the one with the lower melting point is melted first and the rest of the components

are added in the order of increasing melting points. In doing so, the first melted component exerts solvent action on the subsequent components, making them melt at a lower temperature.

Containers: Ointments should be supplied in a suitable containers fitted with a closure which minimizes contamination with microorganisms.

Filling: The tube filling, crimping and coding machine is simple in operation. It consists of an aluminum-rotating disc with interchangeable tube holding sockets for different tube sizes. The filling station is made of SS block, fitted with pneumatic device to control tailing (Fig. 7.1).

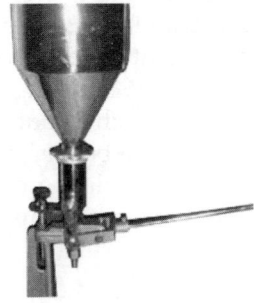

Fig. 7.1: Manual ointment filling and crimping machine

Storage: Ointments should be stored at a temperature not exceeding 25°C.

Labeling: Comply with the general requirements for labeling Fig. 7.2.

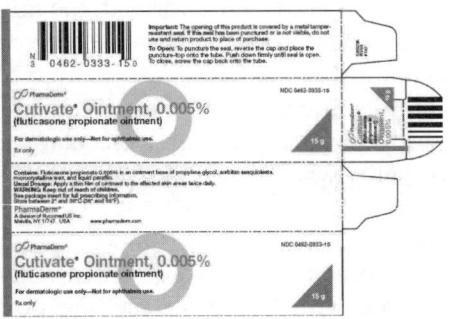

Fig. 7.2: Label of a marketed ointment

Example 1: Paraffin ointment BPC	
Ingredient	**Quantity**
Soft paraffin	50 gm

Method

1. Place an ointment pot on the water bath to warm.
2. Grate the solid ingredients and transfer the required amounts to an evaporating pan.
3. Weigh the soft paraffin on a counterbalance sheet of greaseproof paper; place paper and contents on an ointment tile, so that spillage is easily recovered and remove the paraffin to the basin with a large spatula, taking care to leave the paper virtually clean, an aim that is more easily achieved if the paper is scrapped on a hard surface, rather than from the hand.
4. Place the basin on a water bath, after removing as many rings as the size of the dish will allow and stir to expedite melting and ensure homogeneous admixture.
5. Examine the mixture for foreign matter and decant or strain, if necessary.
6. Pour into the pot; cover loosely with the lid, place on an asbestos pad and leave to set.

Storage: Storing in an airtight or plain amber jar would be most suitable.

Use: Hydrocarbon ointment base.

Example 2: Adsorption ointment base	
Ingredient	**Quantity**
Yellow soft paraffin	50 gm

Method

1. Place an ointment pot on the water bath to warm.
2. Grate the solid ingredients and transfer the required amounts to an evaporating pan.
3. Weigh the soft paraffin on a counter-balance sheet of greaseproof paper; place

paper and contents on an ointment tile, so that spillage is easily recovered and remove the paraffin to the basin with a large spatula, taking care to leave the paper virtually clean, an aim that is more easily achieved, if the paper is scrapped on a hard surface, rather than from the hand.

4. Place the basin on a water bath, after removing as many rings as the size of the dish will allow and stir to expedite melting and ensure homogeneous admixture.

5. Examine the mixture for foreign matter and decant or strain if necessary.

6. Pour into the pot; cover loosely with the lid, place on an asbestos pad and leave to set.

7. If the surface of the wool fat is discolored scrape off the discolored part and use the material below.

Storage: Storing in an airtight or plain amber jar would be most suitable.

Use: Adsorption ointment base.

Example 3: Zinc and castor oil ointment	
Ingredients	Quantity
Zinc oxide finely divided	15 gm
Castor oil	40 ml
Cetosteryl alcohol	25 gm
White beeswax	50 gm
Arachis oil	35 ml

Method

1. Melt together the beeswax, cetosteryl alcohol and arachis oil. Warm the castor oil in a separate dish.

2. Using a warm tile and spatula, levigate the shifted zinc oxide with a suitable quantity of oil until smooth.

3. Transfer the suspension to the dish containing the melted ingredients taking care to leave virtually no materials on the tile. Mix well, add the rest of the castor oil and stir until cold.

Storage: Stored in an airtight or plain amber jar would be most suitable.

Use: Astringent.

Example 4: Whitfield's ointment	
Ingredients	Quantity
Salicyclic acid, in fine powdered	30 g
Benzoic acid, in fine powdered	60 g
Emulsifying ointment	910 g

Method: Triturate the salicylic acid and benzoic acid with a portion of the melted emulsifying ointment until smooth, gradually incorporate the remainder of the melted emulsifying ointment and stir until cold.

Storage: Stored in an airtight or collapsible jar.

Use: Keratolytic.

Example 5: Calamine ointment	
Ingredients	Quantity
Calamine, finely sifted	150 g
White soft paraffin	850 g

Method: Triturate the calamine with part of white soft paraffin until smooth and gradually incorporate the remainder of the white soft paraffin.

Storage: Stored in an airtight or collapsible jar.

Use: Protective.

Example 6: Compound calamine ointment	
Ingredients	Quantity
Calamine, finely sifted	125 g
Zinc oxide, finely sifted	125 g
Strong coal tar solution	25 g
Hydrous wool fat	250 g
White soft paraffin	475 g

Method: Melt together the hydrous wool fat and the white soft paraffin, incorporate the calamine, the zinc oxide and the strong coal tar solution; stir gently until cold.

Storage: Stored in an airtight collapsible jar.

Use: Protective.

Example 7: Cetrimide emulsifying ointment	
Ingredients	Quantity
White soft paraffin	500 g
Cetostearyl alcohol	270 g
Liquid paraffin	200 g
Cetrimide	30 g

Method: Mix together the white soft paraffin, cetostearyl alcohol and liquid paraffin add the cetrimide and stir until cold.

Storage: Stored in an airtight or collapsible jar.

Use: Ointment base.

Example 8: Ichthammol ointment	
Ingredients	Quantity
Ichthammol	100 g
Wool fat	450 g
Yellow soft paraffin	450 g

Method: Melt together the wool fat and the yellow soft paraffin, incorporate the ichthammol and stir until cold.

Storage: Stored in an airtight or collapsible jar.

Use: Minor skin injuries.

Example 9: Macrogol ointment	
Ingredients	Quantity
Macrogol 4000	350 g
Macrogol 300	650 g

Method: Add the macrogol 4000 to the macrogol 300, warm until homogeneous and stir continuously until cold.

Storage: Stored in an airtight collapsible jar or in a wide mouth container.

Use: Water soluble ointment base.

Example 10: Coal tar and salicyclic acid ointment	
Ingredients	Quantity
Coal tar	20 g
Polysorbate 80	40 g
Salicyclic acid	20 g
Emulsifying wax	114 g
White soft paraffin	190 g
Coconut oil	540 g
Liquid paraffin	76 g

Method: Disperse the coal tar in polysorbate 80, incorporate the salicylic acid and mix with the previously melted emulsifying wax. Separately, melt the white soft paraffin and the coconut oil, incorporate the liquid paraffin warmed to same temperature and add with stirring the resulting solution to the coal tar dispersion, mix thoroughly and stir until cold.

Storage: Stored in an airtight container.

Use: Anti-psoriasis.

Example 11: Benzylpenicillin ointment (IP, 1966)	
Ingredients	Quantity
Benzylpenicillin	A sufficient quantity
Liquid paraffin	10 g
Wool fat	10 g
Yellow soft paraffin	80 g

Method

1. Heat together the wool fat, the yellow soft paraffin and the liquid paraffin.
2. Filter while hot through a coarse filter paper placed in a heated funnel.
3. Sterilize by heating for sufficient time to ensure that the entire matter is at 160°C for at least one hour.
4. Allow to cool at room temperature.

5. Add the benzylpenicillin and triturate the mixture.

Storage: Stored in an airtight container and in a dry and cool place.

Use: Antibacterial.

PASTES

Pastes are semisolid preparation usually containing one or more medicaments in suitable bases. They usually contain a high proportion of solids.

Advantages and Disadvantages of Paste

Advantages

- When applied to the skin, they adhere well, forming a thick coat that protects and smooths inflamed surface.
- They are comparatively easy to apply to the diseased areas whereas ointments are suitable for healthy skin.
- They are emollient due to high solid content.
- Addition of powder help in the absorption of exudates for wounded area.
- Pastes with hydrocarbon base are less macerating than ointments.
- Pastes should be supplied in suitable tubes of metal or plastics or in glass or other suitable containers which prevent the evaporation of any volatile ingredient.
- They are less greasy than ointments.

Disadvantages

- Pastes are not suitable for treating scalp conditions because they are difficult to remove from the hair.
- Due to high solid contents, require cautionary appication to open wounds.
- Pastes are not suitable for ophthalmic preparation due to their high solid content.
- Pastes are generally very thick and stiff, limits the rate of drug absorption and they are difficult to remove from the application site.

Bases Used for Pastes

Hydrocarbon, water soluble and water miscible bases are generally used for the preparation of pastes. Table 7.3 includes the properties and types of bases used for the preparation of pastes.

Method of Preparation of Pastes

Pastes are prepared by trituration and fusion methods just like in ointments.

Trituration

In trituration, the different components are mixed together using a spatula on an ointment slab with the help of ointment spatula until a homogeneous product is formed. Add remaining quantity of base until the medicament is uniformly mixed with it.

Fusion

In the fusion method, all the components that can be melted are combined and melted together, and components that cannot be melted are added to the molten mixture while cooling and congealing. The heat-labile and volatile components are mixed toward the end of the preparation. Vigorous stirring should be avoided to obstruct the entrapment of air in the final mass.

Labeling: Comply with the general requirement for labelling

Example 1: Zinc paste BP	
Ingredients	Quantity
Zinc oxide finely divided	150 gm
Starch	50 gm
White soft paraffin	750 gm

Method

1. Melt the base with minimum of heat and sift the powder through separate no. 180 sieves.
2. Using a warm tile and spatula, triturate the shifted zinc oxide with a suitable quantity of base until smooth.

3. The paste is much easier to manipulate in a warm mortar. Pack in a jar. Paste with a semisolid base is often too viscous for easy extrusion from a tube.

Storage: Stored in an airtight container and in a cool place.

Use: Astrigent.

Example 2: Baltimore paste	
Ingredients	Quantity
Aluminum powder	200 g
Zinc oxide	400 g
Liquid paraffin	400 g

Method: Mix the aluminium powder and the zinc oxide with the liquid paraffin until smooth.

Storage: Stored in an airtight container and in a cool place.

Use: Astringent.

Example 3: Dithranol paste	
Ingredients	Quantity
Dithranol or	1 g
Sufficient quantity zinc and salicyclic acid paste	1000 g

Method: Mix the dithranol with a portion of the zinc and salicyclic acid, paste until a smooth even dispersion is obtained and gradually incorporate the remainder of the zinc and salicyclic acid paste.

Storage: Store in an airtight container and in a cool place and the pastes should be protected from light.

Use: Antipsoriatic.

CREAMS

Creams are viscous or semisolid preparations consisting of the solutions or dispersions of one or more medicaments in suitable bases and are formulated so that the preparation is essentially miscible with the skin secretion.

They are used to apply medicaments to the skin for protective, therapeutic or prophylactic purposes especially where occlusive effects not necessary. Creams may contain suitable added antimicrobial preservatives unless the medicaments or basis have sufficient intrinsic bactericidal and fungicidal activities.

Advantages and Disadvantages of Creams

Advantages

- When applied to the skin, they produce emollient and soothing effect.
- Creams are less viscous and easily spread on to the skin.
- They are comparatively less viscous than ointments and pastes, hence more compatible with skin physiology.
- Addition of emulsifier, improve the drug penetration.

Disadvantages

- Creams are not suitable to produce prolong action as they are less viscous and easily washable.
- Due to high moisture content, they require additional preservative for their stability.
- Creams are not suitable for open wounds due to their high surfactant content and are non-sterile.
- Water content of cream limits the compounding of drugs susceptible to hydrolysis.

Ideal Properties of Creams

- They should be stable and have a good appearance.
- They should melt or soften on application to the skin.
- They should spread easily.
- A light emollient film should remain on the skin.
- They should be non-irritant.
- After evaporation of water, the cream residue should not become viscous.

General Method of Preparation

1. All ingredients can be divided into oil phase and aqueous phase.

2. Ingredients of oil phase should be taken in increasing order of their melting point. The material with least melting point should be taken last.

3. Take separately the ingredients of aqueous phase, mix them and heat to the same temperature as oil phase.

4. Mix the two phases with continuous stirring until a smooth cream is formed.

5. Perfume should be added after the primary cream.

Dilution of Creams

Care should be taken in diluting the creams, particularly to prevent microbial contamination. The appropriate diluents should be used and heating should be avoided during mixing. Excessive dilution may affect the stability of some creams. Diluted creams should be used within two weeks of their preparation.

Containers

Creams should be supplied in suitable containers fitted with a closure which minimizes contamination with microorganisms and evaporation while the product is not in use. When issued for use, creams should be supplied in suitable collapsible tubes, wherever practicable.

Storage

Creams should be stored at a temperature not exceeding 25°C unless otherwise authorized. They should not be allowed to freeze.

Labeling

Comply with the general requirements for labeling; in addition on the container states: (1) the date after which the preparation is not intended to be used; (2) the conditions under which it should be stored.

Example 1: Aqueous cream	
Ingredients	Quantity
Emulsifying ointment	300 g
Chlorocresol	1 g
Purified water freshly boiled and cooled	699 g

Method

1. Dissolve the chlorocresol in the purified water with the aid of gentle heat. Melt the emulsifying ointment, add the solution of chlorocresol while still warm, and stir gently until cold.

2. If another antimicrobial preservative replaces chlorocresol in this formulation, the suitability of the cream as diluents should be confirmed before use.

Storage: Stored in an airtight container and they should not be allowed to freeze.

Use: Pharmaceutical aid.

Example 2: Buffered cream	
Ingredients	Quantity
Emulsifying ointment	300 g
Sodium phosphate	25 g
Citric acid monohydrate	5 g
Cholocresol	1 g
Purified water, freshly boiled and cooled	669 g

Method

1. Melt the emulsifying ointment with the aid of gentle heat.

2. Separately, dissolve the sodium phosphate, the citric acid monohydrate and the chlorocresol in the purified water, previously warmed to the same temperature.

3. Mix, and stir gently until cold. If another antimicrobial preservative replaces chlorocresol in this formulation, the suitability of the cream as diluents should be confirmed before use.

Storage: Stored in an airtight container and they should not be allowed to freeze.

Use: Pharmaceutical aid.

Example 3: Aqueous calamine cream	
Ingredients	**Quantity**
Calamine	40 g
Zinc oxide	30 g
Arachis oil	300 g
Emulsifying oil	60 g
Purified water, freshly boiled and cooled	570 g

Method

1. Warm the arachis oil.
2. Dissolve the emulsifying wax in it with the aid of gentle heat.
3. Add 400 g of purified water at the same temperature and stir until cold.
4. Triturate the calamine and the zinc oxide with the remainder of the purified water and incorporate in the cream.

Storage: Stored in an airtight container and they should not be allowed to freeze.

Use: Protective.

Example 4: Cetomacrogol cream	
Ingredients	**Quantity**
Cetomacrogol emulsifying ointment	300 g
Chlorocresol	1 g
Purified water freshly boiled and cooled to produce	1000 g

Method: Melt the emulsifying ointment. Dissolve the preservative in 650 ml of purified water. Mix the solution with the melted ointment at not more than 65°C and add sufficient purified water to produce 1000 g. Mix and stir gently until cool. Cetomacrogol cream should be recently prepared. If another antimicrobial preservative replace those given above in these formulations, the suitability of the cream as diluents should be confirmed before use.

Storage: Stored in an airtight container and they should not be allowed to freeze.

Use: Water soluble ointment base.

Example 5: Cetrimide cream	
Ingredients	**Quantity**
Cetrimide	5 g
Cetostearyl alcohol	50 g
Liquid paraffin	500 g
Purified water, freshly boiled and cooled to produce	1000 g

Method: Dissolve the cetostearyl alcohol in the liquid paraffin with the aid of gentle heat. Dissolve the cetrimide in the purified water at the same temperature and add to the warm oily phase. Stir gently until cold.

Storage: Stored in an airtight container and they should not be allowed to freeze.

Use: Antimicrobial.

Example 6: Chlorhexidine cream	
Ingredients	**Quantity**
Chlorhexidine	Sufficient quantity
Liquid paraffin	100 g
Cetomacrogol emulsifying wax	250 g
Purified water, freshly boiled and cooled to produce	1000 g

Method: Dissolve the cetomacrogol emulsifying wax in the liquid paraffin at 60°C and add, with rapid stirring to the chlorhexidine gluconate solution previously diluted to 500 ml with the purified water at the same temperature. Cool, add sufficient purified water to produce the required weight and mix. Stir gently until cold.

Storage: Stored in an airtight container and they should not be allowed to freeze.

Use: Antimicrobial.

Example 7: Clioquinol cream	
Ingredients	Quantity
Clioquinol in very fine powder	30 g
Cetomacrogol emulsifying cream	300 g
Chlorocresol	1 g
Purified water, freshly boiled and cooled to produce	669 g

Method: Dissolve the chlorocresol in the purified water with the aid of gentle heat. Melt the cetomacrogol emulsifying ointment on a water bath, add the chlorocresol solution at the same temperature, stir under cold, and incorporate the clioquinol. Clioquinol cream may be prepared using any other suitable basis.

Containers: When collapsible tubes are used, they should preferably be made of plastics. If made of aluminium, the inner surface of the tubes should be lacquered.

Storage: Clioquinol cream should be protected from light.

Use: Treating skin inflammation and itching due to certain skin conditions, including eczema.

Example 8: Gamma benzene hexachloride cream	
Ingredients	Quantity
Gamma benzene hexachloride	10 g
Liquid paraffin	80 g
Cetomacrogol emulsifying wax	140 g
Purified water, freshly boiled and cooled to produce	1000 g

Method: Dissolve the cetomacrogol emulsifying wax in the liquid paraffin at a temperature of 60°C. Dissolve the gamma benzene hexachloride in the mixture and gradually add the warm mixture, water at 60°C cool, add sufficient purified water to produce the required weight and mix. Stir gently until cold.

Storage: This cream should be protected from light and stored in an airtight container.

Use: For the treatment of pediculosis capitis or pediculosis pubis.

Example 9: Salicylic acid and sulfur cream	
Ingredients	Quantity
Salicylic acid, finely sifted	20 g
Precipitated sulfur	20 g
Aqueous cream sufficient to produce	1000 g

Method: Triturate the salicylic acid and the precipitated sulphur with part of the aqueous cream until smooth, gradually add the remainder of the aqueous cream.

Storage: Cream should be stored in an airtight container and in a cool place.

Use: Keratolytic.

Example 10: Zinc cream	
Ingredients	Quantity
Zinc oxide finely sifted	320 g
Calcium hydroxide	0.45 g
Oleic acid	5 ml
Arachis oil	320 ml
Wool fat	80 g
Purified water, freshly boiled and cooled sufficient to produce	1000 g

Method: Mix the zinc chloride and calcium hydroxide, triturate to a smooth paste with a mixture of the oleic acid and arachis oil. Incorporate the wool fat and gradually add, with continuous stirring, sufficient purified water to produce 1000 g.

Storage: Cream should be stored in an airtight container and in a cool place.

Use: Preventing and treating diaper rash. It can also be used to treat minor skin irritations (e.g. cuts, burns, and scrapes, poison ivy).

JELLIES

Pharmaceutical gels are transparent semisolid systems that are being increasingly used as pharmaceutical topical formulations. The liquid phase of the gel may be retained within a three-dimensional polymer matrix. Drugs can be suspended in the matrix or dissolved in the liquid phase.

Advantages and Disadvantages of Jellies

Advantages

1. Stable over long periods of time.
2. Good appearance.
3. Suitable vehicles for applying medicaments to skin and mucous membranes giving high rates of release of the medicament and rapid absorption. Gels are usually translucent or transparent and have a number of uses:
   - ❖ Anesthetic gels.
   - ❖ Coal tar gels for use in treatment of psoriasis or eczema.
   - ❖ Lubricant gels.
   - ❖ Spermicidal gels.

Disadvantages

1. Gels made of natural gelling agents like gum tragacanth, pectin, etc. cannot be stored for a longer time.
2. They are susceptible to microbial growth.
3. They vary in viscosity and natural gelling agents are incompatible with a number of drugs, e.g. gums tend to precipitate in alcohol.
4. They lose viscosity beyond pH range 4.5 to 7.0.

Method of Preparation

1. Add the gelling agents to an aqueous solution of drug.
2. The mass is triturated until a homogeneous product is formed by using a glass pestle and mortar.
3. Continue stirring until a clear preparation of uniform consistency is formed.
4. The jellies must be preserved by adding suitable preservatives, e.g. chlorocresol

(0.1 – 0.2%), methylparaben (0.1 – 0.2%). units % w/w or % w/v.

Storage: Jellies are stored in an airtight container to minimize the water evaporation and should be stored in refrigerated conditions.

Example 1: Tragacanth jelly BP	
Ingredients	**Quantity**
Ichthammol	2 gm
Tragacanth in powder	5 gm
Alcohol 90%	10 ml
Glycerol	2 gm
Water, to	100 gm

Method

1. Prepare 60 g to allow manipulation losses.
2. Tare a 100 ml wide mouthed jar and prepare a tragacanth mucilage, using about 35 ml of water.
3. Mix the ichthammol, glycerol and 10 ml of water; add to the mucilage and shake well.
4. Adjust to weight with water and re-shake.
5. Pack in an internally-lacquered aluminum tube.

Storage: Stored in an airtight container and in a cool place.

Use: Antipsoriatic.

POULTICES

Poultices consist of a hydrophilic heat-retentive basis in which solid or liquid active substances are dispersed. They are usually spread thickly on a suitable dressing and heated before application to the skin.

Advantages and Disadvantages of Poultices

Advantages

1. Poultices stimulate body's surface or alleviate an inflame area.
2. They are simple and easy to prepare.
3. They remain on skin for a longer time, producing a sustained therapeutic action.

Disadvantages

1. They are inconvenient to use.
2. They are not suitable for thermoliable drugs.
3. They are not pleasing in appearance.
4. Kaolin used is liable for contamination with bacterial spores.

Containers: Kaolin poultice should be supplied in suitable containers which minimize absorption, diffusion or evaporation of the ingredients.

Example 1: Kaolin poultice (IP, 1966)	
Ingredients	**Quantity**
Heavy kaolin, finely sifted dried at 100°C	527 g
Boric acid finely sifted	45 g
Methyl salicylate	2 ml
Mentha oil	0.5 ml
Thymol	0.5 ml
Glycerin	425 g

Method

1. Mix the heavy kaolin and the boric acid with the glycerin.

2. Heat the mixture at 120°C for one hour, stirring occasionally; allow it to cool.
3. Add the thymol, previously dissolved in the methyl salicylate, followed by the menthe oil.
4. Mix thoroughly.

Storage: Preserve kaolin poultice in a well-closed container.

Use: Anti-inflammatory, counter-irritant.

SUPPOSITORIES AND PESSARIES

Suppositories are solid unit dosage forms suitably shaped for insertion into the rectum. The bases used either melt when warmed to body temperature or dissolve or disperse when in contact with mucous secretions. Suppositories may contain medicaments, dissolved or dispersed in the base, which are intended to exert a systemic effect. Alternatively the medicaments or the base itself may be intended to exert a local action. Suppositories are prepared extemporaneously by incorporating the medicaments into the base and the molten mass is then poured at a suitable temperature into moulds and allowed to cool until set. Suppositories are available in various shapes like cone, torpedo, and bullet (Table 7.4).

Table 7.4: Classification of suppositories		
Type	**Product illustration**	**Description**
Rectal suppositories	Rectal suppository	Rectal suppositories are unit solid dosage form of medicament meant for introduction into the rectum for their systemic activity. They are tapered at one or both ends and usually weighing about 2 g each. They are usually contain drugs like sedatives, tranquilizers and analgesics.
Vaginal suppositories	Vaginal suppositories with mold	Vaginal suppositories are meant for introduction into the vagina. The larger size moulds are usually used in the preparation of pessaries such as 4 g and 8 g moulds. Pessaries are used almost exclusively for local medication, the exception being prostaglandin pessaries that do exert a systemic effect.

contd...

Type	Product illustration	Description
Table 7.4: Classification of suppositories (*contd.*)		
Urethral suppositories	\n\nUrethral suppositories	Urethral suppositories are meant for introduction into the urethra. They are long and cylindrical forms rounded at one or both end to help insertion and weighing about 2–4 g.
Nasal suppositories	\n\nNasal suppositories	They are meant for introduction into the nasal cavity and are also known as nasal bougies. They are usually 10 cm long and weigh about 1 g.
Ear cones	\n\nEar cones	They are meant for introduction into the ear and are also known as aurinaria. They are rarely used. They are weighing about 1 g, ear cones are prepared with theobroma oil.
Rectal capsules	\n\nRectal capsules	Soft gelatin capsules of varying shapes filled with either liquid or suspension of the drug. They are used for rectal and vaginal use.
Compressed tablet suppositories	\n\nTablet suppositories	These are rectal or vaginal suppositories coated with PEG to protect the medicament in the core and also helps in insertion. The compressed tablet for vaginal use is usually almond-shaped to easy insertion. They are usually drugs for topical therapy.
Layered suppositories	\n\nLayered suppositories	Layered suppositories consist of several layers which contain different drugs, this is performed by partial filling of mold. Incompatible drugs may also be prescribed together. Coating delayed disintegration and sustained release of drugs.

Advantages and Disadvantages of Suppositories

Advantages

1. Can exert local effect on rectal mucosa.
2. Used to promote evacuation of bowel.
3. Avoid any gastrointestinal irritation.
4. Can be used in unconscious patients (e.g. during fitting).
5. Can be used for systemic absorption of drugs and avoid first-pass metabolism.

Disadvantages

1. May be unacceptable to certain patients.
2. May be difficult to self-administer by arthritic or physically compromised patients.
3. Unpredictable and variable absorption *in vivo*.

Classification of Suppositories

Classification of suppositories is described in Table 7.4.

Suppository Bases (Table 7.5)

The various types of suppository bases are used to prepare suppositories. An ideal suppository base should have the following properties:

- It should be melt at body temperature.
- It should release the medicament at the desired site.
- It should be stable on storage.
- It should be compatible with large number of drugs and excipients.
- It should be stable, if heating above melting point.
- It should not promote microbial growth.

Table 7.5: Suppository bases		
Vehicle	Melting range (C)	Solidification point (C)
Fatty bases		
Witepsol	32–44	27–38
Cocoa butter	30–35	24
Hard butter	36–45	32–40
Estarinum	29–50	26–40
Suppocire	35–45	30–37
Agrasup A;	35–40	
Water soluble bases		
Myrj 51	39–42	39
PEGa	38–49	38–42
Tween 61	35–49	

- It should be non-toxic and should be economical.

Suppository bases are classified on the basis of their physical characteristics into three main categories:

1. Fatty or oleaginous bases.
2. Water-miscible or water-soluble bases.
3. Miscellaneous bases.

Fatty or Oleaginous Bases

These are the most frequently used suppository bases, e.g. theobroma oil or cocoa butter along with other hydrogenated fatty acids of vegetable oils such as palm kernel oil and cottonseed oil. Fat-based compounds containing compounds of glycerin with high molecular weight fatty acids, such as palmitic acid and stearic acid or various combinations of these ingredients, are used to achieve the desired melting point and hardness to withstand shipping. Suppository bases are also prepared with emulsified fatty materials or with an emulsifying agent to present prompt emulsification when a suppository base makes contact with aqueous body fluids. Cocoa butter NF is a triglyceride of oleopalmitostearin and oleodistearin. Cocoa butter melts between 30 and 36°C; hence it is an ideal suppository base, melting just below body temperature and yet maintaining solidity at room temperature. However, owing to its triglyceride content, cocoa butter exhibits marked polymorphism. Consequently, quick chilling of melted base (cocoa butter) results in a metastable crystalline form with a melting point lower than normal for cocoa butter. A crystal in metastable condition reverts very slowly to the stable form, having a melting point higher than room temperature.

Water-miscible and Water-soluble bases

Water-miscible bases: These bases are primarily composed of glycerinated gelatin. Glycerinated gelatin bases are most commonly used in preparation of vaginal suppositories, where the prolonged localized action is desired. The glycerinated gelatin base is slower to soften and mix with the physiologic fluids than is cocoa butter and, therefore, provides a more prolonged release. The hygroscopic nature of the gelatin explains this slow softening of the base within the rectum. The hygroscopic effect may even cause irritation to the rectal mucosa owing to dehydration, so water is often incorporated in the formula. Such hygroscopic bases need to be protected from atmospheric moisture in order to maintain their shape and consistency. The following is the formula for a glycerinated vaginal suppository:

- Granular gelatin   20%
- Glycerin   70%
- Aqueous drug solution   10%

Water-soluble bases: Polyethylene glycols are polymers of ethylene oxide and water, which can be prepared to various chain lengths to get desired molecular weights and physical states. Polyethylene glycols with average molecular weights of 200, 400, and 600 are clear colorless liquids. Those with average molecular weights of greater than 1000 are wax-like, white solids with the hardness increasing with an increase in molecular weight. Various combinations of polyethylene glycols may be used to prepare a suppository base of desired consistency and characteristics. In the following examples, base 1 exhibits a low melting point, whereas base 2 a high melting point.

- **Base 1:** Polyethylene glycol 1000— 96%, polyethylene glycol 4000— 4%
- **Base 2:** Polyethylene glycol 1000— 75%, polyethylene glycol 4000— 25%

Polyethylene glycol suppositories do not melt at body temperature but dissolve slowly in body fluids, enabling slower release of the drug on insertion into the rectum.

Miscellaneous Bases

Other bases may be mixtures of lipid and water-soluble bases, e.g. polyoxyl 40 stea-rate, which is a mixture of monostearate and distearate esters of mixed polyoxyethylene diols and the free glycols. Recently, hydrogels defined as macromolecular networks that swell but do not dissolve in water have been recommended as bases for rectal and vaginal drug delivery. Rate and extent of drug release from these hydrogel matrices depend on the rate of water migration into the matrix and the rate of drug diffusion out of the swollen matrix.

Factors Affecting Drug Absorption from Suppository

Drug absorption from suppositories is influenced by:

a. Diffusion of the released drug to the site of absorption.

b. Nature of the drug.

c. Presence of a surfactant.

d. Water-lipid partition coefficient of the drug.

e. Physiological state of the colon (amount and chemical nature of the fluids and solids present in it).

f. The state of anorectal membrance.

Preparation of Suppositories

Suppositories are prepared by three methods— molding, compression, and hand rolling and shaping.

Molding

The most commonly used method for producing suppositories on both small and large scale is the molding process. The steps in molding include: (a) melting the base, (b) incorporating required medicaments, (c) pouring the melt into moulds, and (d) allowing the melt to cool and congeal into suppositories and removing the formed suppositories from the mold. The molds in common use today are made from stainless steel, aluminum, brass, and plastic. Molds are of various capacities, depending upon the scale of production. A community pharmacist would have molds capable of producing 6 to 12 suppositories. The mold shown in Fig. 7.3 is a manually operated mold with a capacity of 6 suppositories. Molds are opened longitudinally for cleaning before and after preparation of suppositories. Care must be taken while cleaning molds, as scratches may affect the desired smoothness of the final product. Figure 7.3 shows a suppository mold. Following steps to be followed while preparing suppositories by molding method.

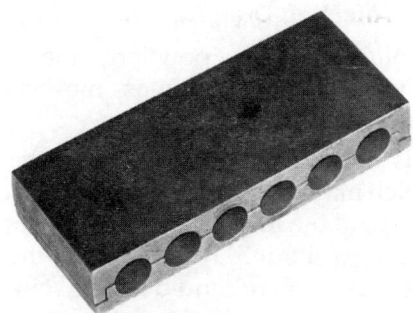

Fig. 7.3: Suppository mold

1. Lubrication of the Mold

This is an important step in the preparation of suppositories. Lubrication is required for clean and easy removal of suppositories. Cocoa butter and polyethylene glycol bases require lubrication, as they do not sufficently contract on cooling within the mold to separate from the inner surfaces and allow their easy removal. Lubrication is not necessary when glycerinated gelatin suppositories are prepared. A thin coating of mineral oil is applied to the molding surface, which provides sufficient lubrication.

2. Calibration of the Mold

It is necessary to account for different densities of different bases. For instance, the weight of suppositories prepared from cocoa butter differs from that of polyethylene glycol for a particular mould. Furthermore, any added medicinal agent alters the density and hence the weight of the resulting suppository. Empty suppositories are prepared from base material alone. The suppositories are weighed and their volume is determined by melting. Thus, the density is computed for that particular base. In the case of extemporaneous preparations, the pharmacist needs to determine the amount of the base required to be incorporated along with the medicaments, so that each suppository provides the required amount of the drug. The volume of the base required is determined by subtracting the volume of the medicaments from the total volume of the mold.

3. Preparing and Pouring the Melt

- The weighed base is melted over a water bath by using the least possible heat. A porcelain casserole is generally used for melting the base, as the melt can be conveniently poured into the cavities of the mold from this utensil.

- Medicaments are usually incorporated into a portion of the melted base by mixing on a porcelain or glass tile with a spatula. This material is then added with stirring to the remaining base, which is cooled almost to its congealing point.

- Any volatile or thermolabile substances should be added to the base with thorough stirring at this point.

- This material is now poured carefully and continuously into the chilled mold. If any undissolved solid materials with a tendency to settle are present, the material should be poured with constant stirring.

- The chilled mold avoids settling of the solids within the mold and also aids in congealing.

- Filling of the suppository cavity should be continuous to avoid layering, which may lead to a product that is easily broken when handled.

- To ensure complete filling of the mold upon congealing, the melt is poured above the level of the mold over each opening.

- After solidification, the excess material is scrapped off evenly with a spatula.

- The mold is usually kept in the freezer to promote hardening of the suppositories.
- When the suppositories are hard, the mold is removed from the freezer, the sections of the mold are separated, and the suppositories are removed with pressure being exerted at the ends.

Compression

Compression molding is a method of preparing suppositories from a mixed mass of grated suppository base and medicaments which is forced into a special compression mold. The method requires that the capacity of the molds first be determined by compressing a small amount of the base into the dies and weighing the finished suppositories. When active ingredients are added, it is necessary to omit a portion of the suppository base, based on the density factors of the active ingredients.

Hand Rolling and Shaping

A plastic-like mass is formed from the base of grated cocoa butter and other ingredients by severe trituration. The mass is rolled into a ball with the palms of the hands. Since the suppository base melts near body temperature, before handling it, hands need to be cooled below body temperature by dipping them in ice water. The mass is shaped into a cylinder with the help of the spatula. The cylinder is cut into appropriate lengths with a knife, each length equal to one suppository. The final shaping of the suppository is done with the fingertips with suppositories rolled in a glassine powder paper to prevent the warmth of the palm melting the base. Alternatively, the cylindrical base can be pushed into a mould to give the suppositories a final uniform shape.

General Method for Suppository Preparation (Using Fatty Bases)

1. Most molds prepare six suppositories, but it is necessary to calculate to include an excess (usually a multiple of 10).

2. Choose a suppository mold to provide the suppositories of the required size (usually a 1 g size). Check that the two halves of the molds are matched (numbers are etched on the sides).

3. Check that the mold is clean and assemble the mold but do not over tighten the screw.

4. For some suppository bases it is necessary to lubricate the mold (e.g. use liquid paraffin BP), but this is not required when using hard fat BP.

5. If the suppository is to contain insoluble, coarse powders, these must be ground down in a glass mortar before incorporation.

6. It is important not to overheat the base, which may change its physical characteristics. Find the melting point of the base and heat it to about 5–10°C less than the melting point. (There should still be some solid base present.) Hold the evaporating basin in the palm of your hand and stir (do not use the thermometer to stir) to complete the melting process.

7. Immiscible liquids and insoluble solids should be incorporated into the fatty base by levigation (wet grinding). The substance should be rubbed into the minimum quantity of molten base on a tile using a spatula. The 'shearing' effect will not be obtained, if too much base is used, resulting in a gritty product.

8. The paste obtained in step 7 above should be returned to the evaporating basin with the remainder of the base, stirring constantly.

9. The molten mass should be poured into the mold when it is just about to solidify.

10. Pour the mass into the molds uniformly in one movement.

11. Allow the mixture to overfill slightly but not to run down the sides of the mold (if this happens, it is likely to be due to the mixture still being too hot).

12. When the suppositories have contracted, but before they have set completely, trim off the excess suppository base. This can easily be achieved by rubbing the flat blade of the spatula over the top of the mold.

13. After further cooling, when the suppositories have set, loosen the screw and tap once sharply on the bench. Remove the suppositories carefully (avoid over handling or damaging the suppositories with your nails).

14. Pack the required number of suppositories individually in foil and place in an amber wide-necked jar.

General Labeling Requirements for Suppository Preparation

Along with the general labeling requirements for semisolid preparation, following points must be considered while labeling suppository:

- Always keep medicines out of the reach of children.

- Always use the medicine according to the printed label or as instructed by your doctor or pharmacist.

- Do not give your medicines to anyone else to use, even if they have the same symptoms as you. They may be harmful to other people.

- If you miss a dose of your medicine, take the dose as soon as you remember, and then go on as before.

- Suppositories are designed only for insertion into the rectum and must not be taken by mouth. If they are accidentally swallowed, tell your doctor at once.

- Do not use your suppositories after the expiry date on the pack.

Displacement Value

Suppositories are prepared by dissolving or dispersing an active medicament in a molten base and pouring the mixture into a suppository mold. Suppository mold are normally available in 1 g, 2 g and 4 g sizes. However, because the density of the medicament may vary considerably from that of the base, the weight of the base required to make a suppository will vary depending on the medicament used. For example, 2 g of a medicament with twice the density of theobroma oil would occupy approximately the same volume as 1 g of the suppository base. The displacement values (DVs) of medicaments are required when calculating the weight of suppository base is required to prepare medicated suppositories.

The displacement value of a medicament is the number of parts, by weight, of a medicament that will displace one part of suppository base (normally theobroma oil). Displacement values of some important medicaments in reference to cocoa butter are summarized in Table 7.6.

Table 7.6: Displacement value of some important drugs	
Boric acid	1.5
Chloral hydrate	1.5
Cocaine hydrochloride	1.5
Codeine phosphate	1.1
Digitalis leaf	1.6
Dimenhydrinate	1.3
Diphenhydramine HCl	1.3
Gallic acid	2.0
Hamamelis dry extract	1.5
Hydrocortisone	1.5
Hydrocortisone acetate	1.5
Ichthammol	1.0
Menthol	0.7
Morphine hydrochloride	1.5
Peru balsam	1.0
Phenobarbital sodium	1.2
Potassium bromide	2.2
Quinidine HCl	3.0
Resorcinol	1.0
Salicylic acid	1.3
Secobarbital sodium	1.2
Tannic acid	1.6
Zinc oxide	5.0
Zinc sulfate	2.8

Importance of Displacement Value

Suppositories are prepared in the mold by incorporating medicament in suppository base. Suppository molds are normally available in 1 g, 2 g and 4 g capacity. Here capacity means equal amount of cocoa butter suppositories can be produced by them with constant volume of the suppository mould. During preparation, we have to add medicament in the suppositories, as the volume of mold is fixed, for addition of medicament into mold we have to displace some amount of base from base required for plain suppositories. However, because the density of medicament may vary considerably from that of base, the weight of base required to make a suppository will vary depending on the medicament used. The displacement value of a medicament is required during the calculation of weight of suppository base required to prepare medicated suppositories.

Calculation of Displacement Value

Displacement value can be calculated by following steps.

Method 1: Weight factor method

- Calculate the weight of base required for plain suppositories = capacity of mold × total number of suppositories required = A.
- Calculate the total weight of medicament required = weight of medicament required for one suppository × total no. of suppositories = B.
- Calculate the weight of base used in medicated suppositories = total weight of suppositories – amount of medicament used = C.
- Calculate weight of base displaced by medicament = total weight of base required for plain suppositories – actual base used = A – C = D.
- Displacement value of medicament = total wt of medicament required/amount of base displaced = (A – C)/B.

The following examples will illustrate the displacement value calculations:

Example 1: If a prescription requires 400 mg of bismuth subgallate per suppository weighing two grams, what would be the displacement value if it is known that six suppositories with required bismuth subgallate weigh 13.6 g?

Solution:

Capacity of mould = 2 gm

Theoretical weight of six cocoa butter suppositories without bismuth subgallate = 12 g

Given weight of six cocoa butter suppositories with bismuth subgallate = 13.6 g

Amount of bismuth subgallate in the suppositories = 0.4 × 6 = 2.4 g

Amount of cocoa butter in the bismuth subgallate suppositories = 13.6 – 2.4 = 11.2 g

Cocoa butter displaced by 2.4 g of bismuth subgallate = 12 – 11.2 = 0.8 g

The displacement value of bismuth subgallate is 2.4/0.8 = 3

Answer: DV = 3

Method 2: Density factor method

- Determine the average blank weight, A, per mold, using the suppository base of interest.
- Weigh the quantity of suppository base necessary for 10 suppositories.
- Weigh 1.0 g of drug. The weight of drug per suppository, B, is then equal to 1 g/10 suppositories = 0.1 g/suppository.
- Melt the suppository base, incorporate the drug, mix, pour into mold, cool, trim, and remove from the mold.
- Weigh the 10 suppositories and determine the average weight (C).
- Determine the density factor as follows:
- Density factor = B/A – C + B

  where A is the average weight of the blank suppository, B is the weight of drug per suppository, and C is the average weight of the medicated suppository.

- Take the weight of the drug required for each suppository and divide it by the density factor of the drug to find the replacement value of the suppository base.
- Subtract this quantity from the blank suppository weight.
- Multiply by the number of suppositories required to obtain the quantity of suppository base required for the prescription.
- Multiply the weight of drug per suppository by the number of suppositories required to obtain the quantity of active drug required for the prescription.

Method 3: Occupied volume method

- Determine the average weight per mold (blank) using the suppository base of interest.
- Weigh the quantity of suppository base necessary for 10 suppositories.
- Divide the density of the active drug by the density of the suppository base to obtain a ratio.
- Divide the total weight of active drug required for the total number of suppositories by the ratio obtained in step 3 (this will give the amount of suppository base displaced by the active drug).
- Subtract the amount obtained in step 4 from the total weight of the prescription (number of suppositories multiplied by the weight of the blanks) to obtain the weight of suppository base required.
- Multiply the weight of active drug per suppository by the number of suppositories to be prepared to obtain the quantity of active drug required.

Storage and Handling

Glycerogelatin suppositories are usually packaged in well-closed screw-capped glass containers, preferably at a temperature below 35°C. Cocoa butter-based suppositories

Table 7.7: Density factors of some medicaments for cocoa butter suppositories

Medicament	Density Factor
Alum	1.7
Aminophylline	1.1
Aspirin	1.3
Balsam peruvian	1.1
Barbital	1.2
Belladonna extract	1.3
Benzoic acid	1.5
Bismuth carbonate	4.5
Bismuth salicylate	4.5
Bismuth subgallate	2.7
Bismuth subnitrate	6.0
Boric acid	1.5
Castor oil	1.0
Chloral hydrate	1.3
Cocaine HCl	1.3
Digitalis leaf	1.6
Glycerin	1.6
Ichthammol	1.1
Iodoform	4.0

are usually packaged by wrapping them individually into partitioned boxes to prevent contact and adhesion (Table 7.7). suppositories containing light-sensitive drugs are generally wrapped in an opaque material such as ametallic foil. Most commercially available suppositories are individually wrapped in either foil or polyvinyl chloride (PVC)—polyethylene. Some suppositories utilize strip-packaging, with individual suppositories being separated by tearing along perforations located between suppositories. Since, suppositories are sensitive to heat, they should be stored in a cool place, but they should not be frozen. Cocoa butter suppositories must be stored below 30°C. preferably in a refrigerator (2 to 8°C). Glaycerinated gelatin suppositories should be stored below 35°F and can be stored at controlled room temperature (20 to 25°C). Polyethylene glycol-based suppositories can be stored at be stored at usual room temperatures. Suppositories are adversely affected by humidity. High humidity causes them to become spongy, whereas an extreme dry environment results in the loss of moisture from suppositories, which makes them brittle.

Example 1: Bismuth subgallate suppositories BPC	
Ingredients	**Quantity**
Bismuth subgallate	300 mg
Whitepsol 45, sufficient for	1 gm mould

Method

1. Calculate the quantity required, taking displacement values into consideration. An excess must be made to compensate the loss.

2. Select a dry, clean mould and place it on a clean tile.

3. Shred the fat with a fine grater. Weigh the required amount, avoiding lumps that will be slow to melt and place in the smallest evaporating basin that will hold it.

4. Finely powdered medicament and pass each through a separate no. 180 sieve. Weigh the required thoroughly afterwards.

5. Heat a small tile until it is comfortable warm to the hand.

6. Mix the powders on the tile with a flexible spatula. Place the base on the water bath until about two-thirds of the content has melted and then remove from the heat.

7. Pour about half of the melted base on to the mixed medicaments and work into a smooth dispersion as quickly as possible by levigating with the spatula. To prevent excessive cooling through spreading over a large area, use as small tile as is consistent with avoidance of spillage.

8. Transfer the dispersion to the dish, leaving virtually none on the tile, and stir to form a homogeneous mixture.

9. Continue stirring until the mixture begins to thicken. Then fill the cavity of the mold to overflowing.

10. Leave in a coolplace for 10 to 15 min then open the mold and remove the suppositories.

Storage: Store your suppositories in a cool dark place, but not in the fridge unless specifically instructed. If they get too warm they may melt and not be firm enough to insert.

Use: Antiseptics/astringents

Example 2: Glycerin suppository (IP, 1966)	
Ingredients	**Quantity**
Gelatin cut small	16 g
Glycerin	70 g
Purified water	A sufficient quantity

Method

1. Soak the gelatin in purified water for minutes or until thoroughly softened.

2. Drain well and add glycerin.

3. Heat on a water bath to effect solution.

4. Evaporate the liquids until the mixture weighs 100 g.

5. Pour the product into suitable mold.

Storage: Store your suppositories in a cool dark place, but not in the fridge unless specifically instructed. If they get too warm, they may melt and not be firm enough to insert.

Use: Rectal evacuant.

PESSARIES

Pessaries are solid preparation each containing one or more medicaments. They are normally administered as a single dose. The shape, volume and consistency of pessaries are such that the preparation is suitable for vaginal insertion. Pessaries usually weigh between 1 g and 15 g. The medicaments are dissolved or dispersed in a suitable bases which may be soluble, dispersible or insoluble in water.

According to the type of pessaries, the excipients may be similar to those described under suppositories or to those described under tablets.

Storage: Molded pessaries and vaginal capsules should be kept in a well-closed container at a temperature not greater than 30°C. Vaginal tablets should be kept in a close container and protected from moisture and crushing.

Labeling: Comply with the general requirements for labeling in addition the label on the container states that the preparation should not be swallowed.

Molded Pessaries

Molded pessaries are prepared using similar excipients and the methods to those described for molded suppositories. Molded pessaries are of various shapes, most commonly being ovoid; their characters corresponds to those of the molded suppositories.

Example 1: Lactic acid pessaries BPC	
Ingredients	**Quantity**
Lactic acid	5 %
Glycerol suppositories	95 %

Method

1. Use about 25 ml of water initially.
2. When the gelatin has dissolved, cover the dish with a large clock-glass and transfer to a gas or electrically heated steamer containing boiling water. Close the lid to ensure that the correct temperature is maintained.
3. After heating, the weight is almost always high. Evaporate to 80 gm on a water bath or on gauze over a bunsen lamp.
4. Since pouring from the very hot dish is difficult and may leave liquid on the outside remove 4 gm with a metal spoon or spatula.
5. Add 4 gm of lactic acid using a pipette to avoid an excess. Note that 4 gm of mass should be replaced by lactic acid; the mass should not be evaporated to 76 g and then the acid added because this would replace 4 g of water.
6. Stir well and pour into a chilled mold.
7. Delay opening the mold as long as possible because lactic acid lowers the setting point of the mass.
8. Individually, wrap the products in metal foil or waxed paper as lactic acid pessaries are very hydrospace. Pack in a well-closed jar.

Storage: Store pessaries in a cool dark place. If they get too warm, they may melt and not be firm enough to insert.

Use: Antimicrobial

Example 2: Acetarsol vaginal tablets (BP, 1988)	
Ingredients	**Quantity**
Acetarsol	250 mg
Anhydrous dextrose	320 mg
Starch	350 mg

Method: Acetarsol pessaries are prepared by compression. They may be prepared using any other suitable basis, including an effervescent basis.

Storage: Store your pessaries in a cool dark place.

Use: Anti-infective.

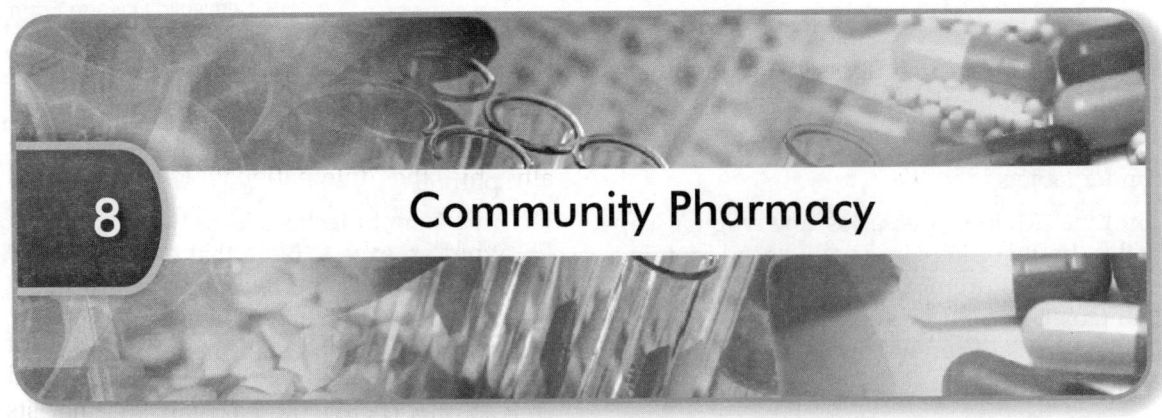

Community Pharmacy

8

INTRODUCTION

Pharmacy is the health profession that links the health sciences with the chemical sciences, and it is charged with ensuring the safe and effective use of pharmaceutical drugs.

The scope of pharmacy practice includes more traditional roles such as compounding and dispensing medications, and it also includes more modern services related to healthcare, including clinical services, reviewing medications for safety and efficacy, and providing drug information.

An establishment in which pharmacy (in the first sense) is practiced is called a pharmacy, chemist's or drug store. A pharmacy is the place where most pharmacists practice the profession of pharmacy. It is the community pharmacy where the dichotomy of the profession exists—health professionals who are also retailers. It is an important link between the doctor, nurse and patients. They play a vital role in ensuring the patient safety and efficacy in therapeutic set up.

Community pharmacies usually consist of a retail storefront with a dispensary where medications are stored and dispensed. The dispensary is subject to pharmacy legislation with requirements for storage conditions, compulsory texts, equipment, etc., specified in legislation. The two symbols most commonly associated with pharmacy are the **mortar** and **pestle** and the Ṙ (recipere) character, which is often written as "Rx" in typed text (Fig. 8.1).

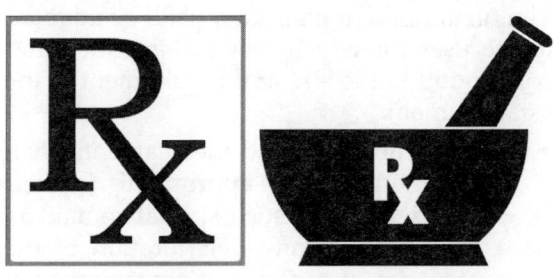

Fig. 8.1: Symbol of pharmacy

Community pharmacy means any place under the direct supervision of a pharmacist where the practice occurs or where prescription orders are compounded and dispensed other than a hospital pharmacy or a limited service pharmacy.

Pharmacists are highly-trained and skilled healthcare professionals who perform various roles to ensure optimal health outcomes for their patients. Many pharmacists are also small-business owners, owning the pharmacy in which they practice.

A community pharmacist is the professional who would be in direct access to the public and whose duties are widely sought after by the public and patients. He/she dispenses medicines with a prescription and in certain cases without a prescription where applicable (OTC drugs). As he/she is the person who will be in direct contact with the public, he/she

has to play an important role in decreasing the mortality and morbidity in the public.

Pharmacists are represented internationally by the International Pharmaceutical Federation (FIP). They are represented at the national level by professional organizations such as the Indian Pharmacy Graduate Association (IPGA), Dutch Pharmacists Association (VNA), Royal Pharmaceutical Society of Great Britain (RPSGB), the Pharmacy Guild of Australia (PGA), the Pakistan Pharmacists Society (PPS) and the American Pharmacists Association (APhA).

ORGANIZATION AND STRUCTURE OF A COMMUNITY PHARMACY (FIG.8.2)

Personnel Present

Managing pharmacist, pharmacists, pharmacy technicians, pharmacy assistants, sales personnel. Staff management includes identifying training needs and providing appropriate training, management to develop a team approach, continuing professional development of professional personnel.

Entrance

The front of a pharmacy shall bear an inscription "Pharmacy" in front.

Premises

Generally, pharmacy premises comprises of areas available for dispensing, storage of medicines, patient counseling and health promotion.

- The premises of a pharmacy shall be separated from rooms for private use.
- Area should be spacious and designed in such a way as to promote communication between pharmacist and patient.
- The premises shall be well built, dry, well lit and ventilated and of sufficient dimensions to allow the goods in stock, especially medicaments and poisons to be

kept in a clearly visible and appropriate manner.

- The area of the section to be used as dispensing department shall be not less than 6 square metres for one pharmacist working therein with additional 2 square metres for each additional pharmacist.
- The height of the premises shall be at least 2.5 metres.
- The floor of the pharmacy shall be smooth and washable. The walls shall be plastered or tiled or oil painted so as to maintain smooth, durable and washable surface devoid of holes, cracks and crevices.
- A pharmacy shall be provided with ample supply of good quality water.
- The dispensing department shall be separated by barrier to prevent the admission of the public.
- Space should be available for patient advice and counseling in privacy.
- Consultation areas should provide for space to carry out point-of-care testing.

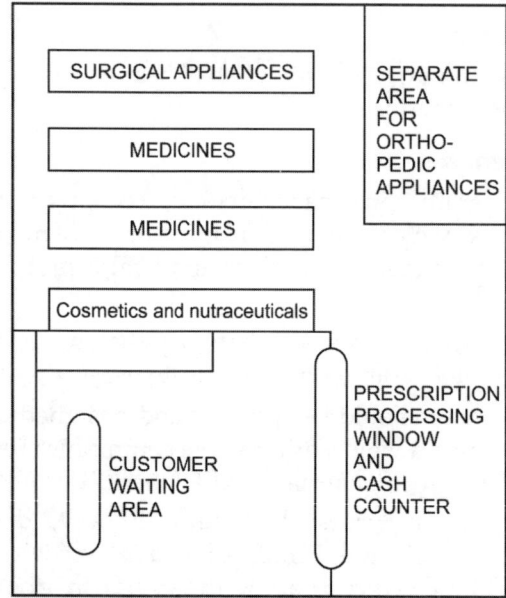

Fig. 8.2: General layout of pharmacy

Storage of Medicines

- Sufficient storage space to store medicines in a dry place.
- Temperature control of areas where medicines are stored.
- Prescription-only medicines not accessible to the public.
- Area available to store medicines that require controlled access.
- Stock rotation, monitoring of expiry dates and systems to ensure that medicines are not damaged.

Furniture

The furniture of a pharmacy shall be adapted to the uses for which they are intended and correspond to the size and requirement of the establishment.

- Drugs, chemicals and medicaments shall be kept in a room appropriate to their properties and in such special containers as will prevent any deterioration of the contents or of contents of containers kept near them.
- Drawers, glasses and other containers used for keeping medicaments shall be of suitable size and capable of being closed tightly to prevent the entry of dust.
- Every container shall bear a label of appropriate size, easily readable with names of medicaments as given in the pharmacopoeias.
- A pharmacy shall be provided with a dispensing bench, the top of which shall be covered with washable and impervious material like stainless steel, laminated or plastic, etc.
- A pharmacy shall be provided with a cupboard with lock and key for the storage of poisons and shall be clearly marked with word "POISON" in red letters on a white background.
- Containers of all concentrated solution shall bear special label or marked with the words "TO BE DILUTED".

Apparatus and Books

A pharmacy shall be provided with the following minimum apparatus and books necessary for making of official preparations and prescriptions.

Apparatus

- Balance, dispensing, sensitivity 30 mg.
- Balance, counter, capacity 3 kg, sensitivity 1 gm.
- Beakers lipped, assorted sizes.
- Bottles, prescription, ungraduated assorted sizes.
- Corks assorted sizes and tapers.
- Cork, extractor.
- Evaporating dishes, porcelain.
- Filter paper.
- Funnel glass.
- Litmus paper, blue and red.
- Measure glasses cylindrical 10 ml, 25 ml, 100 ml and 500 ml.
- Mortar and pestle, glass.
- Mortar and pestles, wedgwood.
- Ointment slab, porcelain.
- Pipettes, graduated, 2 ml, 5 ml, and 10 ml.
- Ring, stand (retort) iron, complete with rings.
- Rubber stamps and pad.
- Scissors.
- Spatulas, rubber or vulcanite.
- Spatulas, stainless steel.
- Spirit lamp.
- Glass stirring rods.
- Thermometer (0 to 200 °C).
- Tripod stand.
- Watch glasses.
- Water bath.
- Water distillation still in case eye drops and eye lotions are prepared.
- Weight guaze.
- Pill finisher, boxwood.
- Pill machine
- Pill boxes.
- Suppository mould.

Books

- **The Indian Pharmacopoeia** (current edition).
- **National Formulary of India** (current edition).
- **The Drug and Cosmetics Act, 1940.**
- **The Drug and Cosmetics Rules, 1945.**
- **The Pharmacy Act, 1948.**
- **The Dangerous Drugs Act, 1930.**

General Provisions

- A pharmacy shall be conducted under the continuous personal supervision of a registered pharmacist whose name shall be displayed conspicuously in the premises.
- The pharmacist shall always put on clean white overall.
- The premises and fittings of the pharmacy shall be properly kept and everything shall be in good order and clean.
- All records and registers shall be maintained in accordance with the laws in force.
- Any container taken from the poison cupboard shall be replaced therein immediately after use and the cupboard locked. The key of the poison cupboard shall be kept in the personal custody of the responsible person.
- Medicaments when supplied shall have labels conforming to the provisions of laws in force.

Maintenance of Drug Store

The purchase and sale of drugs is quite different from the sale of other goods. In case of ordinary goods, the consumer can select the goods according to his/her choice but in case of drugs the choice is in the hands of a physician. Moreover, the sale of drugs is a technical job and requires knowledge and must be performed by a qualified person. Before opening a drug store (whether retail or wholesale), there are certain legal requirements which must be fulfilled which are as follows:

a. Minimum qualification

b. Application for grant of license

c. Duration of license

d. Renewal of license

Legislation

- Pharmacists practising at the pharmacy are registered with a registering body.

- Process of community pharmacy practice is controlled by legislation.

- Legislation classifies medicines according to:
  - Category of medicines that may be sold from other outlets (such as drugstores) not only pharmacies (e.g. general sales list, in countries where this is permitted).
  - Category of medicines that may be sold after being recommended by pharmacists.
  - Category of medicines that require a prescription.
  - Category of medicines that are controlled (e.g. buprenorphine, diamorphine, fentanyl, methadone).

- Pharmacy services must be available for 24 hours, 7 days a week. Rosters are issued for night-time service and for service on Sundays and public holidays.

Minimum Qualification

Qualified person is the essential requirement to start a retail or wholesale drug store. In case of retail drug store, qualified person should be a registered pharmacist. Requirements for qualified person are laid down in the Pharmacy Act which is as follows.

Age: Minimum 18 years

Qualification: Diploma or degree in pharmacy from recognized or PCI approved institute.

He/she should be registered at State Pharmacy Council; registration is required to carry out business in that state.

In case of wholesale drug store, qualified person should have minimum qualification matriculation with 4 years experience in handling of drugs in a chemist shop on permanent basis.

Application for Grant of License

Any person who wants to deal with drugs should have a license issued by the respective licensing authority of the state government. For obtaining the license for sale or purchase of drugs, following documents are required:

1. Application or form no. 19/19B duly filled in and in duplicate.

2. A fees receipt of Rs 3000 to be attached with application form.

3. Layout design 3 copies duly signed by proprietor and attested by registered architect.

4. An attested copy of proof of qualification.

5. Attested copy of registration certificate issued by state pharmacy council.

6. An affidavit from qualified person in case he/she is an employee of a drug store.

7. Attested copy of proof of date of birth.

8. In case of license for wholesale drug store, attested copy of matriculation certificate along with experience certificate.

9. Partnership deed in case of more than one proprietor.

10. Rent receipt with rent deed in case the premises is on rent basis otherwise copy of ownership proof should be attached.

11. Refrigerator purchase bill along with the chassis no. of refrigerator.

All the documents with application form should be submitted to the drug control department of that state. After preliminary scrutiny of the application, the drug control authorities minimum at the level of drug inspector personally visit the premises for which the license for the sale and purchase of drugs is required. After satisfaction of authorities, the license is issued in the form of filled and duly signed certificate.

Duration of License

License for sale and purchase of drug remains valid for 3 years and up to 31st December of the year of expiry.

Renewal of License

Licensee can apply for renewal of license to the licensing authorities before the expiry or within 6 months of the date of its expiry. In case of any change in constitution of licensed firm like change in built up area, rent deed or qualified person, etc., the licensee shall inform to the licensing authorities.

Storage of Drugs

There should be proper storage capacity as well as facilities for drugs at the store. Drugs should be stored in the prescribed manner as per requirement.

TYPES OF DRUG STORE AND DESIGN (FIG.8.3)

Traditional Drug Stores

In these types of drug store, entire area of drug store is exposed to customers. Such a designhas pleasing and professional appearance and is convenient for both workers and customers. With this, maximum sales can be achieved but as well there are chances of theft in such manner.

Personal Service Drug Stores

In these types of drug store, personnel services are provided to the customers, the whole of the area is not exposed to them like traditional drug stores. During the purchasing process, the customer demands his requirement and the personnel provide the same. This service and design enhances the interaction between drug store employee and the customers. The factors which affect the success of the drug store are convenience, friendly service of the personnel at the counter and knowledge of the pharmacist.

Prescription-oriented Drug Store (Fig. 8.4)

These types of drug store are totally prescription oriented. There should be waiting area where the customer is expected to wait during processing of his prescription. In this type of design, drugs and prescription accessories are displayed in the vicinity while orthopedic and surgical and surgical appliances are kept in a separate room. Cosmetics and nutraceuticals are displayed in a suitable manner in the display racks.

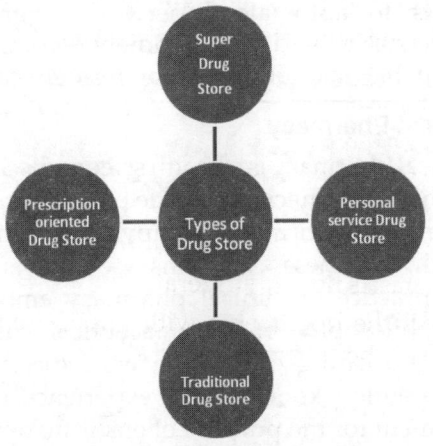

Fig. 8.3: Types of drug store

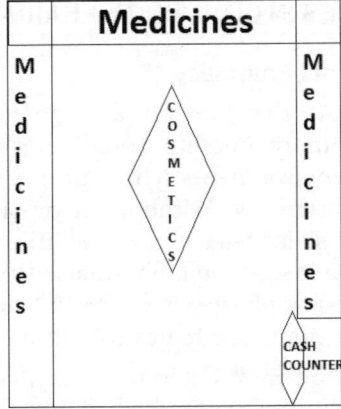

Fig. 8.4: Prescription-oriented drug stores

Super Drugstore (Fig. 8.5)

These types of drugstore are a combination of all above means; these have prescription counter, waiting area, open space for customers and with personnel services. These drug stores have a floor area, ranging from 7500 to 10000 sq ft. The customers have access to almost all the area in the drugstore and can inspect, handle and select articles by themselves except the prescription area which is under the control of pharmacist.

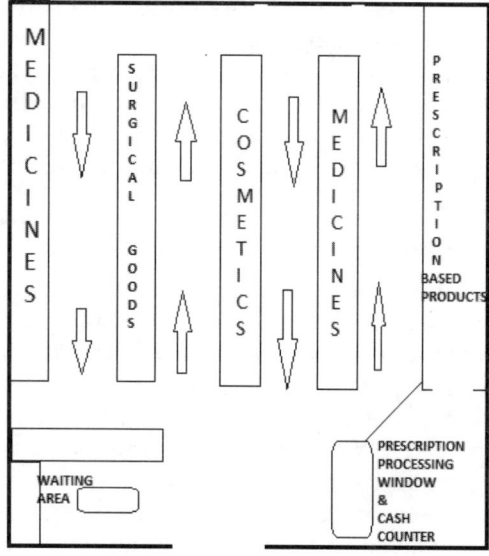

Fig. 8.5: Super drugstores

ADVANCES IN COMMUNITY PHARMACY

Institutional Pharmacy

A pharmacy that provides a range of services to residents of nursing homes, hospitals, or hospice environments which do not have an on-site pharmacy. Without an on-site pharmacy, most long-term care facilities depend instead on institutional pharmacies to provide the necessary pharmacy products and services and to play an integral role in monitoring patient medication.

In addition to providing pharmaceuticals, institutional pharmacies provide consult-

ing services, which include monitoring the control, distribution, and administration of drugs and assisting in compliance with applicable regulations. The pharmacist also plays a role as medication therapy experts. Institutional pharmacists take responsibility for their patients' medication-related needs; ensure that their patients' medications are the most appropriate, most effective, safest possible, and are used correctly; and identify, resolve, and prevent medication-related problems that may interfere with goals of therapy.

Services include special 24-hour delivery and on-call services 365 days a year. The market is dominated by three leading providers. There are many smaller pharmacies as well which belong to purchasing groups to help them to negotiate preferred product pricing. There is a high percentage of medicare residents in these institutions, causing a major concern for profitability and stability in the business model.

Institutional pharmacies are in a key position to help facilities effectively manage these pressures as they relate to prescription drugs, offering services that move beyond simply filling prescriptions. By providing consulting and technology services, institutional phar-macies guide facilities through the complex landscape of pharmaceutical services for seniors. Today's pharmacies work with their clients to automate paperwork, aggregate resident data, and present timely reports with actionable data for improving resident care.

Clinical Pharmacy

Clinical pharmacy is a health science discipline in which pharmacists provide patient care that optimizes medication therapy and promotes health, wellness, and disease prevention. The practice of clinical pharmacy embraces the philosophy of pharmaceutical care; it blends a caring orientation with specialized therapeutic knowledge, experience, and judgment for the purpose of ensuring optimal patient outcomes. As a discipline, clinical pharmacy also has an obligation to contribute to the generation of new knowledge that advances health and quality of life. Clinical pharmacists care for patients in all healthcare settings. They possess in-depth knowledge of medications that is integrated with a foundational understanding of the biomedical, pharmaceutical, sociobehavioral, and clinical sciences.

Within the system of healthcare, clinical pharmacists are experts in the therapeutic use of medications. They routinely provide medication therapy evaluations and recommendations to patients and other healthcare professionals. Clinical pharmacists are a primary source of scientifically valid info-rmation and advice regarding the safe, appropriate, and cost-effective use of medications. Clinical pharmacists are also making themselves more readily available to the public. In the past, access to a clinical pharmacist was limited to hospitals, clinics, or educational institutions. However, clinical pharmacists are making themselves available through a medication information hotline, and reviewing medication lists, all in an effort to prevent medication errors in the foreseeable future.

Chain Pharmacy

Pharmacy chain formats:

Hospital pharmacies: They catered mainly to the requirements of patients admitted in the hospital. They were housed in the hospital building and dispense a limited number of medicines. The average size of such stores is 150–200 sq. ft.

Retail stores/standalone stores: The second category of stores, near the residential areas, provide the benefits of proximity to consumers. Some of these stores offered home delivery. The target customers of the store were the educated middle and upper class households.

Malls/shop-in-shops: The biggest advantage, most retailers say, of having in-store outlets at supermarkets or departmental stores is the fact that popularity of either brand rubs

off on the other. Guardian pharmacy recently signed an agreement to open outlets at Spencer's stores in east India and is negotiating rights for northern India too. Spencer's has tie-up with LifeKen Medicines for store-in-stores at its Daily stores in the South. New-u, retail outlet of H&B Stores Ltd. are located in Malls.

Townships: Many pharmacy chains are planning to set up their pharmacy chain in townships. Apollo is planning to set up Medicity near Pune. Apollo has signed an agreement with Hindustan Construction Co (HCC) to set up the medicity inside the upcoming project named Lavasa near Pune.

The organized pharmacy retail market is dominated by big industrial houses like Ranbaxy's (Fortis), Pantaloon (Tulsi), Reliance Retail's (Reliance Health and Pharma) and Subhiksha as well as healthcare players like Apollo Hospitals Group's (Apollo Pharmacy) , Medicine Shoppe, Zydus Cadilla's (Dial for Health), Sagar Drugs & Pharmaceuticals' (Planet Health), Morepan's (Life Spring), Lifetime Healthcare's (LifeKen), Global Healthline (98.4), Guardian Lifecare's (Guardian Pharmacy), MedPlus to name a few.

Independent Pharmacy

An independent pharmacy is a retail pharmacy that is not directly affiliated with any chain of pharmacies. An independent pharmacy is one which is not owned (or operated) by a publicly traded company. Independent pharmacies are pharmacist-owned, privately-held businesses in varying practice settings. They include single-store operations, pharmacist-owned multiple store locations, franchise, compounding, long-term-care (LTC), specialty, and supermarket pharmacy operation. Independent pharmacy owners generally have high standards of customer service and strive to outperform chain pharmacy competitors.

Wholesale Pharmacy

Anciently, the wholesale drug business were known as drug manufacturing business or apothecary shops or drug stores maintained by good settlers. These first drug stores imported their botanical drugs and chemicals in bulk mostly from Europe and they manufactured their medicine in their retail stores. Gradually some of them specialized as wholesalers in importing and supplying drugs and chemicals to other retailers. Other specialized in manufacturing while still others continued to function primarily as retailers selling directly to the public.

As the years went by, the separation between the function of drug retailing, drug wholesaling and drug manufacturing became distinct. During early days, merchandise handled by drug wholesalers consisted chiefly of crude botanical drugs, medicines, chemicals, essential oils, fixed oils, toiletries and soap all bought in bulk packages which were subdivided by the wholesaler, repackaged and sold in smaller amounts primarily to retail drug stores, partly to industrial users. Today, product handled by the wholesaler consists almost entirely of packed medicines and toiletry articles, surgical and other health supplies, all ready for consumer use. The average wholesale drug house today handles about thousands different items including packaged medicines, prescription specialty items, household remedy, toiletries and other health supplies and various sundry items.

The successful conduct of the wholesale drug business requires an ample warehouse for storing full cases in wholesale quantity and for maintaining a large open stock inventory of all items office for personnel to maintain warehouse records, buying, selling and invoicing. The function of conveying goods from the producer or manufacturer to the retailer who sells to the consumer must be performed by someone.

Direct-to-Pharmacy (DTP) Model

Classical distribution methods of pharmaceutical and medical products via wholesalers can no longer keep up with some of the high and specialised demands of the pharmaceutical industry. Under the new scheme, seen first in the UK, pharmaceutical manufacturers enter into an exclusive agreement with particular wholesalers and make them the sole supplier of its medicines. In effect, the company is selling the drugs directly to pharmacies, and paying the wholesaler a set fee to deliver them.

GlaxoSmithKline pioneered the DTP scheme several years ago, and Pfizer followed suit in March 2007. Several other companies such as Novartis and Eli Lilly are looking at switching to DTP. However, the scheme has come in for its share of criticism as pharmacists fear they will get lower discounts when they buy medicines, which will have the knock-on effect of leading to higher costs for the NHS. There has also been anxiety that service levels might worsen because wholesalers are not competing against each other.

The advantages at a glance:

- Lower distribution costs, among other things, through multi-user solutions.
- Use of existing, validated distribution structures.
- Direct access to pharmacies and their sales data.
- Great transparency along the entire distribution chain – all movements of goods and all storage conditions are recorded precisely and without any gaps.
- To reduce security risks and the insertion of counterfeit products.
- To optimize inventory management.
- To optimize delivery service through shorter response times.
- Single-source service – efficient and comprehensive processing of all activities by one single service provider.

DIRECT TO PATIENT (ONLINE PHARMACIES)

Today, for millions of patient, the internet is the first place they turn for healthcare information. As a result, the advertising and marketing of pharmaceuticals is changing direction — and channels, too — from "direct-to-consumer" to "direct-to-patient," from mass marketing to relationship marketing. Online pharmacies, or internet pharmacies, are pharmacies that operate over the internet. Many such pharmacies are, in some ways, similar to community pharmacies; the primary difference is the method by which the medications are requested and received. Some customers consider this to be more convenient than traveling to a community drugstore, in the same way as ordering goods online rather than going to a shop. While many internet pharmacies sell prescription drugs only with a prescription, some do not require a pre-written prescription. In some countries, this is because prescriptions are not required. Some customers order drugs from such pharmacies to avoid the inconvenience of visiting a doctor or to obtain medications their doctors were unwilling to prescribe.

Many of these websites employ their own in-house physicians to review the medication request and write a prescription accordingly. Some websites offer medications without a prescription or a doctor review. This practice has been criticized as potentially dangerous, especially by those who feel that only doctors can reliably assess contraindications, risk/benefit ratios, and the suitability of a medication for a specific individual. Phar-macies offering medication without requiring a prescription and doctor review or supervision are sometimes fraudulent and may supply counterfeit and ineffective and possibly dangerous medicines.

MAINTENANCE OF RECORDS OF RETAIL AND WHOLESALE

In order to run the business successfully principles of accounting, book keeping and maintaining record properly to identify the expenses and profit is most important. It is imperative that pharmacist and all personnel involved in administration and dispensing of medicines keep permanent records. In addition to specific legal requirements for record keeping, it may be necessary to record reasons for prescribing. All necessary records should be kept in a readily retrievable manner (e.g. a handbook, files, or on a computerised database). Where a computer is used, there must be adequate precautions against inadvertent loss of data. Any discrepancies must be entered into the records. Prescribing cards are a useful aid to record keeping and control of supply.

Maintenance of Records of Retail

Pharmacist must keep records for each incoming transaction concerning products received from wholesalers, manufacturers, etc. along with each outgoing transaction involving the sale of products to clients.

Records should be made within 24 hours of the transaction, kept for a period of at least 2 years, and be available for inspection. In addition, at least once a year a detailed audit of all transactions must be carried out. Incoming and outgoing products should be reconciled with those held in stock and any discrepancies recorded.

Purchase Account

Records of purchase of a drug intended for sale or sold by retail should be maintained by the licensee and such records shall show the following particulars, namely:

- Date of purchase.
- Name and address of the licensed supplier along with his license number.
- Details about the product in connection to its name, quantity, batch number, retail price, wholesale price and its expiry.
- Name of manufacturer.
- The signature of the person under whose supervision the sale was effected.

After receiving the purchase invoice, details of the invoice should be checked with order placed and terms and conditions then only entry is made in the purchase book and ledger. Each amount then written to the suppliers account until the invoices are paid. Once the invoice is correct, then it should be signed for releasing the payment. In case of cash payment, the cash discount should be deducted from the bill. Until the invoices are paid, they are kept in separate file.

Purchase bills including cash or credit memos should be serially numbered by the licensee and maintained by him/her in a chronological order and kept as records at least for 2 years from the date of the last entry therein.

Sales Account

Sale of any drugs on the prescription of a registered medical practitioner shall be recorded at the time of supply in a prescription register especially maintained for the purpose and the serial number of entry in this regard shall be entered on the prescription. The following particulars shall be entered in the register:

- Date of supply or sale.
- Serial number of the cash or credit memo.
- Name and address of the prescriber.
- Name and address of the patient.
- In case of veterinary medicine, name and address of the owner of the animal.
- Details of the product with its name and quantity.
- The name of manufacturer of the drug, the batch number and the date of expiry of potency, if any.
- The signature of the [Registered Pharmacy] by or under whose supervision the medicine was made up or supplied.
- Maintenance of a prescription register or a cash or credit memo book in respect of drugs and medicine which are supplied from or in the original container, should be kept as records at least for 3 years.

Maintenance of Records of Wholesale

Wholesale purchases are made from manufacturer and retailer purchases from manufacturer and sold to the customer. Thus, supply of a drug by wholesale shall be made against a cash or credit memo bearing the name and address of the licensee and his/her licence number under the Drug and Cosmetic Act in which the following particular shall be entered:

- Date of sale.
- Name, address of the licensee and his/her sale licence number.
- In case of supply of drugs to government/hospital/medical/educational/research institute/registered medical practitioner, the name and address of the authority, institution or the registered medical practitioner should be entered.
- Name of the drug, the quantity and the batch number.
- Name of the manufacturer.
- Signature of the competent person under whose supervision the sale was effected.

PATIENT COUNSELING

Patient counseling is a key competency element of the pharmaceutical care process that improves the quality of life of the patients. It is important for pharmacists to provide appropriate, understandable and relevant information to patients about their medication. The pharmacist is in a highly visible and readily available position to answer patient concerns and enquiries about their medications and alternate treatments they may read about or hear from others. Patient counseling not only would serve to help educate patients about their medications, but would also serve to open communication lines further between the pharmacist and the patient. This would allow the pharmacist to give better healthcare as he/she would be better informed of the patients' overall health, and could further help the patient in leading a healthier life.

Counseling may be defined as "a one-to-one interaction between a pharmacist and a patient and/or caregiver. It is interactive in nature. It should include an assessment of whether or not the information was received as intended and that the patient understands how to use the information to improve the probability of positive therapeutic outcomes."

Patient counseling is undertaken by pharmacists:

- During dispensing.
- In disease management.
- In providing advice on self-care: advice on product selection and use, non-drug self-care, referral and health assessment.

The pharmacist should appropriately educate patients on the following:

- Name and class of the drug (e.g. antibiotic, pain reliever).
- Directions for use including education about drug devices.
- Special storage requirements.
- Common or important drug—drug or drug–food interactions.
- The reason for the drug and the intended therapeutic response and associated time frames. (It is recognized that pharmacists do not always have access to the therapeutic indication for the drug.)
- Common or important side effects and associated time frames.
- What the patient should do to monitor his/her therapeutic response or development of side effects.
- Actions the patient should take, if the intended therapeutic response is not obtained or side effects develop.
- When appropriate, the actions the pharmacist will undertake to monitor the patient's progress.

The amount and type of information provided to the patient will vary based on the patient's needs, and practice setting. Ideally, the pharmacist counsels patients on all new and refill prescriptions. If the pharmacist can-not counsel to this extent, it should be defined which patient types, or which medications pharmacists will routinely counsel patients. This will vary depending on the pharmacy clientele and may include:

- Patients receiving more than a specified number of medications.
- Patients known to have visual, hearing or literacy problems.
- Pediatric patients.
- Patients on anticoagulants.

Techniques of Counseling

Several techniques can be adopted for effective counseling. Some of them include providing written information to the patient and the use of audiovisual materials. The use of various compliance aids includes labeling, medication calendars, drug reminder chart and providing special medication containers and caps can also be adopted. The United States Pharmacopoeia (USP) medication counseling behavior guidelines divide medication counseling into the following four stages (USP, 1997).

Stage I: Medication information transfer, during which there is a monologue by the pharmacist providing basic, brief information about the safe and proper use of medicine.

Stage II: Medication information exchange, during which the pharmacist answers questions and provides detailed information adapted to the patients' situation.

Stage III: Medication education, during which the pharmacist provides comprehensive information regarding the proper use of medicines in a collaborative, interactive learning experience.

Stage IV: Medication counseling, during which the pharmacist and patient have a detailed discussion intending to give the patient guidance that enhances problem-solving skills and assists with proper management of medical conditions and effective use of medication.

Communication Skills in Patient Counseling

Communication is the exchange of information, ideas, thoughts and feelings. It involves not just the spoken words, but also what is conveyed through inflexion, vocal quality, facial expression, body posture and other behavioral processes. Effective communication with patients depends greatly on the degree of empathy demonstrated in the course of conversation. Pharmacist should use proper verbal and non-verbal communication skills during the counseling session. Studies repeatedly show that effective patient counseling can significantly reduce patient non-adherence, treatment failure, and wasted health resources. To be good communicators, pharmacist must be attuned to the types of questions asked, the manners in which questions are asked, and the avoidance of repetition. The counseling pharmacist should be well dressed so that the patient feels the pharmacist is a professional. A good counselor is one who listens to the patient carefully and shares the problems intimately so that the patient expresses the emotions underlying the disease. During counseling, pharmacist should be totally involved in the counseling and should not be half minded. Even attending a telephone call while counseling may affect the quality of counseling. An effective counseling will end up with several questions being asked by the patient. Throughout the counseling process, the pharmacist should avoid jargons and slang expressions.

There are some important communication skills required for pharmacist to interact successfully with patients such as active listening, questioning, responding and explaining. Each of these skills is explained below.

Active Listening

During patient counseling, it is important for pharmacist to listen to the patient. Listening is an active process, ensuring not only that all messages are received but also that the speaker knows that the listener has understood the message. It is essential that patient knows that the pharmacist is listening to him/her and taking his/her situation and opinions seriously. This may help to pharmacist to obtain more useful information from the patient, as the patient will find it easier to share such information relating to themselves, enabling the pharmacist to fulfil his/her role more effectively. It is not unusual for a patient to give the pharmacist information that he/she may feel unable to share with his/her doctor or nurse, as many patients perceive pharmacists to be more understanding and approachable.

The three main techniques involved in active listening are:

- Maintaining eye contact – so that the speaker can see you are paying attention.
- Acknowledging what the speaker says – by suitable body language such as nodding and verbal agreement.
- Summarizing or paraphrasing what has just been said (e.g. using a phrase such 'So, what you're saying is. . .').

Questioning

Pharmacists need to use effective questioning in order to obtain information from patients, usually relating to their medication. It is important not to ask leading questions, as patients will sometimes just agree or go along with the lead, because they are afraid to get the question 'wrong'. Moreover, it is also important to get accurate information with regard to a medication history that will help for giving proper and correct medication while they are in hospital.

There are few important points that should always be kept in mind when questioning to the patient:

- Use effective questions by adopting open questions to obtain information that is necessary.
- Ask only one question at a time.

- Structure the flow of questions to follow a logical pattern.
- Use probing questions to follow up patient's response. Patients may not be aware that certain information must be known by the pharmacist to suggest appropriate line of action.
- Encourage patient participation by pausing both after asking a question and after the initial response.

Responding and Explaining

Responding consists of responding to the content, feelings, and meaning of the patient's expression. Responding to contents helps to clarify the basics of the patient's experiences, whereas responding to feelings identifies the affect that is a part of the experience. When explaining something to a patient, such as how to use an inhaler, it is essential to use language and concepts that the patient will understand. Technical words and jargon should never be used, as many patients will not understand such terms, and they might not have the confidence to ask for a further explanation. It also is important to be confident when talking with patients, so they have confidence in what you tell them. It is unlikely that a patient will trust a health professional who is hesitant or does not appear confident about what they are talking about.

It is often necessary to understands following point when responding and explaining to patients.

- Place the most important points at the beginning of the communication session.
- Emphasise key issues.
- Give specific, concrete instructions.
- Limit the information to the essentials to prevent cognitive overload.
- Simplify complicated messages.

Format of Counseling Provided

Counseling should be verbal, and accompanied by written material for the patient to refer to at home. Patients are often stressed and upset from their illness while waiting for their prescription and may not be able to focus on what the pharmacist is discussing with them.

Written material reinforces what the pharmacist says and helps the patient recall what was said. If the patient has forgotten or is unsure of what the pharmacist said, the written material may provide the answer, or stimulate the patient to call the pharmacist. This provides the pharmacist an opportunity to reinforce key points about the medication and assess how the patient is doing. The written material may provide basic information only, or be quite detailed. Pictograms, such as those use for illustrating how to administer eyedrops, are much easier to understand and should supplement a detailed verbal description.

Counseling Area

The patient should be counseled in a semi-private, or private, area away from other people and distractions, depending on the medication(s). The patient should perceive the counseling area as confidential, secure and conducive to learning. This helps ensure that both parties are focused on the discussion, and minimizes interruptions and distractions. It provides an opportunity for patients to ask questions they may be hesitant to ask in public.

Documentation

The counseling session should be documented. This may be as simple as a check list or as detailed as recorded notes in the patients' medication profile. Any follow-up required should be noted. It should also be recorded, if the patient does not wish to be counseled.

When communicating with patients, establishing a good rapport with the patient, active listening, relevant questioning and appropriate body language enhance the process.

Pharmacist counseling programs can be developed focusing on themes such as:

- Lifestyle measures:
  — Counseling on exercise and diet.
  — Monitoring of body weight, lipid profile, glucose levels and blood pressure.

- Smoking cessation:
  — Counseling on nicotine replacement therapy (transdermal nicotine patch, chewing gum, inhalator) and smoking cessation psychological behavior.

- Diabetes:
  — Giving information on condition, advising on proper techniques for insulin storage and administration.
  — Identifying and providing guidance on actions to monitor and compensate for aberrations in glucose levels, dietary and exercise management, and foot care.

- Asthma:
  — Providing information on condition, medicines and pharmaceutical dosage forms.
  — Identifying and providing guidance on actions to compensate for aberrations in peak flow meter readings and exercise management.

- Hypertension:
  — Providing counseling on significance of monitoring blood pressure.
  — Carrying out drug therapy review.
  — Advising patients on lifestyle measures.

- Anticoagulant therapy:
  — Giving information on identification of symptoms indicating hemorrhage.
  — Providing education on anticoagulant–food interactions and drug–drug interactions.

  — Explaining significance of monitoring of prothrombin time.

- Hormone replacement therapy:
  — Providing counseling on impacts of drug therapy, lifestyle measures and requirement for continuous monitoring.

Counseling on Non-prescription Drugs

Effective non-prescription drug counseling requires a thorough description of patient's symptoms. Before advice can be given, the intern will need knowledge on the nature, severity and extenuating circumstances surrounding those symptoms. As well, other aspects of the patient's health, e.g. other diseases, drugs, contraindications, allergies, must be examined. This "information-gathering" stage is most important.

When non-prescription drugs are indicated, the intern must be able to give information to the patient so products are used both safely and effectively. When providing care to patients involving over the counter-medications, it is necessary to perform an adequate mini-assessment of the client's problem, consisting of:

- Properly identifying the person who will be using the product and determining their approximate age.
- Inquiring about any current medical conditions.
- Asking about current non-prescription drug use, including herbal products.
- Asking about current prescription drug use.
- Inquiring about the symptoms and duration of the complaint.
- Asking about whether the client has any medication allergies.
- Asking whether the clients has consulted a healthcare professional about the problem.

- You should refer the client for medical attention if:
  - ❖ Their condition is potentially severe.
  - ❖ They are uncertain about their symptoms.
  - ❖ Their self-diagnosis is likely incorrect.
  - ❖ The condition has not responded to previous appropriate therapy, or
  - ❖ They have other risk factors that should be assessed.
- When you have assessed the client and the problem, and feel that a referral is not necessary, you may recommend an appropriate product or course of action, including non-drug measures. If you recommend a non-prescription drug product, you should discuss:
  - ❖ Directions for use
  - ❖ Expected outcomes of therapy, including a time-frame for a response
  - ❖ Common adverse effects and precautions
  - ❖ Correct storage
  - ❖ When to seek medical attention.
- Ideally, you should document non-prescription drug use on the client's medication profile. This is especially important for clients who have a medical condition and/or are taking prescription medication.

The following are the few selected formulations wherein the patients need proper counseling from the pharmacists, which will enable them to use safely, appropriately and effectively.

- **Proper use of your medicine:** Take medicine only as directed, at the right time, and for the full length of time presented by your healthcare provider. If you are using over-the-counter (non-prescription) medicine, follow the directions on the label, unless otherwise directed by your healthcare provider. If you

feel that your medicine is not working for you, check with your healthcare provider. It is best to keep your medicines tightly capped in their original containers when not in use. Do not remove the label since directions for use and other special information appear on it. To avoid mistakes, do not take medicine in the dark. Always read the label before taking, nothing especially the expiration date, if any of the contents.

- **For oral (by mouth) medicines:** In general, it is best to take oral medicines with a full glass of water. However, follow your healthcare provider's directions. Some medicines should be taken with food while others should be taken on an empty stomach. When taking most long-acting forms of a medicine, each dose should be swallowed whole. Do not break, crush, or chew before swallowing unless you have been specifically told that it is all right to do so. If you are taking liquid medicines, you might consider using a specially marked measuring spoon or other device to measure each dose accurately. Ask your pharmacist about these devices. The average household teaspoon may not hold the right amount of liquid. Oral medicine may come in a number of different dosage forms such as tablets, capsules, and liquids. If you have trouble swallowing the dosage form prescribed for you, check with your healthcare provider. There may be another dosage form that would be better for you.
- **For skin patches:** Apply the patch to a clean, dry skin area with little or no hair and free of scars, cuts, or irritation. Remove the previous patch before applying a new one. Apply a new patch, if the first one becomes loose or falls off. Apply each dose to a different area of skin to prevent skin irritation or other problems. Do not try to trim or cut the adhesive patch to adjust the dosage. Check with your health-

care provider, if you think the medicine is not working, as it should.

- **For nasal (nose) drops:** How to use? Blow your nose gently, without squeezing. Tilt your head back while standing or sitting up or lie down on your back on a bed and hang your head over the side. Place the drips into each nostril and keep your head tilted back for a few minutes to allow the medicine to spread throughout the nose. Rinse the dropper with hot water and dry with clean tissue. Replace the cap right after use. To avoid the spread of infection, do not use the container for more than one person.

- **For nasal (nose) spray:** How to use? Blow your nose gently, without squeezing. With your head upright, spray the medicine into each nostril. Sniff briskly while squeezing the bottle quickly and firmly. Rinse the tip of the spray bottle with hot water. Replace the cap right after cleaning. To avoid the spread of infection, do not use the container for more than one person.

- **For otic (ear) drops:** To prevent contamination of the eardrops, do not touch the applicator tip to any surface (including the ear). How to apply first, wash your hands. Lie down or tilt your head so that the ear into which the medicine is to be placed faces up. (For children, gently pull the earlobe down and back to straighten the ear canal.) Drop the medicine into the ear canal. Keep the ear facing up for several minutes to allow the medicine to run to the bottom of the ear canal. A sterile cotton plug may be gently inserted into the ear opening to prevent the medicine from leaking out.

- **Eye preparations for hospital use:** Preparations for the eye should be sterile when issued. Eyedrops inmultiple-aplication containers include preservative, but care should be taken to avoid contamination of the contents during use.

- Eyedrops in multiple-application containers for domiciliary use should not be used for more than 4 weeks after first opening (unless otherwise stated). Eyedrops for use in hospital are normally discarded 1 week after first opening. Individual containers should be provided for each patient. Containers used before an operation should be discarded at the time of the operation and fresh containers supplied. A fresh supply should also be provided upon discharge from hospital. It may be acceptable in specialist ophthalmology units to issue on discharge eyedrop bottles that have been in use for the patient for less than 36 hours. Eyedrops used in out patient departments should be discarded at the end of each day. In clinics for eye diseases and in accident and emergency departments, where the dangers of infection are high, single application packs should be used, it should be discarded after single use. Diagnostic dyes (e.g. fluorescein) should be used only from single application packs. In eye surgery, it is wise to use single-application containers. Preparations used during intraocular procedures and others that may penetrate into the anterior chamber must be isotonic and without preservatives and buffered if necessary to a neutral pH. Large volume intravenous infusion preparations are suitable for this purpose. For all surgical procedures, a previously unopened container is used for each patient.

- **For ophthalmic (eye) drops:** To prevent contamination, do not let the eye drop applicator tip touch any surface (including the eye) and keep the container tightly closed. How to apply? First, wash hands, tilt you head back and with the index finger pull the lower eyelid away from the eye to form a pouch. Drop the medicine into the pouch and gently close your eyes. Do not blink. Keep your eyes closed for 1 or 2 minutes.

- If your medicine is for glaucoma or inflammation of the eye— with the middle finger of the same hand, apply pressure to the inside corner of the eye (and continue to apply pressure for 1 or 2 minutes after the medicine has been placed in the eye). This will help prevent the medicine from being absorbed into the body and causing side effects. After applying the eye drops, wash your hands to remove any medicine that may be on them. The bottle may not be full; this is to provide proper drop control.

- **For ophthalmic (eye) ointments:** To prevent contamination of the eye ointment. Do not let the applicator tip touch any surface (including the eye). After using, wipe the tip of the ointment tube with a clean tissue and keep the tube tightly closed. How to apply first, wash your hands. Pull the lower eyelid away from the eye to form a pouch. Squeeze a thin strip of ointment into the pouch. A 1-cum (approximately 1/3-inch) strip of ointment is usually enough unless otherwise directed. Gently close your eyes and keep them closed for 1 or 2 minutes. After applying the eye ointment, wash your hands to remove any medicine that may be on them.

- **For rectal cream or ointment:** Bath and dry the rectal area. Apply a small amount of cream or ointment and rub it in gently. If your healthcare provider wants you to insert the medicine into the rectum, first, attach the plastic applicator tip on to the opened tube. Insert the applicator tip into the rectum and gently squeeze the tube to deliver the cream. Remove the applicator tip from the tube and wash it with hot, soapy water. Replace the cap of the tube after use. Wash your hands after you have inserted the medicine.

- **For vaginal medicines:** How to insert the medicine? First, wash your hands. Use the special applicator. Follow any spe-

cial directions that are provided by the manufacturer. However, if you are pregnant, check with your healthcare provider before using the applicator to insert the medicine. Lie on your back with your knees drawn up. Using the applicator, insert the medicine into the vagina as far as you can without using force or causing discomfort. Release the medicine by pushing on the plunger. Wait several minutes before getting up. Wash the applicator and your hands with soap and warm water.

- **For inhalers:** Medicines that come in inhalers usually come with patient directions. Read the directions carefully before using the medicine. If you do not understand the directions or if you are not sure how to use the inhaler, check with your healthcare provider. Since different types of inhalers may not be used in the same way, it is very important to carefully follow the directions given to you.

ROLE OF PHARMACIST IN COMMUNITY HEALTHCARE AND EDUCATION

Health is a word very familiar to us but it also carries a lot of complications and problems. According to the World Health Organization, health is a state of complete physical, mental and social well-being and not merely absence of any illness. To make the above definition of health practical, we have to depend upon a "healthcare team". A healthcare team is the group of people who share a common health goal and common objectives determined by community needs. Community pharmacist is the professional who would be in direct access to the public and whose duties are widely sought after by the public and patients. He/she dispenses medicines with a prescription and in certain cases without a prescription where applicable (OTC drugs). As he/she is the person who will be in direct contact with the public, he/she has to play an important role in decreasing the mortality and morbidity in the public.

The community pharmacist can take part in health promotion campaigns, locally and nationally, on a wide range of drug-related and health-related topics. The role of pharmacist is to act in an important and responsible manner for the propagation of national health programs.

Pharmacist Interventions in the Healthcare System

- *Ensuring rational use of medicines:* Participation in the development of formularies, clinical guidelines and protocols, and analysis of prescribing information and drug use evaluation data.
- *Disease management:* Contributing towards enhancement of compliance, adherence to evidence-based clinical guidelines and monitoring patient outcomes.
- *Management of drug therapy:* Ensuring that safe and effective drug products are used and are accessible, collaboration with health professionals to ensure that prescribing is carried out for definite objectives, accessing patients' profiles and medical records, undertaking counseling about safe use of drugs, patient monitoring to identify problems and suggest actions to solve problems.

Actions of Community Pharmacists in Society

- Procurement of medicines that are suitable for human consumption.
- Storage of medicines in appropriate conditions (temperature, humidity, cleanliness, stock monitoring).
- Dispensing of medicines chosen by patient or as pharmacist-recommended products or on presentation of a prescription.
- Compounding and ensuring quality of compounded products.

- Patient medication review, advise patients on use of medicines and participate in adverse drug reaction reporting.
- Ensuring rational and safe use of medicines by patients, developing care plans and collaborating with prescribers to establish a therapeutic plan, implement it and monitor patient outcomes.
- Monitoring of self-care, responding to symptoms and identifying cases warranting referral.
- Point-of-care testing.
- Health promotion and promotion of healthy lifestyles (nutrition, physical activity, smoking cessation, sexual and reproductive health).
- Ensuring safe disposal of unwanted or expired medicines.
- Signposting patients to other healthcare providers and support agencies.
- Participating in national health service schemes to provide social pharmacy services.
- Other responsibilities: Nutritional supplements, special foods (e.g. gluten-free products, food for diabetic people), colostomy care and urinary incontinence devices, disability and mobility aids (e.g. wheelchairs, walking aids), oxygen supplies and ventilation equipment, veterinary medicines.

As a Quality Drug Supplier

The pharmacist must ensure that the purchased products are from reputed sources and of good quality. The pharmacist must ensure the proper storage of these products. The pharmacist should not purchase any drug which is sold without bill.

As a Communicator

The pharmacist is the person who is in direct contact with the patient so he/she should initiate the dialogue with the patient to obtain sufficiently detailed medication history before dispensing the drugs. In order to address the condition of the patient appropriately, the pharmacist must ask the patients key questions and pass on relevant information to him or her.

- The pharmacist must provide objective information to him/her.
- The pharmacist must be able to use and interpret additional sources of information to satisfy the needs of the patient.
- The pharmacist should be able to help the patient to undertake appropriate and responsible self-medication.
- The pharmacist must ensure confidentiality concerning details of patient's condition.

As a Trainer and Supervisor

The pharmacist provides training to non-pharmacist subordinate staff regarding establishment of standards of practice. Trained non-pharmacist staff with matric qualification can become eligible to run a wholesale drug store.

As a Social Worker

In India, rural population form a major part of our population so by working as a social worker in these areas, pharmacist can help in improving the hygienic conditions of these areas and thus can play role in prevention and spread of infections.

Family Planning

One of the greatest needs of the hour is to control the tremendously increasing population in India. Pharmacist is a link between physician and patient. A community pharmacist is the one who can explain, educate, motivate and implement family planning in population by:

- Counseling with people.
- Arranging seminars/programs which exhibit the problems related with large families.

- Educating the people regarding various families planning measures that are available in the market.
- Convincing the people regarding advantages of small families.
- Encouraging people to take advantage of government schemes like free sterility operations and low cost family planning appliances(condoms, cooper-T), etc.

Nutrition Counseling

Nutrition is a science that examines the relationship between diet and health. Deficiencies, excesses and imbalances in diet can produce negative impact on health. Community pharmacist can educate people including his patients about adequate nutrition and also regarding the balanced diet. He can advice efficiently about special diet instructions for diabetic patients, people with food allergy and intake during pregnancy. The community pharmacist could explain the nutraceuticals/dietary supplements which are considered to provide medical or health benefits.

Women Welfare—Pregnancy and Infant

A woman goes through different stages throughout her life, each of which has specific need and the presence of a counselor is needed in each one of them. The pharmacist who understands the normal course of pregnancy and infancy is at a distinct advantage as he or she can guide the mother in simple matters of hygiene and management. The community pharmacist can:

- Guide about the adequate nutrition during pregnancy, encourage breastfeeding.
- Play a major role by guiding the mother for the protection of the child by following proper immunization schedule.

Rational Use of Drugs

A community pharmacist can provide information on the proper usage and storage of the medication. Drug information, aware-ness programs should be conducted to make people aware of side effects of certain OTC drugs. A community pharmacist should have a sound knowledge of drug–drug reactions and adverse drug reactions. A community pharmacist is one of the important members of the healthcare team who can help to achieve the goal of rational use of drugs by:

- Giving proper information to patient regarding possible side effects, allergic reactions and ADRs.
- By properly examining and dispensing the prescriptions.
- By providing proper information to the patient about time and way of administ-ration of prescribed medicament(s).

Sexually Transmitted Diseases—AIDS

India has about 4 million HIV positive cases and this disease has become a pandemic. A community pharmacist can help in prevention and spread of infection by exhibiting the post-ers and distributing literature on preventive measures against the disease. Explaining to what HIV is, its transmission, risk reduction, patient counseling are the components of the counseling that a community pharmacist can provide.

Alcohols, Drug Abuse and Smoking Cessation

The pharmacist has a key role to help indi-viduals who become dependent upon alcohol, smoking and drug abuse. It is the responsibility of a community pharmacist to take an active role in helping these type of people by written information and posters side effects of these. The pharmacist can advise on the products available to assist the patient in giving up smoking. Counseling sessions can be made by the community pharmacist to stop smoking.

In nut shell, a pharmacist should spare time for patient counseling regarding pharmaco-economics, drug information, pharmacovigilance, alternative therapy, moral supporting, etc. A pharmacist can set up a consultation room and provide counseling to the patient. He can store the details of biochemical investigations of patient, patient history, allergies and other details necessary for therapy. The future ideal pharmacists will have seven principal roles to play like care-giver, decision-maker, communicator, leader, manager, lifelong learner and a role model.

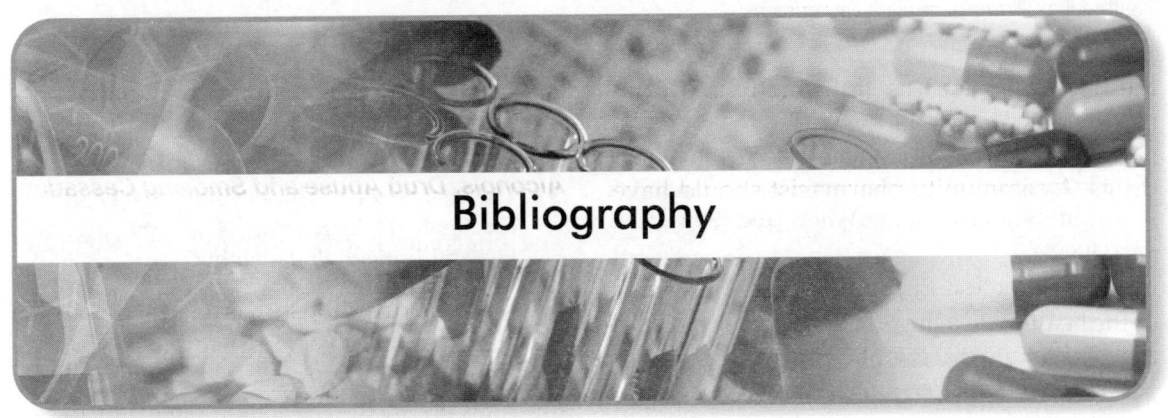

Bibliography

- A Practical Guide from Candidate Drug Selection to Commercial Dosage Form (Gibson M, ed.), Informa Healthcare, London.
- A treatise on Pharmacy for students and pharmacists (Caspari C, ed.) Lea and Febiger, Philadelphia.
- Advanced Pharmaceutics: Physicochemical Principles (Kim CJ, ed.), CRC Press, New York.
- Applied Pharmaceutical Practice (Langley CA, Belcher D, eds), Pharmaceutical Press, 2009.
- British Pharmaceutical Codex.
- Clinical Pharmacy: A text for Dispensing Pharmacy, Jenkins, Sperandio and Latiolais, Mc-Graw-Hill Book Company, London.
- Compend of Pharmacy (Stewart FE, ed.), P. Blakiston Son and Co., Philadelphia.
- Cooper and Gunn's Dispensing for Pharmaceutical Students (Carter SJ, ed.), Pitman Medical Publishing Co. Ltd., London.
- Dispensing of medication, formerly Husa's pharmaceutical Dispensing (Martin EW and Husa WJ, eds), Mack Publishing Co., Pennsylvania.
- Drugs and the Pharmaceutical Sciences (Alderborn G, Nystrom C, eds), Marcel Dekker, New York.
- Emulsions and Emulsion Stability (Sjoblom J, ed.), Marcel Dekker, New York.
- Encyclopedia of pharmaceutical technology (Swarbrick J eds), Informa Healthcare USA, Inc. 270 Madison Avenue, New York.
- Extra Pharmacopoeia Martindale.
- Fifty-fifth report. WHO Technical Report Series (www.who.int/biologicals).
- Flick EW, Cosmetic and Toiletry Formulations, Noyes Publications/William Andrew Publishing, New York, 1999.
- Ghosh TK, Jasti BR (eds), Theory and Practice of contemporary pharmaceutics, CRC Press, LLC, Florida.
- Handbook of Pharmaceutical Excipients (Wade A, Weller PJ, eds), Pharmaceutical Press, Washington, DC.
- Handbook of Pharmaceutical Excipients, Pharmaceutical Press, UK, 5th ed, 2006.
- Handbook of Pharmaceutical Excipients (Kibbe AH, ed.), American Pharmacists Association, Washington, DC.
- Handbook of Pharmacy-Theory and Practice of Pharmacy (Coblentz, V. ed.), P. Blakiston Sons and Co., Philadelphia, 1894.
- Modern Pharmaceutics (Banker GS, Rhodes CT, eds), Marcel Dekker, Inc. New York.
- National Formulary of India.
- Opportunities in Pharmacy Careers (Gable FB, eds), NTC Contemporary, Illinois, USA, 1998.
- Pharmaceutical Compounding and Dispensing (Langley C, Belcher D, eds), Pharmaceutical Press, London.
- Pharmaceutical Compounding and Dispensing (Marriott JF, Wilson KA, Langley CA, Belcher D, eds), Pharmaceutical Press, London.

- Pharmaceutical Dosage Forms (Avis KE, Lieberman HA, Lachman L, eds), Marcel Dekker, New York.
- Pharmaceutical Manufacturing Handbook (Gad SC, eds), John Wiley and Sons, Inc. Hoboken, New Jersey.
- Pharmaceutical Preformulation and Formulation (Gibson M., ed.), CRC Press, Florida.
- Pharmacy: What It Is and How It Works (Kelly WN, ed.), CRC Press, LLC, Florida, 2002.
- Physicians' Desk Reference, Medical Economics, New York.
- Remington's Pharmaceutical Sciences (Gennaro AR, ed.), Mack Publishing Company, Pennsylvania.
- The Art of Dispensing (Macewan P, ed.), The Chemist and Druggist, London, 1915.
- The British Pharmacopoeia.
- The Pharmacopoeia of India.
- The Pharmacopoeia of USSR.
- The Pharmacopoeia of United States.
- The Prescription (Wall OA, ed.), C. V. MOSBY Company, St. Louis.
- The Theory and Practice of Industrial Pharmacy (Lachman L, Lieberman HA, Kanig JL, eds), Lea and Febiger, Philadelphia.
- The Theory and Practice of Industrial Pharmacy, Lea and Febiger, Philadelphia.
- Therapeutics Index and Prescription writing practice (Barton WM. ed.), The Copp. Clark Co., Limited, Boston, 1917.
- US Food and Drug Administration, Code of Federal Regulations, Office of the Federal Register, National Archives and Records Administration.
- United States Pharmacopeia-National Formulary, The United States Pharmacopeial Convention, Rockville, MD.
- Walter KA (ed), Dermatological and Transdermal Formulations, Informa Healthcare USA, Inc.

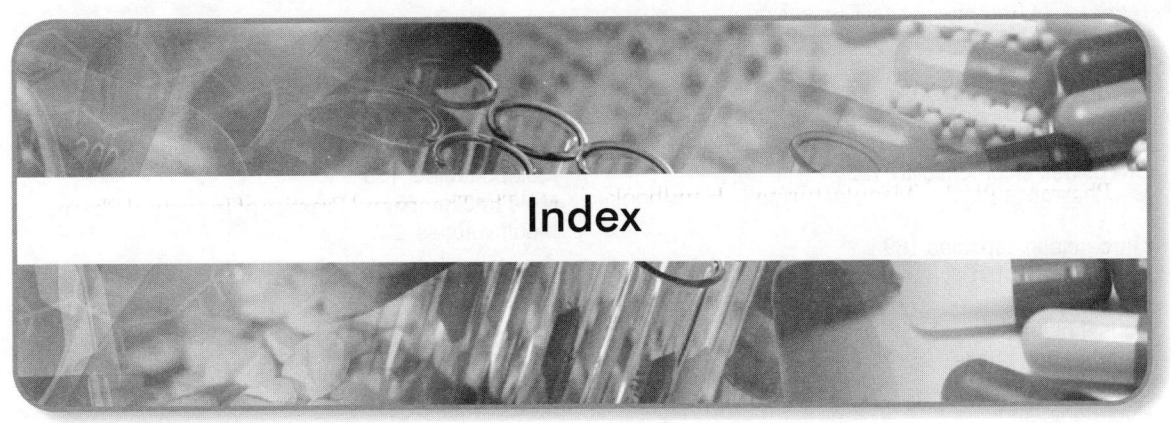

Index